Modern Contraception

Updates from
The Contraception Report

Published by
Emron
Totowa, New Jersey
1997

Emron is a company of IMS America, Ltd. and the Cognizant Corporation.

Acknowledgments

The editors wish to thank all the clinicians who have contributed to *The Contraception Report* since its inception. We would also like to thank the staff members at Emron who provided invaluable help in preparing the material for this book. Finally, we acknowledge the ongoing support and commitment of Wyeth-Ayerst Laboratories, which generously provided the unrestricted educational grant that made this book possible.

Library of Congress Catalog Card Number: 97-060969

ISBN: 0-9651745-1-4

First Edition, First Printing

Printed in the United States of America

Table of Contents

Editors

David A. Grimes, MD
Professor and Vice Chairman, Department of Obstetrics, Gynecology and
 Reproductive Sciences, University of California, San Francisco
Professor, Department of Epidemiology and Biostatistics,
 University of California, San Francisco
Chief, Department of Obstetrics, Gynecology and Reproductive Sciences,
 San Francisco General Hospital — San Francisco, California

Melinda Wallach, RN
Managing Editor, *The Contraception Report* — Emron, Totowa, New Jersey

Associate Editors

Ernie J. Chaney, MD
Professor, Department of Family and Community Medicine, The University
 of Kansas School of Medicine, Wichita — Wichita, Kansas

Elizabeth B. Connell, MD
Professor Emeritus, Department of Gynecology and Obstetrics, Emory University
 School of Medicine — Atlanta, Georgia

S. Jean Emans, MD
Chief, Division of Adolescent/Young Adult Medicine, Children's Hospital
Associate Professor of Pediatrics, Harvard Medical School — Boston, Massachusetts

Joseph W. Goldzieher, MD
Distinguished Professor, Department of Obstetrics and Gynecology, Texas Tech
 University Health Sciences Center — Amarillo, Texas

Paula J. A. Hillard, MD
Associate Professor, Department of Obstetrics and Gynecology and Department of
 Pediatrics, University of Cincinnati College of Medicine — Cincinnati, Ohio

Luigi Mastroianni, Jr., MD
William Goodell Professor of Obstetrics and Gynecology
Director, Division of Human Reproduction, Hospital of the University of
 Pennsylvania — Philadelphia, Pennsylvania

■ Preface

Contraception and related fields of women's health are rapidly evolving. Products and techniques are entering (eg, the female condom) and exiting the market (eg, the contraceptive sponge). New health benefits of contraception are emerging, such as sturdier bones in women who use oral contraceptives (OCs), while others are disappearing, such as protection against functional ovarian cysts. The long-held notion that the progestin content of oral contraceptives has no effect on the small risk of blood clots has been challenged—and hotly debated. In addition, in the era of managed care, a broader array of health care professionals is providing these services to women and their families. Traditional textbooks often give superficial coverage to these issues, and the long publication times mean that information may be stale.

Because of these concerns, in 1990 we began to publish a continuing medical education periodical entitled *The Contraception Report*. Each issue has focused on an important and timely subject; we have provided evidence-based reviews of current knowledge on issues ranging from the effects of OCs on breast cancer to strategies for counseling teens about abstinence, contraception and prevention of sexually transmitted disease. In addition, we have commented on important articles appearing in the scientific literature and in newspapers, and we have responded to questions from readers of *The Contraception Report*.

Requests from readers of *The Contraception Report* led to this book, a compilation of updated highlights from the first 7 years. In this volume, you will find timely, practical, evidence-based guidance for clinical care. Where evidence is lacking, the authors share with you their advice, based on years of clinical experience. Patient counseling strategies are also included.

The book is divided into chapters and the chapters into sections. Each section has been designed so that it can be read independently of other sections or chapters. The material has been updated wherever new data have become available. Over the years, many clinicians and researchers contributed to our publication. The titles of these persons, as stated in this book, are those at the time the interview was completed and may not be reflective of their current positions.

Contraception and related services are preventive medicine at its best. Indeed, every clinician's office needs to be a family planning facility if we are to meet the health needs of the patients whom we serve.

— David A. Grimes, MD
San Francisco, California
May 1997

Note to Readers on Interpretation of Risk

Throughout this book, the editors use several terms that measure risk. These terms include *relative risk*, *odds ratio* and *confidence interval*. For those unfamiliar with these concepts, the following brief explanation and sample graphic should help in interpretation of various study data reported in this book.

A relative risk (RR) is a measure of association that can be obtained from prospective studies. An RR of 1.0 indicates no association between the exposure (eg, oral contraceptives) and the outcome (eg, stroke). A relative risk greater than 1.0 indicates an increased risk; an RR lower than 1.0 indicates a decreased risk. An odds ratio (OR) is a measure of association derived from case-control studies and is a good approximation of relative risk for infrequent diseases.

A relative risk must be interpreted in light of its confidence interval (CI). Confidence intervals indicate how precise the RR estimate is. A narrow confidence interval implies good precision, and vice versa. Confidence intervals that exclude 1.0 are considered statistically significant at the p<0.05 level.

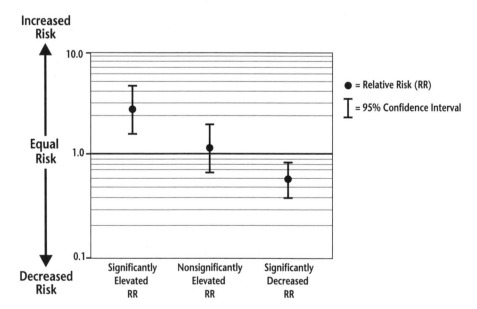

Examples of Relative Risks with 95% Confidence Intervals

1 Oral Contraceptives

Oral contraceptives (OCs) are among the most intensely studied drugs of all time. Early investigations focused on cardiovascular disease associated with OC use. Later, the focus shifted to the potential relationship between the pill and breast cancer. More recently, much attention has been given to such metabolic effects as lipid changes and so-called "androgenic" effects of the progestational agent. Then, in late 1995, the potential for venous thromboembolism (VTE) with OC use again was raised by some controversial data on the risk of VTE with the progestins desogestrel and gestodene.

This chapter explores these and other important issues concerning women's reproductive health and OCs: the substantial health benefits conferred by the pill, use in women over the age of 35 years, a reassessment of cardiovascular risks with use of modern formulations, trends in development and utilization, the relationship of OCs to cervical cancer, and suggestions for helping women take the pill correctly and consistently.

In addition, we look at some of the common myths regarding OCs. Do women really need to take a "rest" from the pill? Does the pill cause weight gain? Will it cause teenagers to engage in early sexual activity? The evidence suggests none of these myths is true.

Women and their clinicians need scientifically balanced information in order to assess both the benefits and risks of OCs when deciding on a method of contraception. The various sections contained in this chapter attempt to provide such an overview.

1.1: Health Benefits

Ongoing studies of the effects of oral contraceptives have added to the already extensive list of "good news" health benefits that are attributable to OC use (Figure 1). In addition to their protective effect against ovarian and endometrial cancers, OCs provide well-documented protection against benign breast disease, salpingitis, ectopic pregnancy, dysmenorrhea and iron deficiency anemia.[1] Growing evidence also suggests that OCs may help prevent osteoporosis by slowing or preventing loss of bone mineral density in the premenopausal years. Protective effects against other conditions—colorectal cancer, uterine fibroids, toxic shock syndrome (TSS) and rheumatoid arthritis—also have been suggested. Pending the outcomes of further studies, however, these latter findings remain controversial.

Clinicians providing family planning counseling need to communicate the full spectrum of health benefits afforded by OCs. Since more than 10 million American women use OCs, the positive public health impact could be large. Yet, health benefits rarely rank among the list of factors women consider when selecting a method of birth control. Despite the strong evidence, awareness of the pill's advantageous effects among women remains low. According to Gallup polls commissioned by the American College of Obstetricians and Gynecologists, most American women believe the pill presents serious health risks, while health benefits of OC use remain virtually unknown. These negative public perceptions stem, in part, from an undue media emphasis on adverse effects of the pill (for further discussion, see Chapter 9). The latest data demonstrate that for most women:

- Relatively small health risks are associated with current pill formulations, particularly for those who are healthy and do not smoke.
- Health benefits of OCs clearly outweigh the risks.

Well-Established Noncontraceptive Benefits

FACT: Ovarian cancer causes nearly 15,000 deaths a year—more deaths than any other cancer of the female reproductive system—but has virtually no early warning signs or method of early detection.[2]

FACT: Endometrial cancer is the most common cancer of the reproductive tract, affecting about 34,000 women a year. Approximately 6,000 women a year die from endometrial cancer.[2]

FACT: Oral contraceptives help prevent both ovarian and endometrial cancers.

Ovarian and Endometrial Cancers

The protection provided by OCs against endometrial and ovarian cancers are two of the best documented and least controversial noncontraceptive benefits of the pill. Women using OCs or considering starting OCs need to know the health implications of this protection. Because of its insidious onset, lack of early warning signs and symptoms, and absence of methods for early detection, ovarian cancer has already metastasized at the time of diagnosis in approximately 75% of women. Consequently, outcomes are poor: 5-year survival is only about 40% to 45%.[2]

Clearly established risk factors for ovarian cancer include age, race, nationality, nulliparity, few completed pregnancies and a family history of the disease. The biological mechanism of protection from ovarian cancer afforded by OCs is thought to involve avoidance of "incessant" ovulation or suppression or reduction of pituitary gonadotropin levels.

Figure 1

Noncontraceptive Health Benefits of OCs

Well Documented, Noncontroversial

Protection against:
Life-Threatening Diseases
- Ovarian Cancer
- Endometrial Cancer
- Salpingitis
- Ectopic Pregnancy

Diseases Affecting Quality of Life
- Benign Breast Disease
- Dysmenorrhea
- Iron Deficiency Anemia

Growing Evidence

Protection against:
- Osteoporosis

Still Controversial

Protection against:
- Colorectal Cancer
- Uterine Fibroids
- Toxic Shock Syndrome
- Rheumatoid Arthritis

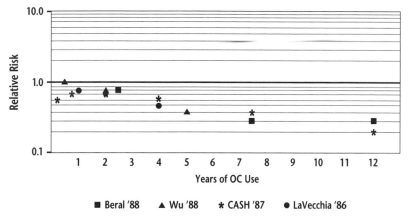

Figure 2

Relative Risk of Epithelial Ovarian Cancer in Women <60 Years of Age by Years of Oral Contraceptive Use, Selected Studies

■ Beral '88   ▲ Wu '88   ∗ CASH '87   ● LaVecchia '86

Source: Schlesselman JJ. Cancer of the breast and reproductive tract in relation to use of oral contraceptives. Contraception 1989;40:1-38. Reproduced with permission of the publisher, Elsevier Science, Inc.

Users of oral contraceptives are less likely to develop ovarian cancer than never-users (Figure 2).[3,4] The largest investigation to date, the Cancer and Steroid Hormone study (CASH), found an average 40% decrease in the future likelihood of ovarian cancer in women who had ever taken OCs. A protective effect has been observed with as little as 3 to 6 months of OC use, with further declines in risk accompanying longer periods of use. In addition, the duration-of-use effect persists for at least 15 years after the oral contraceptives are stopped. The finding that the reduction of ovarian cancer risk persists 15 years after last OC use is important in view of the increased incidence of this disease in older women.

Protective Effects of Oral Contraceptives in Ovarian Cancer

Summary of Findings

- Risk reduced approximately 40% in ever-users.
- Protective effect increases with duration of use.
- Protective effect apparent even with short-term use.
- Protective effect lasts at least 15 years after last use of pill.

Risks of each of the four main histologic subtypes of epithelial ovarian cancer—serous, mucinous, endometrioid and clear cell—are similarly reduced. The CASH investigators also found no difference in the amount of protection afforded by different OC formulations, including low-dose pills (<50 mcg of estrogen).[4]

Endometrial Cancer

Although ovarian cancer is responsible for more deaths than other gynecologic cancers, endometrial cancer represents the most common gynecologic cancer affecting American women.[2] With OC use for 12 months or longer, however, researchers have found a reduced risk of each of three major histological subtypes of

Figure 3

Selected Case-Control Studies of Oral Contraceptives and Endometrial Cancer

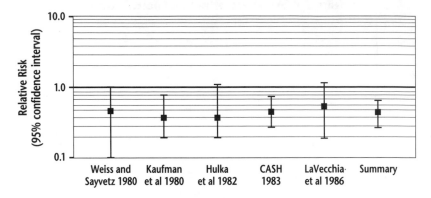

Source: Prentice RL, et al, 1987 (see reference 6).

endometrial cancer—adenocarcinoma, adenoacanthoma and adenosquamous carcinoma.[5] The overall risk of endometrial cancer is about 50% lower in pill users than in never-users (Figure 3).[6]

The CASH study found further declines in risk with extended duration of OC use, persisting for at least 15 years after discontinuation.[5] The lasting nature of the protective effect is important because most endometrial cancers occur in women over 50 years of age.

The mechanism of the effect of OCs on the endometrium presumably is mediated by progestin. Protection may vary by formulation, with OCs containing larger amounts of progestin providing the greatest benefit.

Benign Breast Disease

A reduced incidence of benign breast lumps—including both fibrocystic lumps and fibroadenomas—is among the most consistently demonstrated benefits of OC use.[7,8] The pill's favorable effects on benign breast disease have been attributed to inhibition of breast cell proliferation normally occurring in the first half of an ovulatory menstrual cycle.

Two prospective studies from the United Kingdom found risk reduction to be greater with formulations containing larger amounts of progestin.[9,10] One of these, the Oxford Family Planning Association study, also found decreasing risk of benign breast disease (both fibroadenomatous and chronic cystic disease) with increasing years of OC use (Figure 4).[10]

Protective Effects of Oral Contraceptives in Endometrial Cancer

Summary of Findings
- Risk reduced approximately 50% in ever-users.
- Risk declines further with longer-term use.
- Use for 12 months or longer conferred protection against all three major histologic subtypes.
- Protective effect apparent even with short-term use.

Figure 4

Relative Risk of Benign Breast Disease by Years of OC Use

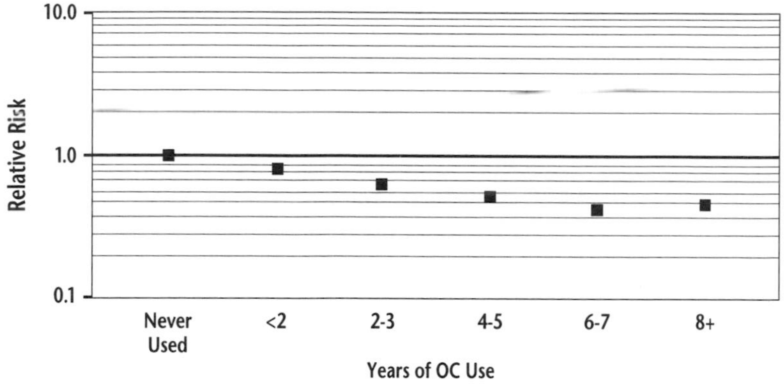

Source: Brinton LA, 1981 (see reference 10).

Studies note significant decreases in fibrocystic changes beginning after 1 to 2 years of OC use.[8] Current users appear to be at lowest risk of developing benign breast disease, with protection persisting for at least 1 year following pill discontinuation. A reduced risk of benign breast disease has been established across all age groups.

Salpingitis

OCs offer important protection against hospitalization for salpingitis or pelvic inflammatory disease (PID). Protection against salpingitis may be a result of OC-related changes in cervical mucus, which becomes thick, viscous and less penetrable by both spermatozoa and bacteria. These progestin-mediated changes impede ascent of infectious organisms into the upper reproductive tract.

Data from a United States multicenter, case-control study of salpingitis analyzed by the Centers for Disease Control and Prevention (CDC) indicate that women with no history of salpingitis using OCs have a 50% lower risk of being hospitalized for the disease than nonusers.[1] Protection was concentrated among women using the pill for at least 1 year, in whom the risk was reduced 70%. Protection, particularly in the age group at greatest risk for salpingitis—sexually active women between the ages of 15 and 24 years—can considerably reduce associated consequences of PID, such as blockage of the fallopian tubes and subsequent increased risk of infertility or ectopic pregnancy.

Ectopic Pregnancy

By inhibiting ovulation, OCs protect against ectopic pregnancy and associated mortality and morbidity. Case-control studies demonstrate 90% protection from ectopic pregnancy with current OC use.[1,6]

5

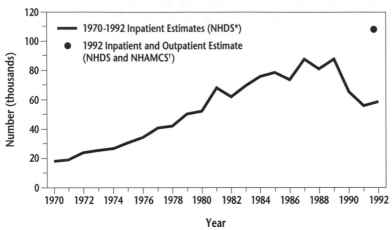

Figure 5

Number of Ectopic Pregnancies — United States, 1970-1992

*National Hospital Discharge Survey.
†National Hospital Ambulatory Medical Care Survey.
Source: Centers for Disease Control and Prevention, 1995 (see reference 11).*

The number of ectopic pregnancies in the U.S. has been on the rise since 1970 (Figure 5).[11] Data from the CDC indicate that since 1989, the number of hospitalizations for ectopic pregnancy has decreased; however, this may be due to a rise in the number of cases treated on an outpatient basis. When recalculated to take outpatient treatments into consideration, the number of ectopic pregnancies in 1992 reached a 20-year high. The CDC attributes this rise to the trend in increased prevalence of such risk factors as chlamydial infection and other sexually transmitted diseases (STDs).

Functional Ovarian Cysts

Older epidemiologic studies found the risk of functional ovarian cysts decreased with the use of OCs.[1,6] Newer data suggest, however, that this effect is attenuated by the lower estrogen dosage in currently used pills (for further discussion, see section 1.8, *Trends in Development and Utilization*, in this chapter).

Iron Deficiency Anemia

Combination OCs decrease menstrual blood loss, which reduces the likelihood of development of iron deficiency anemia. Both current and past OC use have been associated with a protective effect.[1]

Menstrual Cycle Benefits

Fewer menstrual disorders—eg, menorrhagia, irregular menstruation or intermenstrual bleeding—occur in OC users than in women having spontaneous menstrual cycles.[8] OC use also improves primary dysmenorrhea in most women and premenstrual tension in some. This effect may particularly benefit teenage patients, among whom dysmenorrhea is a very common complaint. Studies have found that about

60% of adolescents report dysmenorrhea, and of those, 14% missed school as a result.[12] While these conditions seldom pose any serious threat to health, they frequently impair quality of life and the ability to participate in activities.

Growing Evidence

During the past decade, evidence has accumulated to suggest that OCs may also help protect against osteoporosis.

Osteoporosis

Estrogen replacement therapy is one approach to reducing the risk of post-menopausal osteoporosis. More recently, however, a positive effect of combination OCs on preserving bone density has been demonstrated. Whether these effects persist into the age span when maximal protection would be most valuable, however, remains unestablished. (For further discussion, see the following section on OCs and bone density in this chapter.)

Still Controversial

Colorectal Cancer

Some evidence suggests that OCs may protect women against the later development of colorectal cancer. In North America and Europe, incidence and mortality of large bowel cancer have been consistently lower among women than among men. Although some of this difference may be explained by dietary factors or a healthier lifestyle, another possible explanation involves exposure to endogenous or exogenous sex hormones.

One recent investigation found a 40% reduction in risk among women who had ever used OCs (odds ratio [OR]=0.6; 95% confidence interval [CI], 0.4-0.9).[13] Use for 2 or more years conferred a 50% reduction in risk (OR=0.5; 95% CI, 0.3-1.0). Although several studies have found similar protection with OC use,[14,15] others have not.[16,17] Also, the relationship between duration of use and reduction of risk has been inconsistent; therefore, caution is warranted in interpretation of these findings. Further research is needed to confirm or dispute this potential health benefit of OCs.

Uterine Fibroids

The Oxford Family Planning Association researchers noted a reduced risk of uterine fibroids in OC users.[18] Increasing protection correlated with a longer duration of pill use; 10 years of use conferred a 30% risk reduction. Uterine fibroids are the most common pelvic neoplasm in women; thus, confirming evidence of a protective effect could mean substantial prevention of surgeries and hospitalizations. A large case-control study from Italy found no effect.[19]

Toxic Shock Syndrome

Five studies of TSS (reviewed and summarized by Gray in 1987) reported an overall 50% reduction in risk associated with OC use.[20] However, two more recent, large case-control studies—one of menstrual TSS and the other of nonmenstrual TSS—failed to demonstrate such an effect of OCs.[21,22] The latter findings may be explained by subsequent changes in tampon composition, absorbency and usage. It appears plausible that because of decreased menstrual bleeding, OC users were less likely to use highly absorbent tampons than were other women. Thus, the lower risk of TSS seen in OC users could be considered an indirect effect of OC use.

Rheumatoid Arthritis

Two studies conducted before 1982 demonstrated a 40% to 50% reduction in the risk of premenopausal rheumatoid arthritis in OC users.[23,24] Since that time, 12 studies —eight case-control and four cohort—have yielded conflicting results. Biases in these observational studies subsequently have been identified, however, which complicate attempts to correlate OC use and risk of rheumatoid arthritis. A meta-analysis of all studies published through 1996 found no conclusive evidence of a protective effect of OCs; additional work is needed before any firm conclusions can be drawn.[25]

Summary

When counseling women about oral contraception, it is important to give a balanced perspective on both the benefits and the risks. Often, women are frightened of hormonal contraception, believing that hormones cause cancer and other serious health risks. Thus, counseling and education about the many health benefits conferred by OC use are necessary to help women put the advantages and disadvantages of birth control methods in perspective. Clinicians should stress with patients the immediate benefits of the pill, such as decreased menstrual flow, relief of dysmenorrhea and cycle control, as well as longer-term health benefits, such as reduction in ovarian and endometrial cancers and possible protection against bone loss and colorectal cancer.

References

1. Peterson HB, Lee NC. The health effects of oral contraceptives: misperceptions, controversies, and continuing good news. *Clin Obstet Gynecol* 1989;32:339-355.

2. American Cancer Society. *Cancer Facts and Figures-1996.* Atlanta: American Cancer Society;1996.

3. Schlesselman JJ. Cancer of the breast and reproductive tract in relation to use of oral contraceptives. *Contraception* 1989;40:1-38.

4. The Cancer and Steroid Hormone Study of the Centers for Disease Control and the National Institute of Child Health and Human Development. The reduction in risk of ovarian cancer associated with oral contraceptive use. *N Engl J Med* 1987;316:650-655.

5. The Cancer and Steroid Hormone Study of the Centers for Disease Control and the National Institute of Child Health and Human Development. Combination oral contraceptive use and the risk of endometrial cancer. *JAMA* 1987;257:796-800.

6. Prentice RL, Thomas DB. On the epidemiology of oral contraceptives and disease. *Adv Cancer Res* 1987;49:285-401.

7. Ory HW. The noncontraceptive health benefits from oral contraceptive use. *Fam Plann Perspect* 1982;14:182-184.

8. Mishell DR. Noncontraceptive health benefits of oral steroidal contraceptives. *Am J Obstet Gynecol* 1982;142:809-816.

9. Royal College of General Practitioners' Oral Contraception Study. Effect on hypertension and benign breast disease of progestagen component in combined oral contraceptives. *Lancet* 1977;1:624.

10. Brinton LA, Vessey MP, Flavel R, et al. Risk factors for benign breast disease. *Am J Epidemiol* 1981;113:203-214.

11. Centers for Disease Control and Prevention. Ectopic pregnancy—United States, 1990-1992. *MMWR* 1995;44:46-48.

12. Klein JR, Litt IF. Epidemiology of adolescent dysmenorrhea. *Pediatrics* 1981;68:661-664.

13. Fernandez E, La Vecchia C, D'Avanzo B, et al. Oral contraceptives, hormone replacement therapy and the risk of colorectal cancer. *Br J Cancer* 1996;73:1431-1435.

14. Potter JD, McMichael AJ. Large bowel cancer in women in relation to reproductive and hormonal factors: a case-control study. *J Natl Cancer Inst* 1983;71:703-709.

15. Furner SE, Davis FG, Nelson RL, et al. A case-control study of large bowel cancer and hormone exposure in women. *Cancer Res* 1989;49:4936-4940.

16. Kune GA, Kune S, Watson LF. Oral contraceptive use does not protect against large bowel cancer. *Contraception* 1990;41:19-25.

17. Weiss NS, Daling JR, Chow WH. Incidence of cancer of the large bowel in women in relation to reproductive and hormonal factors. *J Natl Cancer Inst* 1981;67:57-60.

18. Ross RK, Pike MC, Vessey MP, et al. Risk factors for uterine fibroids: reduced risk associated with oral contraceptives. *BMJ* 1986;293:359-362.

19. Parazzini F, Negri E, LaVecchia C, et al. Oral contraceptive use and risk of uterine fibroids. *Obstet Gynecol* 1992;79:430-433.

20. Gray RH. Toxic shock syndrome and oral contraception. *Am J Obstet Gynecol* 1987;156:1038.

21. Schwartz B, Gaventa S, Broome CV, et al. Nonmenstrual toxic shock syndrome associated with barrier contraceptives: report of a case-control study. *Rev Infect Dis* 1989;11(suppl):S43-S48.

22. Reingold AL, Broome CV, Gaventa S, et al. Risk factors for menstrual toxic shock syndrome: results of a multi-state case-control study. *Rev Infect Dis* 1989;11(suppl):S35-S41.

23. Wingrave SJ. Reduction in incidence of rheumatoid arthritis associated with oral contraceptives: Royal College of General Practitioners' oral contraception study. *Lancet* 1978;1:569-571.

24. Vandenbroucke JP, Boersma JW, Festen JJM, et al. Oral contraceptives and rheumatoid arthritis: further evidence for a preventive effect. *Lancet* 1982;2:839-842.

25. Pladevall-Vila M, Delclos GL, Varas C, et al. Controversy of oral contraceptives and risk of rheumatoid arthritis: meta-analysis of conflicting studies and review of conflicting meta-analyses with special emphasis on analysis of heterogeneity. *Am J Epidemiol* 1996;144:1-14.

1.2: Bone Density

Can the use of oral contraceptives (OCs) prior to menopause help prevent bone loss and possibly slow the progression of or prevent osteoporosis? This question has taken on greater importance as women live longer. Given the fact that women in ever-increasing numbers are living well into their 70s, 80s and beyond, it is a matter of great importance for them to reach the time of their menopause with the maximum bone density possible. This section explores the growing body of evidence that suggests that OCs, in fact, do help women retain bone mass during the period of decline, which normally starts between the ages of 30 and 40 years.

It has long been known that postmenopausal estrogen helps to prevent osteoporosis; it is biologically plausible that OCs may exert a similar effect, but, until recently, the evidence was conflicting.

Several studies of both college-aged and postmenopausal women published over the past several years provide further evidence that OCs can prevent loss of bone mass.[1-3] A cross-sectional, retrospective study by Kleerekoper et al investigated risk factors for low bone mineral density in a group of 2,297 women, 76% of whom were postmenopausal.[1] Thirty percent of the women in the study reported prior OC use.

The investigators found that a history of OC use was protective against low bone mineral density (odds ratio [OR]=0.4; 95% confidence interval [CI], 0.2-0.5). Further analyses demonstrated an increasing protective effect with increasing duration of use—women who reported using OCs for 10 years or longer were afforded the greatest protection (OR=0.2; 95% CI, 0.1-0.7) when compared with women who had never used OCs. These results were true whether the measurements were taken from the distal radius and ulna or lumbar spine. Because the mean age of the study participants was high (54 years), it is likely that most OC users took higher-dose pills. More work needs to be done to examine the effect of low-dose pills on postmenopausal bone density.

A longitudinal, prospective study of 156 college-aged women sought to determine whether bone mass increases in healthy, nonpregnant, white women during early adult life after cessation of linear growth.[2] The study also looked at whether physical activity, nutrient intake and OC use influenced increase in bone mass. A bivariate analysis showed that the use of OCs was associated with greater gain in total body bone mass (p=0.01). The study concluded that increased activity and calcium intake, as well as use of OCs, may significantly reduce the risk of osteoporosis late in life.

The third investigation—a large, community-based sample of older postmenopausal women—also examined the relationship between OC use and bone mineral density.[3] The study of 239 women ages 55 to 69 years found that those who used OCs for 6 or more years had significantly greater spine and femoral neck bone densities than women who never used them. Higher bone densities were not found, however, in the ultradistal wrist or midshaft radius. Even when such potential confounding factors as age, body mass index, parity, cigarette smoking, number of years postmenopausal, or use of estrogen and thiazide medications were taken into consideration, the association between OC use and greater spine and femoral neck bone densities persisted. The investigators noted that the association was strong enough to be detected despite the small sample of long-term OC users (n=21). The authors concluded, "If use of oral contraceptives for 6 or more years reduces the risk of postmenopausal bone loss, the public health impact could be large."[3]

In a 1996 review of the literature, DeCherney weighed the evidence for and against OCs protecting against bone loss.[4] Overall, the weight of the evidence suggests that premenopausal use of OCs is beneficial for preserving bone mass; eight studies supported an association while four did not. While it is unclear just how much estrogen is optimal, DeCherney suggests that "It appears that in the premenopausal woman, oral contraceptives that will provide bone-sparing effects while minimizing long-term complications should contain the equivalent of ≥20 mcg/day."

References

1.   Kleerekoper M, Brienza RS, Schultz LR, et al. Oral contraceptive use may protect against low bone mass. *Arch Intern Med* 1991;151:1971-1976.

2. Recker RR, Davies M, Hinders SM, et al. Bone gain in young adult women. *JAMA* 1992;268: 2403-2408.

3. Kritz-Silverstein D, Barrett-Connor E. Bone mineral density in postmenopausal women as determined by prior oral contraceptive use. *Am J Public Health* 1993;83:100-102.

4. DeCherney A. Bone-sparing properties of oral contraceptives. *Am J Obstet Gynecol* 1996;174:15-20.

1.3: Use in Women over Age 35 Years

In early 1990, the Food and Drug Administration (FDA) accepted the recommendation of its Fertility and Maternal Health Drugs Advisory Committee to revise the labeling for oral contraceptives (OCs). In a letter to manufacturers, the FDA requested that the language of the patient information be modified.[1] Specifically, reference to increased cardiovascular mortality risks among healthy, nonsmoking women ages 40 years and older was deleted.

The guidelines reflect the growing body of evidence that the benefits of OCs for healthy, nonsmoking women over 40 may outweigh the risks. The FDA has never identified age as a mandatory contraindication to OC use. However, the earlier labeling often determined *de facto* age limits; that is, limits that were adhered to by physicians unwilling to prescribe outside of labeling.

The Fertility and Maternal Health Drugs Advisory Committee met on October 26, 1989, and thoroughly reviewed the data on the use of oral contraceptives by older women. The committee concluded that "...there are greater potential health risks associated with pregnancy in older women and with the alternative surgical and medical procedures which may be necessary if such women do not have access to effective and acceptable means of contraception." Elizabeth B. Connell, MD, Associate Editor of *The Contraception Report*, noted that "epidemiological data clearly show the substantial health benefits of OCs, particularly prevention of ovarian and endometrial cancers. Of course, as the revised labeling states, all women, especially older women, are cautioned to use the lowest-dose pill that is effective."

Since 1985, the American College of Obstetricians and Gynecologists has taken the position that OCs, particularly low-dose OCs, are safe and appropriate contraception for healthy, nonsmoking women over 35.[2] Low-dose OCs, which are the most widely used preparations today, cause very few side effects and are highly effective.[3] The use of low-dose pills, containing 35 mcg or less of estrogen combined with lower doses of progestin, has reduced the incidence of certain adverse effects previously associated with OCs.

Origins of Age Limitations

Early British studies that initially raised concern about the cardiovascular risks associated with OCs were done in the 1970s, when high-dose pills were being used. At that time, little was known about screening women for risk factors, such as smoking. Virtually every woman who wished to use OCs was allowed to do so. These early studies were eventually reanalyzed and the side effects initially attributed to OCs were determined to be largely the result of a critical confounding factor—smoking. Unfortunately, the smoking factor led to a distorted perception of the safety of OCs.

The original data from the Royal College of General Practitioners' Oral Contraception Study, for example, found an increased risk of death from vascular disease with increasing duration of OC use.[4] Other studies published in 1975 found that OC users were at increased risk of fatal and nonfatal myocardial infarction. The risk was seen for women ages 30 to 39, and increased for women ages 40 to 44.[5,6]

In a review of the literature, Realini and Goldzieher found that serious epidemiologic flaws were present in the early studies by Mann et al, which suggested an increased cardiovascular risk.[7] Joseph W. Goldzieher, MD, Associate Editor of *The Contraception Report*, comments that "the age restriction limiting OC use was a mistake in the first place. It was based on early British studies that did not take smoking into consideration. When the confounding smoking factor was removed, there was no cardiovascular pill risk at any age. And, this was true at a time when mostly over-50 mcg pills were being used. Furthermore, an increased risk in very light smokers (<15 cigarettes per day) was not detectable. The risk absolutely increases, however, in women who smoke more than 15 cigarettes per day."

OCs Chosen Infrequently by Women over Age 35

Pill use declines markedly with advancing age. The 1988 National Survey of Family Growth (NSFG) documents low utilization of the pill in the 35 to 39 and 40 to 44 age groups among women using contraception (Figure 1).[8] Among women ages 20 to 24, 68% use the pill. Pill use declines until, at age 35, the percentage of women who choose to use OCs is a mere 5%. For women ages 40 to 44, the percentage using the pill is 3%, up slightly from 1982, when the percentage relying upon OCs was 1%. These data clearly indicate that pill use is uncommon among older women.

Consequences of Pill Discontinuation

Perceived risks lead to discontinuation of OCs, method switching and an important consequence—increased risk of unintended pregnancy. Pratt and Bachrach (1987) analyzed data from the 1982 NSFG with regard to method switching and found that when women discontinued using OCs, many did not immediately use another method of birth control (Figure 2).[9] Four-fifths of women discontinuing the pill were at an increased risk of pregnancy by using less-effective contraception, such as barrier methods or no method at all. If women had a break between methods, the rate of unintended pregnancy was 26%. Still, even if a new method was adopted in the same month or the next month after pill discontinuation, an unintended pregnancy occurred in 10% of these women. In order to avoid unnecessary OC discontinuation because of misperceptions and decrease the potential for unintended pregnancy, women need to be better informed about the safety of OCs. This is particularly true for healthy, nonsmoking women ages 35 years and older, in whom pill use is still infrequent.

Figure 1

Use of Oral Contraceptives by Age: United States, 1982 and 1988

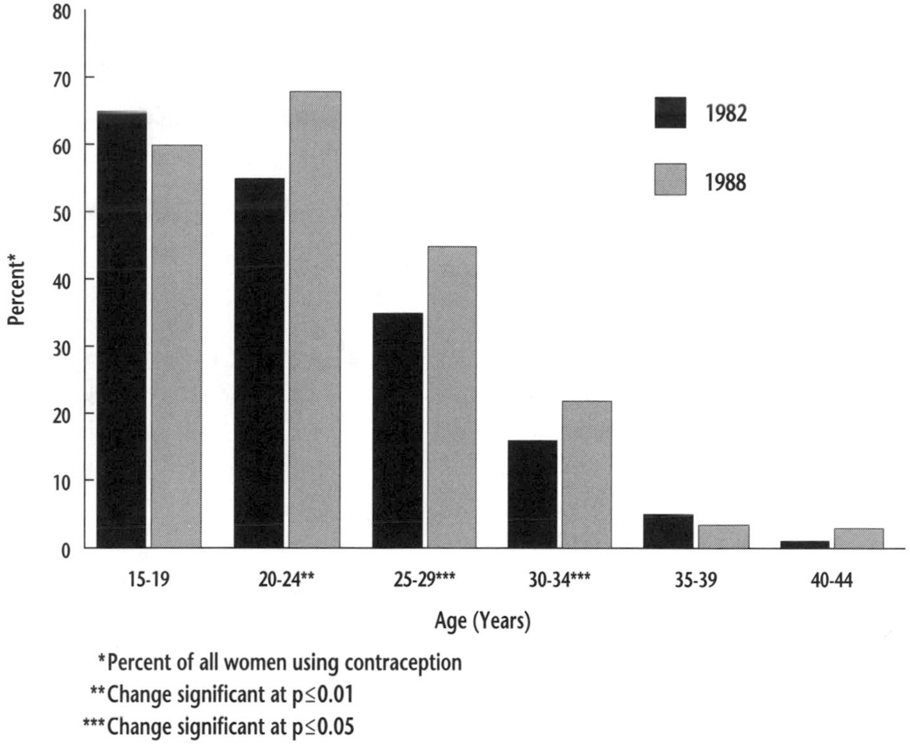
80
70
60
50
40
30
20
10
0
Percent*
1982
1988
15-19
20-24**
25-29***
30-34***
35-39
40-44
Age (Years)
*Percent of all women using contraception
**Change significant at p≤0.01
***Change significant at p≤0.05

Source: Mosher WD, 1990 (see reference 8).

Can Women Take OCs until Menopause?

For healthy, nonsmoking women without contraindications, the pill is a safe and effective birth control method up to menopause. Cardiovascular events, in particular, seem to occur primarily in OC users with other risk factors, such as cigarette smoking and hypertension, both of which appear to work synergistically with OCs to enhance risk. Furthermore, the pill provides many noncontraceptive benefits that must be weighed against possible risks. Cycle control may be an especially important benefit for older women, in whom irregular cycles are likely to become more frequent.

Screening for Women Ages 40 and Older

Current recommendations concerning the screening of women ages 40 and older when prescribing OCs vary among practitioners and health organizations, such as the World Health Organization and the American Diabetes Association. Recommendations differ depending upon family history of cardiovascular diseases, diabetes, age and whether or not the patient smokes. Many clinicians prescribe OCs for healthy, nonsmoking women ages 40 years and older without additional screening, while others may opt for such tests as a lipid profile. There is considerable debate as to whether or not such tests are cost-effective. In addition, the clinical relevance of altered lipid profiles in OC users is unproven (see section on metabolic effects of OCs in this chapter).

OCs Can Benefit Perimenopausal Women

The multiple consequences of unwanted pregnancies in older women are reasons to consider use of a highly effective method, such as OCs, in this age group. Some of the reasons why an unintended pregnancy can be particularly traumatic in this age group are the increased incidence of Down syndrome and the potential need for an abortion. Besides preventing unintended pregnancies, OCs can prove helpful in maintaining regular bleeding cycles and a consistent hormonal pattern right up to menopause.

When Can Hormone Replacement Therapy (HRT) Begin?

In order to determine when HRT can begin, one approach is to discontinue OCs for 2 weeks and counsel the patient to use a nonhormonal contraceptive method. Follicle-stimulating hormone (FSH) levels should be tested once or twice. If these levels are consistently at or above the menopausal range given by the laboratory, it is safe to switch to HRT. For the woman who is not taking the pill, clinical symptoms should be evaluated. Women in their late 40s to early 50s who are having symptoms of menopause should have an FSH level done; when levels are at or above menopausal levels, HRT can begin.

One small study found that FSH levels did not always rise in postmenopausal women after discontinuing OCs.[10] On the other hand, basal estradiol levels remained unchanged before and after OC use. Thus, the authors suggest that measuring E_2 levels in addition to FSH may be helpful to determine when to switch from OCs to standard HRT.

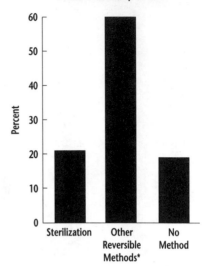

Figure 2

Choice of Contraception after Discontinuing Oral Contraceptives: United States, 1982

*Includes IUD, diaphragm, condom, foam, creams, jellies, periodic abstinence, withdrawal, douche and others.

Source: Pratt WF, et al, 1987 (see reference 9).

References

1. *F-D-C Reports.* February 5, 1990; T&G-8.

2. American College of Obstetricians and Gynecologists. Contraception for women in their later reproductive years. *ACOG Committee Opinion* 1985;41.

3. Mishell DR Jr. Contraception. *N Engl J Med* 1989;320:777-787.

4. Beral V. Mortality among oral contraceptive users: Royal College of General Practitioners' Oral Contraception Study. *Lancet* 1977;2:727.

5. Mann JI, Vessey MP, Thorogood M, et al. Myocardial infarction in young women with special reference to oral contraceptive practice. *BMJ* 1975;2:241-244.

6. Mann JI, Inman WHW. Oral contraceptives and death from myocardial infarction. *BMJ* 1975;2:245.

7. Realini JP, Goldzieher JW. Oral contraceptives and cardiovascular disease: a critique of the epidemiologic studies. *Am J Obstet Gynecol* 1985;152:729-798.

8. Mosher WD. Contraceptive practice in the United States, 1982-1988. *Fam Plann Perspect* 1990;22:198-205.

9. Pratt WF, Bachrach CA. What do women use when they stop using the pill? *Fam Plann Perspect* 1987;19:257-266.

10. Castracane VD, Gimpel T, Goldzieher JW. When is it safe to switch from oral contraceptives to hormonal replacement therapy? *Contraception* 1995;52:371-376.

1.4: Breast Cancer

Endogenous hormones play a role in the etiology of human breast cancer. In particular, the timing of different hormonal events in a woman's life, such as menarche, first birth and menopause, impact her subsequent chance of getting breast cancer. Hormones are implicated in the etiology of the disease, though they are believed to be tumor promoters rather than initiators. Therefore, it is reasonable to ask whether exogenous hormones affect a woman's risk of developing breast cancer. This presumed hormonal link is the basis for the concern about whether oral contraceptives (OCs) may increase a woman's risk of developing the disease.[1]

i. Overview

Incidence of Breast Cancer

Over half a million women in the United States are diagnosed each year with cancer; the most common is breast cancer, followed by lung/larynx and colon/rectal cancers.[1,2] Over 180,000 new cases of breast cancer are diagnosed and over 40,000 women die of the disease annually. Breast cancer is relatively rare in women under 35 years of age. However, the incidence rises sharply at ages 35 to 40 and then continues to rise less steeply thereafter. Over a lifetime, approximately one in eight women will develop breast cancer.[2]

Risk Factors for Breast Cancer

A woman's chance of getting breast cancer varies, depending upon her risk factor profile. For example, her risk of developing breast cancer is directly related to age. Younger women are least likely, while older women are most likely to develop the disease. The risk factors related to endogenous hormones are early age at menarche, late age at menopause, nulliparity and advanced age at birth of first child (Figure 1).[3] Conversely, premenopausal oophorectomy, late age at menarche and early age at first birth are associated with a reduction in risk. Some of the other risk factors for developing breast cancer are Caucasian race, Northern American or Northern European ethnic origin, excess exposure to ionizing radiation, family history of breast cancer (a particularly strong association), presence of the BRCAI gene and presence of biopsy-proven benign breast disease with cellular atypia.[3]

Figure 1

Selected Risk Factors for Breast Cancer that Implicate Hormones in Etiology

Factor	Higher Risk	Lower Risk
Age at menarche	Early	Late
Age at menopause	Late	Early
Oophorectomy (early age protective)	No	Yes
Nulliparity	Yes	No
Age at first birth	Older than 30	Younger than 20
Genetics	BRCAI gene	No BRCAI gene

Source: Adapted from Kelsey JL, et al, 1988 (see reference 3).

Studies Show No Overall Increased Risk of Breast Cancer in OC Users over Lifetime

A 1991 review of the literature summarized the data from 15 case-control studies of breast cancer and OC use in women of all ages in developed countries.[4] Relative risk (RR) estimates are shown by year of study in Figure 2. A summary relative risk of 1.0 in women who ever used OCs was estimated from the published results of these studies. Only one study (Ravnihar et al, 1988) found a significant trend of increasing risk with duration of exposure.

Figure 2

Relative Risk of Breast Cancer in Women in Developed Countries Who Have Ever Used OCs: Case-Control Studies of Women of All Ages at Risk of Exposure

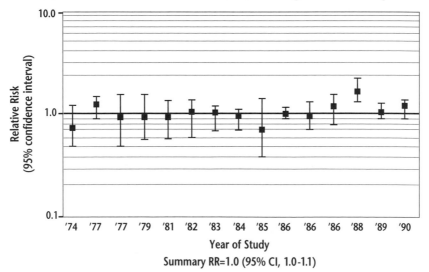

Year of Study
Summary RR=1.0 (95% CI, 1.0-1.1)

Source: Adapted from Thomas DB, 1991 (see reference 4).

16

The review also estimated the relative risk from the published results of five cohort studies (Figure 3). A summary relative risk of 1.1 (95% confidence interval [CI], 1.0-1.2) in women who ever used OCs was found. The conclusion derived from this overview of both case-control and cohort studies was that there appeared to be no overall association between use of OCs and breast cancer.

Several of the studies shown in Figures 2 and 3 are large and sophisticated. One of these, a population-based case-control study, was the Cancer and Steroid Hormone (CASH) study conducted by the Centers for Disease Control and Prevention.[5] The CASH study evaluated nearly 4,700 women with breast cancer and an equal number of controls. The study identified cases of breast, endometrial and ovarian cancers occurring among women ages 20 to 54 in 10 regions of the U.S. The relative risk of developing breast cancer for OC users versus never-users was 1.0, indicating no overall increased risk of developing the disease.[5]

In addition, the Royal College of General Practitioners' (RCGP) study, a long-term, prospective cohort study started in 1968, also found no increased risk of breast cancer for OC users compared with never-users.[6] The study evaluated 23,000 women who used OCs and an equal number of women who had never used OCs. Though the data from CASH and RCGP were later reanalyzed by subgroups and suggested some increased risk in certain populations, the overall risk for women up to age 55 was not elevated.

A more recent analysis (1989) of a large cohort study, the Nurses' Health Study, confirmed the lack of an association between OC use and breast cancer for all users when compared to never-users.[7] The analysis included data on over 118,000 female nurses. For all users, the relative risk was 1.1 (95% CI, 1.0-1.2). The authors concluded

Figure 3

Relative Risk of Breast Cancer in Women Who Have Ever Used OCs: Cohort Studies

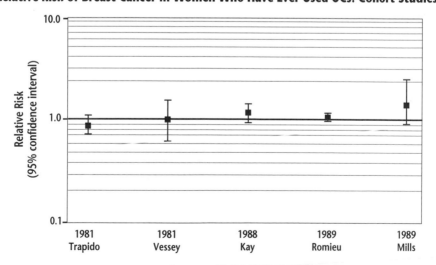

Summary RR=1.1 (95% CI, 1.0-1.2)

Source: Adapted from Thomas DB, 1991 (see reference 4).

that, overall, past use of OCs was not associated with an increased risk of breast cancer.

In 1990, the World Health Organization (WHO) released the results of the WHO Collaborative Study of Neoplasia and Steroid Contraceptives.[8] Based on data collected on 2,116 women with newly diagnosed breast cancer and 12,077 controls, the study found a relative risk of 1.1 (95% CI, 0.9-1.3) for women in developed nations (not statistically significant). For women in developing countries, the relative risk estimate was statistically significant, 1.2 (95% CI, 1.1-1.5).

Furthermore, a 1990 comprehensive review and meta-analysis by Romieu et al[9] of OCs and breast cancer again confirmed the findings of earlier studies. There was no increased risk of breast cancer in women who had ever used OCs, even after a long duration of use. A 1996 analysis that pooled worldwide data from 54 case-control studies on breast cancer and use of OCs found similar results.[10] The overall relative risk of breast cancer with OC use was 1.1 (95% CI, 1.0-1.1); current users had a relative risk of 1.2 (95% CI, 1.2-1.3). (For more complete discussion, see *Worldwide Data Reassuring* in this section on page 24.)

Subgroups Are the Focus of Intensive Study and Conflicting Results

Even though most studies have found no overall increased risk of breast cancer with OC use, investigations into the possibility have continued. In addition to the publication of new results, many studies, including CASH and RCGP, were reanalyzed to examine special groups of OC users.

Family History of Breast Cancer, Benign Breast Disease and Latency

OC users with a family history of breast cancer or existing benign breast disease do not seem to have a further increased risk due to their use of OCs (Figure 4).[11,12] The CASH study also found no evidence of an increased risk associated with a particular OC formulation.[5] Furthermore, though it has been suggested that a latency effect could exist, a review by Schlesselman has shown that none of the studies directly examining this issue supported a long-term latent effect.[11]

Age and Parity

The results of subgroup analyses have been conflicting. For example, a reanalysis (1988) of the original RCGP report found that the risk of breast cancer was significantly increased only in British women 30 to 34 years of age when compared to never-users (RR=3.3; 95% CI, 1.3-8.8).[13] However, no evidence of a dose response by duration of use was apparent. The authors also found OC users with a parity of 1, but not parity of 0 or ≥2, to be at increased risk of developing breast cancer. Importantly, in confirmation of earlier studies, the risk of breast cancer was not increased in OC users over 35 years of age.

In contrast, CASH study reanalyses found a suggestion of an increased risk for women who were nulliparous long-term users of OCs (>8 years) who had an early menarche (age <13 years).[14,15] However, older women (ages 45 to 54) in this subgroup had a decreased risk of breast cancer, although this was not statistically significant (RR=0.9; 95% CI, 0.8-1.0). The United Kingdom National Case-Control Study Group, on the other hand, found an increased risk in *both* young parous and nulliparous OC

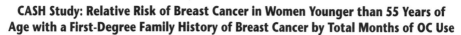

Figure 4

CASH Study: Relative Risk of Breast Cancer in Women Younger than 55 Years of Age with a First-Degree Family History of Breast Cancer by Total Months of OC Use

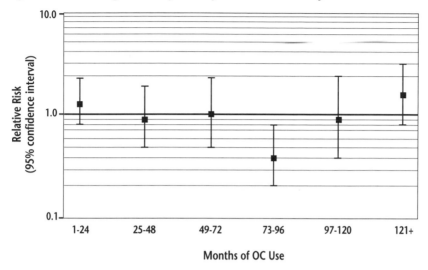

Months of OC Use

Source: Adapted from Murray PP, et al, 1989 (see reference 12).

users.[16] The WHO Collaborative Study found a relative risk of 1.5, which was of borderline statistical significance (95% CI, 0.98-2.3), for women who had used OCs for more than 2 years prior to age 25. A steady trend of increasing risk with years of use was not evident.

A U.S. case-control study published in 1996 suggests that OC use has not resulted in an excessive risk of breast cancer in middle-aged women (those 50 to 64 years of age between 1988 and 1990).[17] Researchers interviewed 537 women diagnosed with breast cancer identified through the Cancer Surveillance System, a population-based cancer registry operating as part of the National Cancer Institute's Surveillance, Epidemiology and End Results program. These women were likely to have started using OCs in the 1960s and 1970s, when higher-dose pills were more commonly prescribed. Despite this, the adjusted relative risk of breast cancer was 1.1 (95% CI, 0.8-1.4) for ever use of OCs. No trends were evident with regard to total duration of OC use, time since last use, or age at first or last use. While the study supports the absence of any strong association between OC use and breast cancer risk during middle age, a very small percentage of users took the pill for long durations at a young age—a subgroup under intense scrutiny.

Long-Term Use before First-Term Pregnancy

In a 1990 review of the breast cancer literature, Schlesselman found that nine studies looked at the risk of breast cancer in relation to duration of OC use before first-term pregnancy (Figure 5).[11] There is a suggestion of a possible increase in risk, with a relative risk of 1.5 at 4 to 6 years of use, and a relative risk of 2.0 at 8 to 10 years of use.

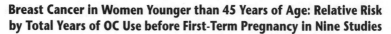

Figure 5

Breast Cancer in Women Younger than 45 Years of Age: Relative Risk by Total Years of OC Use before First-Term Pregnancy in Nine Studies

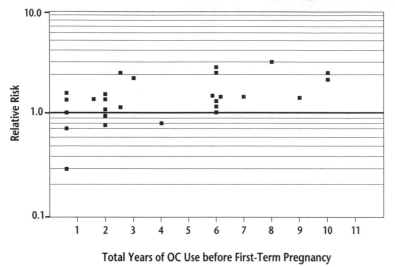

Total Years of OC Use before First-Term Pregnancy

Source: Schlesselman JJ. Oral contraceptives and breast cancer. Am J Obstet Gynecol 1990;163: 1379-1387. Reproduced with permission of the publisher, Mosby-Yearbook, Inc.

Only three of these studies, however, individually show a gradient of risk. Dr. Schlesselman states, "The absence of any compelling explanation for the striking inconsistencies among these studies prevents any certain conclusion with regard to cause and effect."

Long-Term Use in Young Women

The most consistent results are for an increase in risk in young women after long-term use. David B. Thomas, MD, DrPH, combined results from 12 case-control studies that reported data for young, long-term users and found the overall relative risk for young women who used OCs for ≥4 years to be 1.4 (95% CI, 1.3-1.6) (Figure 6).[4] Dr. Thomas is Head of the Program in Epidemiology at the Fred Hutchinson Cancer Research Center in Seattle, Washington.

According to Dr. Thomas' analysis, "Selective reporting of only positive results does not appear to be a likely explanation for the relative consistency of findings among studies. Only two case-control studies...that have specifically addressed the issue of oral contraceptive use and risk of breast cancer in young women have not shown some evidence of an enhanced risk. ...If the estimate of approximately a 40% increase in risk in young women who were long-term users is correct, a few studies could have failed to detect such a small enhancement in risk because of chance or insufficient statistical power."[4]

Figure 6

Relative Risk of Breast Cancer in Women under 45 Years of Age with Long-Term OC Use: Summary of Results from 12 Case-Control Studies

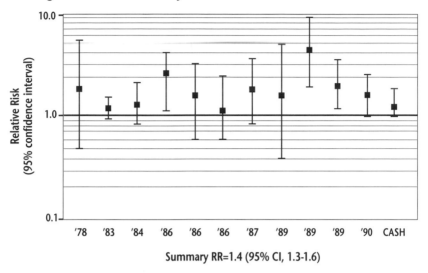

Summary RR=1.4 (95% CI, 1.3-1.6)

Source: Adapted from Thomas DB, 1991 (see reference 4).

It is not known why many studies disagree on the nature and degree to which OCs may affect a woman's risk of breast cancer. One hypothesis is that OCs may accelerate the growth of undetected breast tumors so that they are diagnosed earlier than they would have been otherwise (growth stimulation). Another explanation is that OC users are likely to be screened more often and therefore may have their tumors detected earlier (screening bias). A third possibility is that OCs act as tumor promoters to cause an actual increase in the risk of breast cancer. It is possible that the proportion of cases under age 45 in most of the studies have been relatively small, and thus the increased risk may have contributed too little to the overall relative risk to elevate it appreciably above unity. The risk, if it is a true association, appears to be a subtle one, possibly enhancing the risk of developing breast cancer early in life, but not resulting in an aggregate increased risk over a lifetime.

According to Dr. Thomas, "...it appears that there may be a small increase in risk for young women who used OCs for a prolonged period of time; however, I don't think there is a definitive interpretation of these recent study results. We will need to monitor these young, long-term users to determine whether or not this apparent increase in risk continues at later ages or whether it is present only during a particular age. It will be some time before that type of data is available. In addition, it is important to remember that these results are largely for women who have used high-dose pills. The effect of low-dose pills is unknown and will not be known for many years."

Interpreting the Subgroup Data

In order to interpret study results and try to determine whether there is a cause-effect relationship, epidemiologists evaluate several factors. These include the strength of the reported association, consistency of results among studies, whether a dose response is apparent and whether there is biologic plausibility.

For the breast cancer investigations to date, particularly the subgroup analyses reported since 1986, the following limitations must be taken into consideration: one, the studies are conflicting; two, the strength of the association has, in general, been weak; three, there is a limitation in many subgroup analyses in that the number and type of women studied are small; four, if there is an increased risk of breast cancer with OC use, then a dose response over time should be seen. Studies have not confirmed the presence of a dose response for all users, although long-term use confers the greatest risk in young women.

FDA and Institute of Medicine Report Recommend No Change in Use of OCs

In the U.S., the Food and Drug Administration thoroughly reviewed all the evidence through 1989 on breast cancer and recommended no change in labeling, use or prescribing practices.[18] The Institute of Medicine's Committee on the Relationship Between Oral Contraceptives and Breast Cancer also does not recommend any change in prescribing practices of OCs.[4]

In the U.K., no change in prescribing practices has been recommended; however, in July of 1990, statements regarding OCs and cancer were added to labeling. The following statement now appears on OC data sheets (equivalent to package inserts) in the *U.K. Data Sheet Compendium* (similar to the *Physicians' Desk Reference*): "The evidence linking combined oral contraceptive use and breast cancer remains inconclusive. The results of some studies suggest an increased risk of breast cancer presenting below the age of about 35, the risk rising with duration of use. Any possible increased risk of breast cancer with combined oral contraceptives is, however, likely to be small and may be expected to be less with low-dosage pills. This possible risk should be weighed against the many benefits of combined oral contraceptives, including their protective effects against ovarian and endometrial cancers."[19]

The health benefits of OCs include not only protection from endometrial and ovarian cancers, but also reductions in the incidence of dysmenorrhea, iron-deficiency anemia, pelvic inflammatory disease, benign breast disease and ectopic pregnancy. An Alan Guttmacher study reports that the risk of developing

---

Epidemiologic Overview: Oral Contraceptives and Breast Cancer

- No overall increased risk for women up to age 55

- No firm evidence of latency effect

- No apparent difference in risk noted with different pill formulations

- No increased risk for women with:
  – A family history of breast cancer
  – Existing benign breast disease

- Possible increased risk in long-term users under age 45 years

---

cancer (either breast, endometrial, ovarian or liver) over an OC user's lifetime may actually be less than if she never used OCs.[20] The greatest protection is conferred after age 40.

Summary

The data indicate that there is no overall increased risk of developing breast cancer for OC users up to age 55 when compared to those who never used OCs. In addition, it does not appear that OCs increase the risk for women with other risk factors for breast cancer, such as a family history of breast cancer or nulliparity. There remain some unanswered questions regarding early, long-term OC use and the risk of breast cancer; however, on balance, the evidence available at this time does not warrant any change in prescribing practices for OCs. Furthermore, the potential risks must always be weighed against the known health benefits of OCs and prevention of unwanted pregnancy.

References

1. Committee on the Relationship Between Oral Contraceptives and Breast Cancer. *Oral Contraceptives and Breast Cancer*. Institute of Medicine, Division of Health Promotion and Disease Prevention. Washington, DC: National Academy Press; 1991.

2. American Cancer Society. *Cancer Facts & Figures—1996*. American Cancer Society, Atlanta, Georgia;1996.

3. Kelsey JL, Berkowitz GS. Breast cancer epidemiology. *Perspect Cancer Res* 1988;48:5615-5623.

4. Thomas DB. Oral contraceptives and breast cancer: review of the epidemiological literature. In: *Oral Contraceptives and Breast Cancer. Committee on the Relationship Between Oral Contraceptives and Breast Cancer*. Institute of Medicine, Division of Health Promotion and Disease Prevention. Washington, DC: National Academy Press; 1991.

5. Cancer and Steroid Hormone Study of the Centers for Disease Control and the National Institute of Child Health and Human Development. Oral contraceptive use and the risk of breast cancer. *N Engl J Med* 1986;315:405-411.

6. Royal College of General Practitioners. Breast cancer and oral contraceptives: findings in Royal College of General Practitioners' study. *BMJ* 1981;282:2089-2093.

7. Romieu I, Willett WC, Colditz GA, et al. Prospective study of oral contraceptive use and risk of breast cancer in women. *J Natl Cancer Inst* 1989;81:1313-1321.

8. The WHO Collaborative Study of Neoplasia and Steroid Contraceptives. Breast cancer and combined oral contraceptives: results from a multinational study. *Br J Cancer* 1990;61:110-119.

9. Romieu I, Berlin JA, Colditz G. Oral contraceptives and breast cancer: review and meta-analysis. *Cancer* 1990;66:2253-2263.

10. Collaborative Group on Hormonal Factors in Breast Cancer. Breast cancer and hormonal contraceptives: collaborative reanalysis of individual data on 53,297 women with breast cancer and 100,239 women without breast cancer from 54 epidemiological studies. *Lancet* 1996;347:1713-1727.

11. Schlesselman JJ. Oral contraceptives and breast cancer. *Am J Obstet Gynecol* 1990;163(pt 1): 1379-1387.

12. Murray PP, Stadel BV, Schlesselman JJ. Oral contraceptive use in women with a family history of breast cancer. *Obstet Gynecol* 1989;73:977-983.

13. Kay CR, Hannaford PC. Oral contraceptives and the pill—a further report from the Royal College of General Practitioners' oral contraception study. *Br J Cancer* 1988;58:675-680.

14. Stadel BV, Lai S, Schlesselman JJ, et al. Oral contraceptives and premenopausal breast cancer in nulliparous women. *Contraception* 1988;38:287-299.

15. Stadel BV, Schlesselman JJ, Murray PA. Oral contraceptives and breast cancer. *Lancet* 1989;1: 1257-1258.

16. UK National Case-Control Study Group. Oral contraceptive use and breast cancer in young women. *Lancet* 1989;1:973-982.

17. Rossing MA, Stanford JL, Weiss NS, et al. Oral contraceptive use and risk of breast cancer in middle-aged women. *Am J Epidemiol* 1996;144:161-164.

18. *F-D-C Reports*. January 9, 1989; T&G-13.

19. *ABPI Data Sheet Compendium*. London: Datapharm Publications Limited; 1990.

20. Harlap S, Kost K, Forrest JD. *Preventing Pregnancy, Protecting Health: A New Look at Birth Control Choices in the United States*. New York, NY: The Alan Guttmacher Institute; 1991:65.

ii. Worldwide Data

The largest-ever epidemiologic analysis provides strong evidence that OCs do not cause breast cancer. The Collaborative Group on Hormonal Factors in Breast Cancer gathered data on over 53,000 women with breast cancer and over 100,000 controls from 54 studies conducted in 26 countries. The researchers compiled their information from 90% of the known studies regarding the relationship between OCs and breast cancer. The findings were first published in Lancet.[1] *Detailed analyses then appeared in a supplement to the journal* Contraception.[2]

Two main findings emerged. One, current users and those who have taken OCs within the past 10 years have a small increased risk of having breast cancer diagnosed (RR for current use =1.24; 99% CI, 1.20-1.28).[2] Two, women have no significant excess risk of having breast cancer diagnosed 10 or more years after stopping use (RR at 10 years=1.0; 99% CI, 0.97-1.07).

The risk was essentially unchanged despite numerous analyses for factors hypothesized to impact breast cancer risk with OC use. These factors included: duration of use, age at first use, type of formulation, high-dose versus low-dose preparations, parity, age, age at menarche, reproductive history, family history of breast cancer, ethnic origin, height, weight, menopausal status or alcohol use.

The lack of an association between duration of use, dose and breast cancer risk supports the hypothesis that OCs do not cause the disease. According to the authors, "The risk increases soon after first exposure, does not increase with duration of exposure [or higher dosage], and returns to normal 10 years after cessation of exposure. Such a pattern seems incompatible with a genotoxic effect."[1] Instead, the likelihood of diagnosis may be enhanced by closer surveillance of women who take OCs. Or, it may be that women taking OCs access health care services more frequently.

Importantly, breast tumors diagnosed in OC users were more likely to be localized to the breast (RR=1.24; 99% CI, 1.18-1.30).[2] Two explanations are possible. First, users of OCs may have their cancers diagnosed earlier than never-users. Second, OCs might affect the rate of growth of tumors and their tendency to metastasize. The authors acknowledge that their analysis was unable to "infer from these data whether the patterns of risk observed are due to an earlier diagnosis of breast cancer in ever-users, the biological effect of hormonal contraceptives or a combination of both factors."

Young users are not at greater risk than women who begin using OCs at a later age. According to the authors, "Women who began use before age 20 had higher relative risks of having breast cancer diagnosed while they were using combined oral contraceptives and in the 5 years after stopping than women who began use at older ages, but the higher relative risks apply at ages when breast cancer is rare and, for a given duration of use, earlier use does not result in more cancers being diagnosed than use beginning at older ages."

Joseph Goldzieher, MD, Associate Editor of *The Contraception Report*, commented, "This analysis, using 99% confidence intervals, is now the gold standard. The fact that the risk of cancer was unrelated to duration of use, unrelated to dose and then disappears is not what you would expect from a carcinogenic effect. Everything points to the fact that any small increased risk of breast cancer in women taking OCs is due to diagnostic bias or random chance. These findings are very reassuring." In fact, the study group emphasized, "The conclusion from these calculations can be only that up to 20 years after cessation of use there is little difference in the cumulative incidence of breast cancer between women who have used and have not used oral contraceptives."

References
1. Collaborative Group on Hormonal Factors in Breast Cancer. Breast cancer and hormonal contraceptives: collaborative reanalysis of individual data on 53,297 women with breast cancer and 100,239 women without breast cancer from 54 epidemiological studies. *Lancet* 1996;347:1713-1727.
2. Collaborative Group on Hormonal Factors in Breast Cancer. Breast cancer and hormonal contraceptives: further results. *Contraception* 1996;54:1S-106S.

1.5: Cervical Cancer

Does the use of oral contraceptives (OCs) have an effect on the development of cervical cancer? A concrete answer to this question has eluded epidemiologists for more than 2 decades, largely due to the disease's complex etiology. Cervical cancer has been linked to factors other than OC use, including human papillomavirus (HPV), cigarette smoking, sexual behavior, lower socioeconomic status and parity. Furthermore, biases and confounding variables have often been present in studies of cervical cancer in relation to OC use.[1]

Incidence

Invasive cervical cancer develops in about 1% of American women and is the result of a series of changes in the cervical epithelium.[2] The disease is hypothesized to begin as cervical dysplasia, progress to carcinoma *in situ* and develop finally into invasive cancer. When detected early, Stage I invasive cervical cancer is one of the most curable types of cancer; cases diagnosed with localized disease have a 5-year relative survival rate of 90%.[2] Appropriate evaluation and treatment of preinvasive cervical dysplasia markedly decrease the risk of progression to invasive cancer.

Bias and Confounding Variables

Research on OCs and cervical cancer is subject to a variety of possible biases and confounding factors. The following summarizes some of the major potential confounding variables that have influenced study results over the years.

Sexual History—Studies have provided strong evidence in support of the hypothesis that cervical cancer is associated with one or more sexually transmitted diseases (STDs).[3] Intercourse at an early age, multiple sexual partners and sexual behavior of partners have been associated with cervical cancer development.[3,4] Both HPV and herpes simplex virus type 2 have been implicated as etiologic agents, although the evidence for the latter is weak.

On the other hand, the evidence is much stronger that HPV causes cervical cancer. One study of 500 women with cervical intraepithelial neoplasia and 500 disease-free women attributed about 76% of cases to HPV infection.[5] The researchers also found that subjects smoked more and had more sexual partners, an earlier age at first intercourse and lower socioeconomic status. These researchers also found an association of cervical cancer with parity, even after adjustment for HPV status. Since women who use OCs may be more sexually active than users of other methods, information regarding past STD infection, age at first coitus and number of sexual partners must be obtained in order for studies to assess accurately the relationship between OCs and cervical cancer.

Parity—The likelihood of developing invasive cervical cancer has been shown in some studies to increase with number of births. In one study, the risk was found to double after just one birth; women with five or more births were four times more likely to develop cervical cancer than were nulliparous women.[6]

Smoking History—There is now a large body of research regarding the possible effect of smoking on the development of cervical cancer. In a 1990 review of the literature, Winkelstein reported that almost 80% of the 33 cited studies supported an association.[7] Although smoking may not be the main cause of cervical cancer, Winkelstein concluded that carcinogens in tobacco smoke appeared to be responsible for a substantial proportion of the overall incidence of the disease.

Barrier Methods—The use of barrier methods of contraception has been shown to provide a protective effect against the development of cervical cancer.[8] Methods such as the condom or diaphragm provide a physical barrier to viruses suspected of causing the disease. Spermicidal agents inactivate these viruses and may also be protective, but the evidence for this is weaker. Use of either barrier or spermicidal methods by more controls than cases could result in a spurious association between OCs and cervical cancer.[9]

Pap Smear Frequency—In studies of the effect of OC use on cervical dysplasia and carcinoma *in situ*, frequency of Pap smears can be a source of bias that inflates relative risk estimates. OC users may receive Pap smears more regularly than nonusers. Since both can be detected by Pap smear, OC users may more likely be diagnosed with these two conditions than nonusers, resulting in a spuriously elevated relative risk.[1] Conversely, OC users may be less likely to have their disease reach the invasive stage because of their more frequent screening, and this could result in spuriously low relative risk observed in OC users.

Cervical Dysplasia and Carcinoma in situ

Studies of OCs and cervical intraepithelial neoplasia need to consider each stage of the disease separately, as OCs could act at any one stage to influence progression along the continuum of lesions from mild dysplasia to severe dysplasia to carcinoma *in situ* to invasive cancer.[10] Many researchers have failed to assess individual stages and studies have often included a mixture of lesion types. Furthermore, there is uncertainty regarding the relevance of findings from studies of preinvasive conditions to the risk of invasive cervical cancer because many preinvasive lesions do not progress to the final stage.[10] Examining studies of OC use and cervical cancer performed since 1980, Schlesselman concluded in a 1989 review that collective data regarding both cervical dysplasia and carcinoma *in situ* were difficult to interpret, and that evidence of an association between OCs and these two disease stages was weak.[9]

Invasive Cervical Cancer

Studies focusing on invasive cervical cancer and OCs have yielded conflicting results, although two reports from the World Health Organization (WHO), published in 1993 and 1996, confirm an increased risk of invasive cervical cancer with OC use.[8,11-16] All studies attempted to adjust relative risk findings for potential confounding factors and sources of bias. However, studies have varied in the number of items that were included in the adjustment process.

The Royal College of General Practitioners' Oral Contraception Study has followed 47,000 women since 1968. A 1988 review of the study reported a relative risk of invasive cervical cancer of 1.8 (95% confidence interval [CI], 1.0-3.3) in OC users; however, current use of protective methods by controls was not considered in the study. Certain confounding factors relating to sexual history were also excluded from relative risk adjustment. The researchers reported that "residual confounding" might still be influencing their results.[12]

A 1986 case-control study by Brinton involving over 1,200 American women found an adjusted relative risk of 1.5 (95% CI, 1.1-2.1) associated with the use of OCs.[13] While allowing for all confounding variables related to sexual history, the researchers stated that smoking, parity, and use of protective methods were not found to be significant confounders and, therefore, were not included in their adjustment of relative risk. They concluded that their findings raised some concern and are continuing to collect data regarding the association.

Brinton et al subsequently published results of a case-control study in developing countries.[14] This study included adjustments for age, number of sexual partners, age at first sexual intercourse, years since last Pap smear, parity, HPV types 16 and 18, and years of education. The researchers again found recent users at a slightly higher, but nonsignificant, risk of invasive cervical cancer (RR=1.3; 95% CI, 0.9-1.9). Recent long-term users were at highest risk (RR for 5+ years use=1.7; 95% CI, 1.1-2.6). Interestingly, this investigation found that the risk associated with OC use was nonsignificant for squamous cell tumors (the more common type of cervical cancer) (RR=1.1; 95% CI, 0.9-1.5), whereas the risk was significantly elevated for adenocarcinomas (RR=2.4; 95% CI, 1.3-4.6).

Possible Sources of Confounding in Case-Control Studies of Oral Contraceptives and Cervical Cancer

- History of STDs
- Number of previous sexual partners
- Sexual behavior of partners
- Age at first coitus
- Number of previous births
- History of smoking
- Use of barrier contraceptive methods
- Pap smear frequency

Epidemiologic Overview: Oral Contraceptives and Cervical Cancer

- Definitive causal relationship cannot be confirmed
- HPV subtypes are likely etiologic agents
- Other possible risk factors:
  - Number of sexual partners
  - Age at first coitus
  - Smoking
  - Parity
- Recommendations:
  - Annual Pap smear screening
  - Use of barrier methods with multiple or serial partners

Both the WHO's 1985 collaborative study and a 1988 study by Irwin included confounding variables of sexual history and parity in relative risk adjustment and excluded smoking and use of protective methods.[11,15] Relative risk assessments were 1.2 (95% CI, 1.0-1.4) and 0.8 (95% CI, 0.5-1.3), respectively. WHO reported that although its results were of borderline significance, the slightly elevated relative risk could be explained on the basis of incomplete control of confounding variables.[15] Irwin likewise concluded that no association between OCs and invasive cervical cancer could be found.[11]

A study by Celentano did not include STD history, relying instead upon adjustment for other sexual history variables. The researchers also included an adjustment for the use of protective methods. Adjustment for possibly confounding variables produced an odds ratio of 0.7 (95% CI, 0.3-1.9). The researchers suggested that this was due to the increased likelihood of Pap smear detection prior to the invasive stage by users of OCs.[8]

In his 1989 review of the literature, Schlesselman concluded that the risk of invasive cervical cancer did not appear to be elevated during the first 5 years of oral contraceptive use.[9] An association was more likely to exist with durations of use greater than 5 years, with about a two-fold increased risk at 10 years (Figure 1). WHO investigations support the idea that long-term use, in particular, increases the risk of cervical cancer in women taking OCs.[16,17] The ongoing WHO Collaborative Study of Neoplasia and Steroid Contraceptives recruited 2,361 cases and over 13,000 controls from 11 centers in nine countries. This hospital-based, case-control investigation found that the relative risk of invasive squamous cell cervical carcinoma was 1.3 (95% CI, 1.2-1.5). Duration of use was associated with an increased risk of the disease "4 to 5 years from first exposure and declined with the passage of time after cessation of use to that of nonusers in about 8 years."[16]

Figure 1

**Invasive Cervical Cancer in Women under Age 60 Years:
Relative Risk by Years of OC Use — Eight Studies**

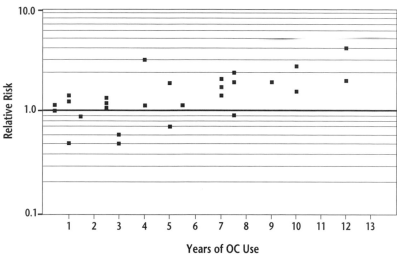

Source: *Schlesselman JJ. Cancer of the breast and reproductive tract in relation to use of oral contraceptives. Contraception 1989;40:1-38. Reproduced with permission of the publisher, Elsevier Science, Inc.*

In later analyses of adenocarcinomas, WHO investigators found similar results. The adjusted relative risk in ever-users for adenocarcinomas was 1.6 (95% CI, 1.2-2.1) and for adenosquamous carcinomas, 1.1 (95% CI, 0.7-1.8). The researchers did not find HPV infection to be a confounder in this study; controlling for multiple sexual variables did not appreciably alter the results. They concluded, "For both types [of adenocarcinomas] combined, risk increased with duration of oral contraceptive use, was highest in recent and current users, and declined with time since cessation of use."[17]

Summary and Recommendations

Results of existing studies are inconclusive with regard to cervical dysplasia and carcinoma *in situ*. The risk of invasive cervical cancer may be elevated with longer durations of use; however, bias and confounding factors have plagued studies of this disease stage, as well. Present evidence is insufficient to warrant a change in prescribing habits. Use of barrier methods should be advised for patients at risk for acquiring STDs and Pap smear screening should be performed periodically in all sexually active women at risk.

The frequency of Pap smear screening continues to be debated. The American College of Obstetricians and Gynecologists and the American Cancer Society recommend annual screening. On the other hand, the U.S. Preventive Services Task Force recommends screening at least once every 3 years. Clinicians may wish to perform frequent Pap smears in women with multiple risk factors for cervical cancer.

References

1. Swan SH, Petitti DB. A review of problems of bias and confounding in epidemiologic studies of cervical neoplasia and oral contraceptive use. *Am J Epidemiol* 1982;115:10-18.

2. National Cancer Institute. *Annual Cancer Statistics Review, Including Cancer Trends: 1950-1985.* Bethesda: National Institutes of Health, 1988.

3. Slattery ML, Overall JC Jr., Abbott TM, et al. Sexual activity, contraception, genital infections, and cervical cancer: support for a sexually transmitted disease hypothesis. *Am J Epidemiol* 1989;130:248-258.

4. Berget A. Relation of dysplasia and carcinoma of the uterine cervix to age at onset of sexual life and number of coital partners. *Dan Med Bull* 1978;25:172-176.

5. Schiffman MH, Bauer HM, Hoover RN, et al. Epidemiologic evidence showing that human papillomavirus infection causes most cervical intraepithelial neoplasia. *J Natl Cancer Inst* 1993;85:958-964.

6. Parazzini F, La Vecchia C, Negri E, et al. Reproductive factors and the risk of invasive and intraepithelial cervical neoplasia. *Br J Cancer* 1989;59:805-809.

7. Winkelstein W Jr. Smoking and cervical cancer—current status: a review. *Am J Epidemiol* 1990;131:945-957.

8. Celentano DD, Klassen AC, Weisman CS, et al. The role of contraceptive use in cervical cancer: the Maryland cervical cancer case-control study. *Am J Epidemiol* 1987;126:592-604.

9. Schlesselman JJ. Cancer of the breast and reproductive tract in relation to use of oral contraceptives. *Contraception* 1989;40:1-38.

10. Prentice RL, Thomas DB. On the epidemiology of oral contraceptives and disease. *Adv Cancer Res* 1987;49:285-401.

11. Irwin KL, Rosero-Bixby L, Oberle MW, et al. Oral contraceptives and cervical cancer risk in Costa Rica: detection bias or causal association? *JAMA* 1988;259:59-64.

12. Beral V, Hannaford P, Kay C. Oral contraceptive use and malignancies of the genital tract. Results from the Royal College of General Practitioners' Oral Contraception Study. *Lancet* 1988;2:1331-1335.

13. Brinton LA, Huggins GR, Lehman HF, et al. Long-term use of oral contraceptives and risk of invasive cervical cancer. *Int J Cancer* 1986;38:339-344.

14. Brinton LA, Reeves WC, Brenes MM, et al. Oral contraceptive use and risk of invasive cervical cancer. *Int J Epidemiol* 1990;19:4-11.

15. WHO Collaborative Study of Neoplasia and Steroid Contraceptives. Invasive cervical cancer and combined oral contraceptives. *BMJ* 1985;290:961-965.

16. WHO Collaborative Study of Neoplasia and Steroid Contraceptives. Invasive squamous-cell cervical carcinoma and combined oral contraceptives: results from a multinational study. *Int J Cancer* 1993;55:228-236.

17. Thomas DB, Ray RM, and The World Health Organization Collaborative Study of Neoplasia and Steroid Contraceptives. Oral contraceptives and invasive adenocarcinomas and adenosquamous carcinomas of the uterine cervix. *Am J Epidemiol* 1996;144:281-189.

1.6: Cardiovascular Risks

Oral contraceptive use confers little or no increased risk of cardiovascular disease, especially among healthy, nonsmoking women.[1] This understanding of the relationship between oral contraceptives (OCs) and cardiovascular disease has emerged as new evidence has appeared and old data have been reanalyzed. In the late 1960s and early 1970s, study findings indicated that OC use resulted in an increased risk of myocardial infarction (MI), stroke and venous thromboembolism (VTE).[2] The subsequent press coverage concerned many women, practitioners and regulatory agencies. Newer analyses point to cigarette smoking as the real culprit, however, and suggest that early conclusions about OCs and cardiovascular disease were mistaken.

Three developments may explain why little or no cardiovascular risk now exists.[1,2] First, screening is better. Clinicians generally urge older women who smoke and women with other predisposing cardiovascular risk factors to use another form of contraception. Second, more sophisticated epidemiologic analysis available today can help to sort through the many factors that influence cardiovascular disease. As a result, researchers now recognize smoking as an important confounding factor in early studies. Third, some hypothesize that lowering the estrogen dose in OCs helped to decrease the risk of cardiovascular disease.

Questions about cardiovascular disease arose early. In 1961 in Los Angeles, two deaths from pulmonary embolism (PE) occurred among women using an oral contraceptive (Enovid®).[2] The press widely covered these cases. In 1962, physicians reported single cases of PE and stroke in women using Enovid. Subsequently, the manufacturer gathered 132 reports of thromboembolic disease associated with the product and presented them to a panel of experts for review. In 1963, the Food and Drug Administration (FDA) commissioned the Wright Committee to investigate the matter.

Then, in 1967, a British case-control study associated the use of OCs and a diagnosis of thrombophlebitis.[3] This further added to the concern about OCs and thromboembolic events. However, researchers have found detection bias and diagnostic inaccuracy largely to be responsible for this association. Given the publicity, physicians were more likely to diagnose thrombophlebitis when they knew that the patient was on OCs. The clinical diagnosis of thrombophlebitis "is now known to be plagued by a high degree of false positives when the physician is aware that the patient has been using OCs."[2,4] Two additional papers published in 1968 also suggested an association between thromboembolic disease and OCs.[5,6]

In 1970, Inman and colleagues concluded that high-dose OCs (which at that time contained 150 mcg of estrogen) were less safe than lower-dose OCs.[7] The special report, prepared for the Committee on the Safety of Drugs, the United Kingdom's counterpart to the FDA, stated that there appeared to be a dose-response relationship, even though the relationship was not statistically significant. Nonetheless, the report unleashed an international flurry of negative publicity. Unfortunately, a firm link formed in the minds of practitioners and the general public between thromboembolic events and the pill.

More reliable data from prospective investigations were needed. Early studies linking pill use to cardiovascular disease were largely case-control studies, which suffer from certain limitations. Case-control studies are observational studies that look backward in time.[1] Researchers begin by looking at a group who have experienced the medical event (eg, heart attack) and choose controls who have not suffered the medical event. Case-control studies are particularly useful for gaining insight into rare events and events that take a long time to develop; however, selection bias in choosing appropriate controls is often a problem.[1]

Prospective Studies

The first large prospective study appeared to support the hypothesis that pill use is related to thromboembolic disease.[8] The 1977 report of the Royal College of General Practitioners (RCGP) found a 4.7 times increased relative risk (RR) of death from circulatory disease (primarily subarachnoid hemorrhage) among ever-users of OCs. The authors found an increased risk in OC users with advancing age and, later, with smoking.

RCGP updates have found lower morbidity and mortality risks from cardiovascular disease for OC users.[9,10] In addition, the data consistently support a link between smoking and an increased risk of cardiovascular disease. Mant et al found no increased risk of myocardial infarction among current pill users, but did find that the overall incidence of MI and angina pectoris for women who smoked was more than three times that of nonsmoking women.[11]

The second large prospective study found that smoking increased mortality risk with OC use.[12] This investigation followed patients in 17 clinics of the British Family Planning Association. According to Sturtevant's review, "Reporting on mortality after 20 years of follow-up, Vessey et al found no difference between OC users and nonusers [in overall mortality risk], and suggested that the RCGP assessment of cardiovascular risk may have been overestimated. Of the 18 deaths due to ischemic heart disease, all but one woman had been a smoker and only two were using OCs at the time of death. Of the 10 deaths due to cerebrovascular disease, six were smokers and only two were current OC users. The rates of death from these two causes were not significantly different for OC users and nonusers."[2] Vessey et al stated, "Interestingly, the mortality from circulatory disease associated with oral contraceptive use (RR=1.5; 95% confidence interval [CI], 0.7-3.0) was substantially less than that found in [the 1981 update of] the Royal College of General Practitioners' study (RR=4.2; 95% CI, 2.3-7.7)."[12]

The National Institutes of Health (NIH) supported a third prospective study.[13] The Walnut Creek study began with "the express purpose of confirming the initial findings of increased risk reported by the two prospective British studies. When, at the end of 8 years, confirmation was not forthcoming, the NIH withdrew its support and the study was ended. The NIH included in the published report a commentary by Vessey that sought to explain the differences between the British and American experiences.

"Having observed firsthand the procedures employed at the RCGP and at Walnut Creek, I was impressed by the rigorous scientific approach taken by Dr. Ramcharan [the primary investigator for Walnut Creek], and therefore considered the American data more reliable. Time and subsequent reanalyses of the British experience have, I believe, tended to support the Walnut Creek findings that there was 'no evidence of an increased risk of [ischemic heart disease] in past or current users of OCs.'"[2]

The authors reported an increased risk of subarachnoid hemorrhage associated with OC use, but admit this association was based on small numbers. They also stated that since "national mortality statistics in both the United States and the United Kingdom showed no increases in death rates such as would be expected if the risk for circulatory disease or subarachnoid hemorrhage were high, it is possible that the association with OCs might be due to undetermined confounding factors. Understanding these factors might have to await the development of further knowledge about the precipitating causes of subarachnoid hemorrhage other than [congenital vascular malformations], hypertension and perhaps smoking."

The Walnut Creek study found few cases of MI, cerebral thrombosis or PE in nonsmoking OC users. "Thus, among 33 cases of IHD [ischemic heart disease] in the smoking subgroup, only five occurred among current OC users; among 42 cases in the nonsmoking subgroup, only one occurred in a current user," Dr. Sturtevant reported.[2] "There were seven cases of subarachnoid hemorrhage, two of which were in current users, both of whom smoked. There were 24 cases of cerebral thrombosis, three of which were in current users, two of whom smoked. There were 25 cases of pulmonary embolism, two of whom were current users, one of whom smoked. In summary, in the 8-year Walnut Creek study, among current OC users who did not smoke, there was but a single case each of myocardial infarction, cerebral thrombosis and pulmonary embolism."

A fourth prospective study used discharge diagnoses from hospitals of the Group Health Cooperative of Puget Sound linked to computerized pharmacy records.[14] Summarizing the findings, Sturtevant stated, "In their first publication, the authors analyzed the experience of over 40,000 women ages 20 to 44 over a period of 3 years. There were 10 discharge diagnoses of venous thromboembolism, seven in OC users and three in nonusers, which was a statistically significant difference [risk ratio=8.3; 90% CI, 3-23]. Seven women had a stroke; none had been an OC user. No cases of myocardial infarction were recorded for this age group. An update was published 3 years later.[15] This covered over 65,000 women over a new 3-year period. This time, there were nine cases of VTE, only three of which were in OC users; there were eight strokes, only one being in a user. There was only one myocardial infarction and that was in a nonuser."[2] A later analysis of mortality found 11 cardiovascular deaths, all in nonusers of OCs.[16]

Some researchers believe the evidence does not clearly support a cause-and-effect relationship between cardiovascular disease and oral contraceptives. According to a critique of the epidemiologic literature by Realini and Goldzieher, many sources of potential bias and methodologic deficiencies preclude a definitive answer as to the validity of the observed association between OC use and cardiovascular disease.[17] In addition, three factors have been ignored that may explain why recent analyses do not find cardiovascular complications among women using OCs.[2] "What tends to be ignored is that: (1) statistical analysis is now able to control for confounding variables by computerized multivariate analysis, such as by multiple logistic regression; (2) physicians are increasingly cautious about prescribing OCs for women with predisposing risk factors; (3) diagnostic accuracy has improved."

Low-Dose OCs and Stroke

Several studies published in 1996 on the risk of stroke with OCs are reassuring. One study of 1.1 million women enrolled in the Kaiser Permanente Medical Care Programs of Northern and Southern California in the U.S. found no increased risk of stroke among healthy, nonsmoking women using low-dose OCs (RR=1.2; 95% CI, 0.7-1.9).[18] Data on women from European and developing nations gathered by the World Health Organization were similar.[19,20] Researchers found no significant increased risk of either ischemic or hemorrhagic stroke among European users of low-dose OCs. For women in developing countries, on the other hand, odds ratios for both types of stroke were more likely to be significantly elevated. The investigators attributed the elevated risk of stroke to undetected cardiovascular risk factors and differences in prescribing practices. Independent risk factors, such as smoking and hypertension, increased the risk of stroke both among OC users and nonusers.

VTE Risk with OCs Containing Desogestrel or Gestodene

In late 1995, a media and scientific debate erupted about the possible link between OCs containing the progestins desogestrel or gestodene and VTE. The concern originated after several studies found a similar twofold increased risk of VTE with OC formulations containing these two progestins compared to levonorgestrel-containing pills.[21-24]

The debate began prior to publication of the studies. In October 1995, the United Kingdom's Committee on the Safety of Medicines issued an urgent warning to clinicians advising them against using OCs containing these progestins. The media scare that followed concerned clinicians and frightened women, many of whom immediately stopped taking their pills.

While some believe the link is based on firm evidence, others dismiss the concerns, citing probable biases.[25-29] For example, selection or prescribing bias may have occurred if clinicians steered women at higher risk of thromboembolic complications, such as obese women, toward the newer pills, believing newer pills to be safer.

Another type of bias is "attrition of susceptibles" or the "healthy user effect." This type of bias may have occurred because women taking levonorgestrel-containing pills were longer-term users. Long-term users as a group tend to include fewer women likely to experience problems with the pill, as those women who have side effects discontinue OC use early. Younger, first-time users are thus at greater risk of experiencing VTE. Some evidence suggests that young, first-time users were more likely to have taken the newer pills. Furthermore, one analysis also found that the risk of VTE for different OC formulations increased linearly and significantly with recency of market introduction.[25]

Even if real, the increased risk of VTE associated with OCs containing desogestrel or gestodene is still less than that associated with pregnancy (Figure 1).[30] Pregnancy results in about 60 cases of VTE per 100,000 users per year; use of these third-generation pills would result in about 30 cases, versus about 15 cases for users of pills containing older progestins, versus about 4 cases among healthy, nonpregnant women not using the pill. Mortality risk associated with VTE is low; the estimated increased rate of fatal VTE among users of desogestrel- or gestodene-containing pills is 1 to 1.5 deaths per 1 million women-years.

The controversy elicited regulatory responses from governments around the world. In the U.S., the FDA advised that "the risk is not great enough to justify switching to

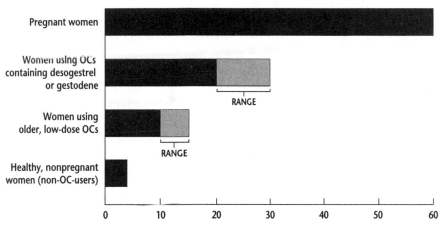

Figure 1

**Estimated Average Risk of Nonfatal Venous Thromboembolism
per 100,000 Women per Year, United States**

Source: U.S. Food and Drug Administration, 1995 (see reference 30).

other products. ...The agency...does not recommend that women using the deso-gestrel-containing products stop using them or change to another oral contraceptive. Women who are taking these products are advised to discuss these contraceptives with their health care providers and make an informed choice based on the benefits and risks and individual preferences."[30]

Despite the FDA's position, in 1996, manufacturers of desogestrel-containing products (gestodene is not available in the U.S.) amended package labeling to include a warning about a possible increased risk of VTE. The American College of Obstetricians and Gynecologists' Committee on Gynecologic Practice did not recommend that patients already taking desogestrel-containing products switch.[31] It did recommend, however, that other pills be considered first-line choices in most circumstances. More research is needed to determine whether the enhanced VTE risk was a true association or the result of biases.

Smoking, Myocardial Infarction and OC Use

Several investigations have found a correlation between smoking, OC use and increased risk of myocardial infarction. Rosenberg et al, for example, performed a case-control analysis of 555 women under the age of 50 years who survived their first MI.[32] Nonsmoking OC users had no increased risk of MI; however, smoking substantially increased the risk of MI in general and among women using OCs. Light smokers (<25 cigarettes/day) using OCs had three times the risk of MI, while heavy smokers (≥25 cigarettes/day) using OCs had 23 times the risk of nonsmoking OC users.

Data from the Royal College of General Practitioners' study also support these findings. Croft and Hannaford found an association between smoking, hypertension,

Figure 2

Relative Risk of Myocardial Infarction in Women by Number of Cigarettes Smoked and Current, Past or Never-Use of Oral Contraceptives

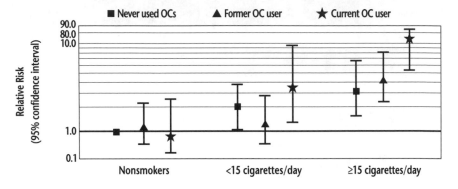

Source: Croft P, et al, 1989 (see reference 33).

toxemia of pregnancy, diabetes mellitus and risk of MI.[33] Current use of the pill increased the risk of MI only among women who also smoked (Figure 2). In fact, the risk was 21 times greater for OC users who smoked heavily. Previous use of the pill did not influence the risk of MI. According to Croft and Hannaford, "Overall, smoking was the most important independent risk factor and had a strong influence on risks associated with other factors."

Goldbaum et al studied the prevalence of smoking and OC use among U.S. women.[34] Using telephone surveys from 28 states and the District of Columbia from 1981 through 1983, they estimated that about 7% of U.S. women ages 18 to 44 years smoked and used OCs. About 1% reported smoking 25 or more cigarettes per day while using OCs. The authors found that young women, those ages 18 to 24 years, were most likely to smoke and use OCs. "Our calculations suggest that while combined smoking and OC use accounts for a disproportionate number of the excess cases of nonfatal myocardial infarction, most excess cases among U.S. women ages 35 to 44 years can be attributed solely to smoking. ...However, in the long run, pregnancy carried to term is more dangerous than combined smoking and OC use, except for women ages 35 years and older. ...Therefore, when considering whether to prescribe OCs, health care providers should generally base the decision on factors other than smoking."

Patients should be encouraged to stop smoking rather than discontinue OCs. Women under the age of 35 years who smoke may use OCs, but should be warned about the dangers of smoking. Women over 35 years of age who smoke and are unable to quit should be encouraged to use another method of birth control.

Active counseling from clinicians can help patients quit smoking. (For more information on a Stop Smoking Kit from the American Academy of Family Physicians, refer to the end of Chapter 9.)

Figure 3

Cardiovascular Mortality and Past Use of Oral Contraceptives

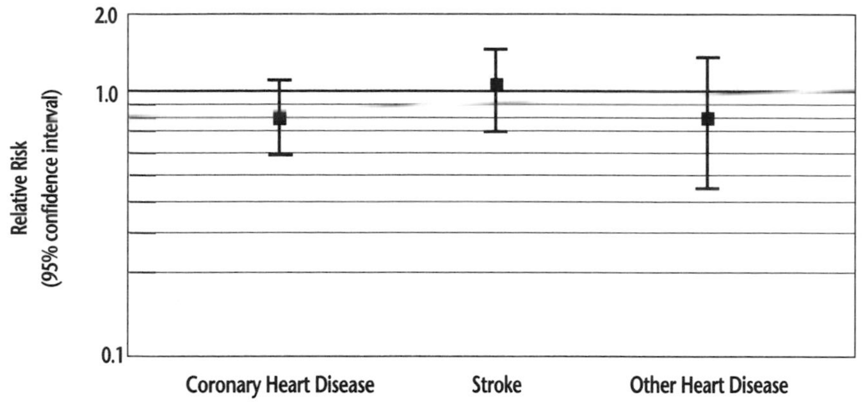

Source: Colditz GA, 1994 (see reference 35).

Past Use of OCs

Past use of OCs does not increase the risk of any cardiovascular disease. Recent data from the Nurses' Health Study confirm these findings.[35] The Nurses' Health Study, a large, prospective, cohort study of 121,700 women who were ages 30 to 55 years in 1976, followed participants through 1988 (1.3 million person-years of follow-up). No difference in overall mortality was found among women who had ever used oral contraceptives compared with women who had never used OCs. When adjusted for age, body mass index and cigarette smoking, the overall mortality RR was 0.9 (95% CI, 0.9-1.0). Long durations of OC use conferred no added risk. Women who had used OCs for 10 or more years had an RR of 1.1 (95% CI, 0.8-1.4).

A multivariate analysis found no increased risk for coronary heart disease, stroke or other heart disease (Figure 3). This confirmed previous findings from the Nurses' Health Study and a meta-analysis of 13 additional studies that past use of oral contraceptives, even long durations of use, does not confer increased risk of cardiovascular disease.[36,37]

OCs, Lipids and Atherogenesis

Alterations in lipids from OCs do not increase the risk of atherosclerotic heart disease. Some researchers have theorized that alterations in LDL (low-density lipoprotein) and HDL (high-density lipoprotein) profiles may influence long-term risk of coronary atherosclerosis in women using OCs. Data on the long-term effects of OC use in women and in experimental animals do not support such a belief, however. In fact, some evidence from monkeys suggests the opposite effect.[38]

If alterations in lipids induced by OCs did cause an increased risk of atherogenesis, then an increased risk of disease should be seen in women who used OCs, especially for long durations. No such association is evident. According to Joseph Goldzieher, MD, Associate Editor of *The Contraception Report*, "Much discussion has focused on the supposed 'adverse' lipid profile effects of oral contraceptives, but this focus is misguided. The fundamental flaw in this line of reasoning is that any cardiovascular risk associated with OCs has always been believed to be due to the estrogen component and has been thrombotic, rather than atherogenic, in nature. If cardiovascular risk were increased by an atherogenic mechanism, then long-term use should confer an increased risk. Yet, analyses of the Nurses' Health Study by Stampfer and colleagues found no increased risk of subsequent cardiovascular disease among former OC users, even with prolonged previous use.[35-37] In addition, most so-called adverse lipid effects are within normal limits and have not been shown to be clinically relevant.[39] The concern regarding lipid effects is unwarranted." (For further discussion of the relationship between OCs and lipids, see the section on metabolic effects of OCs in this chapter.)

Summary

New data and reanalyses of older data confirm that pills are safe for healthy, non-smoking women of any age. Past use of oral contraceptives presents no increased risk of cardiovascular disease, although current use of OCs may pose some increased risk of thromboembolic disease for women over age 35 years who smoke. Women who smoke should be counseled to quit. No evidence supports a relationship between atherogenic disease and use of OCs.

Early studies of OCs and cardiovascular disease, which first linked pill use to heart attack, stroke and embolism, had many limitations, including not accounting for smoking as a confounding factor. Women should be informed about the health benefits of the pill and reassured as to their cardiovascular safety in healthy, non-smoking women up to menopause.

References

1.   Grimes DA. The safety of oral contraceptives: epidemiologic insights from the first 30 years. *Am J Obstet Gynecol* 1992;166:1950-1954.

2.   Sturtevant FM. Cardiovascular safety of oral contraceptives: a critical commentary. *Int J Fertil* 1991;36(suppl):32-36.

3.   Royal College of General Practitioners. Oral contraception and thromboembolic disease. *J R Coll Gen Pract* 1967;13:267-279.

4.   Barnes RW, Krapf T, Joak JC. Erroneous clinical diagnosis of leg vein thrombosis in women on oral contraceptives. *Obstet Gynecol* 1978;51:556-558.

5.   Inman WHW, Vessey MP. Investigation of deaths from pulmonary, coronary, and cerebral thrombosis and embolism in women of child-bearing age. *BMJ* 1968;2:193-199.

6.   Vessey MP, Doll R. Investigation of relation between use of oral contraceptives and thromboembolic disease. *BMJ* 1968;2:199-205.

7.   Inman WHW, Vessey MP, Westerholm B, et al. Thromboembolic disease and the steroidal content of oral contraceptives. A report to the Committee on the Safety of Drugs. *BMJ* 1970;2:203-209.

8.   Royal College of General Practitioners' Oral Contraception Study. Mortality among oral contraceptive users. *Lancet* 1977;2:727-732.

9.   Royal College of General Practitioners' Oral Contraception Study. Further analyses of mortality in oral contraceptive users. *Lancet* 1981;1:541-546.

10. Royal College of General Practitioners' Oral Contraception Study. Incidence of arterial disease among oral contraceptive users. *J R Coll Gen Pract* 1983;33:75-82.

11. Mant D, Villard-Mackintosh L, Vessey MP, et al. Myocardial infarction and angina pectoris in young women. *J Epidemiol Commun Health* 1987;41:215-219.

12. Vessey MP, Villard-Mackintosh L, McPherson K, et al. Mortality among oral contraceptive users: 20-year follow-up of women in a cohort study. *BMJ* 1989; 299:1487-1491.

13. Ramcharan S, Pellegrin FA, Ray RM, et al. The Walnut Creek Contraceptive Drug Study. Volume III, an interim report: a comparison of disease occurrence leading to hospitalization or death in users and nonusers of oral contraceptives. *J Reprod Med* 1980;25(suppl):347-372.

14. Porter JB, Hunter JR, Danielson DA, et al. Oral contraceptives and nonfatal vascular disease— recent experience. *Obstet Gynecol* 1982;59:299-302.

15. Porter JB, Hunter JR, Jick H, et al. Oral contraceptives and nonfatal vascular disease. *Obstet Gynecol* 1985;66:1-4.

16. Porter JB, Jick H, Walker AM. Mortality among oral contraceptive users. *Obstet Gynecol* 1987;70:29-32.

17. Realini JP, Goldzieher JW. Oral contraceptives and cardiovascular disease: a critique of the epidemiologic studies. *Am J Obstet Gynecol* 1985;152:729-798.

18. Petitti DB, Sidney S, Bernstein A, et al. Stroke in users of low-dose oral contraceptives. *N Engl J Med* 1996;335:8-15.

19. WHO Collaborative Study of Cardiovascular Disease and Steroid Hormone Contraception. Ischaemic stroke and combined oral contraceptives: results of an international, multicentre, case-control study. *Lancet* 1996;348:498-505.

20. WHO Collaborative Study of Cardiovascular Disease and Steroid Hormone Contraception. Haemorrhagic stroke, overall stroke risk, and combined oral contraceptives: results of an international, multicentre, case-control study. *Lancet* 1996;348:505-510.

21. World Health Organization Collaborative Study of Cardiovascular Disease and Steroid Hormone Contraception. Venous thromboembolic disease and combined oral contraceptives: results of an international multicentre case-control study. *Lancet* 1995;346:1575-1582.

22. World Health Organization Collaborative Study of Cardiovascular Disease and Steroid Hormone Contraception. Effect of different progestagens in low oestrogen oral contraceptives on venous thromboembolic disease. *Lancet* 1995;346:1582-1588.

23. Jick H, Jick SS, Gurewich V, et al. Risk of idiopathic cardiovascular death and nonfatal venous thromboembolism in women using oral contraceptives with differing progestagen components. *Lancet* 1995;346:1589-1593.

24. Spitzer WO, Lewis MA, Heinemann LAJ, et al. Third generation oral contraceptives and risk of venous thromboembolic disorders: an international case-control study. *BMJ* 1996;312:83-88.

25. Lewis MA, Heinemann LAJ, MacRae KD, et al. The increased risk of venous thromboembolism and the use of third generation progestagens: role of bias in observational research. *Contraception* 1996;54:5-13.

26. Westhoff CL. Oral contraceptives and venous thromboembolism: should epidemiologic associations drive clinical decision making? *Contraception* 1996;54:1-3.

27. Jamin C, de Mouzon J. Selective prescribing of third generation oral contraceptives (OCs). *Contraception* 1996;54:55-56.

28. Farley TMM, Meirik O, Poulter, et al. Oral contraceptives and thrombotic diseases: impact of new epidemiological studies. *Contraception* 1996;54:193-195. Letter to the editor.

29. Lidegaard O, Milsom I. Response to the editor. *Contraception* 1996;54:195-198.

30. Food and Drug Administration. Oral contraceptives and risk of blood clots. *FDA Talk Paper* Nov. 24, 1995.

31. American College of Obstetricians and Gynecologists. *ACOG Newsletter* 1996;40:1,4.

32. Rosenberg L, Kaufman DW, Helmrich SP, et al. Myocardial infarction and cigarette smoking in women younger than 50 years of age. *JAMA* 1985;253:2965-2969.

33. Croft P, Hannaford PC. Risk factors for acute myocardial infarction in women: evidence from the Royal College of General Practitioners' Oral Contraceptive Study. *BMJ* 1989;298:165-168.

34. Goldbaum GM, Kendrick JS, Hogelin GC, et al. The relative impact of smoking and oral contraceptive use on women in the United States. *JAMA* 1987;258:1339-1342.

35. Colditz GA and The Nurses' Health Study Research Group. Oral contraceptive use and mortality during 12 years of follow-up: The Nurses' Health Study. *Ann Intern Med* 1994;120:821-826.

36. Stampfer MJ, Willett WC, Colditz GA, et al. A prospective study of past use of oral contraceptive agents and risk of cardiovascular diseases. *N Engl J Med* 1988;319:1313-1317.

37. Stampfer MJ, Willett WC, Colditz GA, et al. Past use of oral contraceptives and cardiovascular disease: a meta-analysis in the context of the Nurses' Health Study. *Am J Obstet Gynecol* 1990;163:285-291.

38. Adams MR, Clarkson TB, Koritnik DR, et al. Contraceptive steroids and coronary artery atherosclerosis in cynomolgus macaques. *Fertil Steril* 1987;47:1010-1018.

39. Hoppe G. The clinical relevance of oral contraceptive pill-induced plasma lipid changes: facts and fiction. *Am J Obstet Gynecol* 1990;163:388-391.

1.7: Metabolic Effects

Concerns about the metabolic effects of oral contraceptives (OCs) have traditionally centered on two areas: carbohydrate and lipid metabolism. Most recently, speculation has centered on the "androgenic" properties of progestins. Innumerable studies have examined these issues; the results suggest changes in these metabolic processes have little or no relevance to clinical practice.

OCs and Carbohydrate Metabolism

The effects of estrogen and progestin on carbohydrate metabolism are complex and not fully elucidated.[1,2] Early studies demonstrated that high-dose OCs induced changes in various aspects of carbohydrate metabolism. Some of the changes observed included decreased glucose tolerance, hyperinsulinemia and changes in the binding affinity of insulin receptors. Researchers now believe the progestin component is primarily responsible for altering carbohydrate metabolism by elevating peripheral insulin resistance.

Several issues must be considered when assessing what impact changes in glucose tolerance should have on clinical practice. One: What are the short- and long-term consequences for patients of these changes? Two: Will OCs accelerate the progression of diabetes in women who are glucose intolerant or diabetic? Three: Do alterations in carbohydrate metabolism accelerate or interact with other metabolic effects, such as lipid changes, to increase cardiovascular complications among healthy women or among diabetics?

Studies indicate that the majority of healthy women, women with a history of gestational diabetes and women with insulin-dependent diabetes may safely use OCs. Importantly, modern low-dose OCs have less impact than older formulations on carbohydrate metabolism, as this effect is dose-dependent. In insulin-dependent diabetic women, a careful risk-to-benefit assessment is especially warranted because pregnancy carries risks for both mother and fetus.[3,4]

Effect of OCs on Glucose Tolerance in Healthy Women

One early survey found slightly impaired glucose tolerance in OC users versus nonusers, but attributed little clinical relevance to the finding.[5] The second National Health and Nutrition Examination Survey (1976 to 1980), conducted by the National

Center for Health Statistics, reported results of 75 g oral glucose tolerance tests in over 700 OC users and nonusers 20 to 44 years of age. The survey estimated a decreased glucose tolerance after adjustment for age and body mass index of 15% in OC users (95% confidence interval [CI], 8%-23%) compared to 6% in nonusers (95% CI, 5%-8%). Although OC use was associated with elevation in 1- and 2-hour plasma glucose concentrations, the nonsignificant mean adjusted differences between OC users and nonusers at 1 and 2 hours were only 14 mg/100 ml and 13 mg/100 ml, respectively.

Investigators noted the transient nature of the effect and its probable lack of clinical significance. Women who had recently discontinued OCs had the lowest mean plasma glucose levels at 1 and 2 hours after testing. The authors suggest, "Given that mean fasting glucose values in OC users are about the same as those of nonusers after adjustment, and given that increases in mean 1- and 2-hour glucose values appear to be reversible after discontinuation of the pill, the clinical significance of these findings would appear to be minimal. ...If the metabolic effects are transient and reversible, one would have to question whether the role of the OC pill in diabetes and cardiovascular disease pathogenesis, if it exists, might not be small compared to the role of diet, genetics and other nonreversible factors."[5]

OCs do not increase a woman's chance of developing diabetes mellitus. This is the finding of several large prospective studies. The initial report from the Royal College of General Practitioners' (RCGP) Oral Contraception Study and the Oxford Family Planning Association study found no difference in the occurrence of diabetes mellitus among current users, past users and women who never used the pill.[6] These findings were based on over 317,000 women-years of observation.

It is important to note that the findings from both the National Health and Nutrition Examination Survey and the RCGP were for women using high-dose pills (50+ mcg). Since alterations in glucose metabolism are dose-dependent, any finding of an increased risk of diabetes mellitus would be more likely in a population of women using the higher-dose pills. Neither study supported such an association.

The latest findings from the RCGP confirm previous results (Figure 1).[7] Based on almost 106,000 women-years of current OC use and almost 175,000 women-years of former OC use, the researchers found no evidence of an increased risk of developing diabetes mellitus among current users (relative risk [RR]=0.8; 95% CI, 0.5-1.3). This was true even for long durations of use (10 years or more). Former pill use also conferred no additional risk (RR=0.8; 95% CI, 0.6-1.1).

The Nurses' Health Study also found no increased risk of non-insulin-dependent (type 2) diabetes mellitus in current or former OC users (Figure 2).[8] The Nurses' Health Study is a large prospective, cohort survey that has followed almost 122,000 female nurses since 1976. During over 1 million person-years of follow-up, 2,276 women were diagnosed with type 2 diabetes. Among these women, current users had no increased risk of type 2 diabetes mellitus (RR=0.9; 95% CI, 0.5-1.6) when compared to women who had never used OCs. In addition, former users of the pill also had no increased risk (RR=1.1; 95% CI, 1.0-1.2). The investigators found no difference in risk after a multivariate adjustment for age, body mass index, family history of diabetes, cigarette smoking, menopause and postmenopausal hormone use. In addition, the

Figure 1

Relative Risk of Diabetes Mellitus in Past and Current Users of Oral Contraceptives vs Never-Users — Royal College of General Practitioners' Oral Contraception Study, 1989

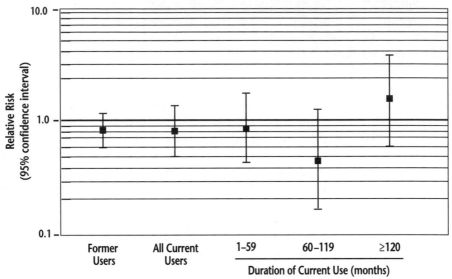

Source: Hannaford PC, et al, 1989 (see reference 7).

researchers noted that surveillance bias, if present, would have resulted in an inflated diagnosis rate in the population because OC users are regularly screened by their physicians. Yet, "current users of oral contraceptives had no increased risk and possibly even a reduced risk of type 2 diabetes as compared to never-users or past users in our population. Furthermore, restricting the analyses to symptomatic cases of diabetes did not appreciably alter the findings."[8]

Women with Glucose Intolerance or Gestational Diabetes

The Walnut Creek study also found no evidence that high-dose OCs lead to impaired glucose tolerance or diabetes.[9] Duffy and Ray administered a 1-hour glucose screening test to 8,652 healthy women. Of these, 593 had an abnormal glucose tolerance test. These women were given a standard oral glucose tolerance test and then classified as normal, as having impaired glucose tolerance or as having diabetes mellitus. The women were followed for an average of 8.5 years. According to Duffy and Ray, "No permanent change in glucose status as a result of oral contraceptive use was found in an analysis for impaired glucose tolerance, diabetes mellitus, diabetic symptoms, or use of oral agents and/or insulin. Increased glucose intolerance was observed for women who were older, had a positive family history of diabetes or were of greater relative weight. Diabetic symptoms correlated most closely with the onset of persistent fasting hyperglycemia [rather than OC use]."

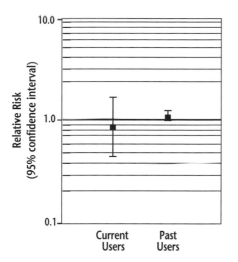

Figure 2

Relative Risk of Non-Insulin-Dependent Diabetes Mellitus among Past and Current Users of Oral Contraceptives — Nurses' Health Study, 1976 to 1988

Source: Rimm EB, et al, 1992 (see reference 8).

Women with gestational diabetes also do not appear at increased risk of developing diabetes mellitus from use of OCs. Kjos and colleagues studied 230 women with previously diagnosed gestational diabetes who used low-dose OCs for up to 13 months of treatment.[10] The researchers randomly assigned patients to use an OC containing either ethinyl estradiol (EE) plus norethindrone or EE plus levonorgestrel. A 75 g, 2-hour glucose tolerance test and fasting lipid profile were performed at entry, after 3 months and after 6 to 13 months of treatment. Kjos et al found no difference in the prevalence of diabetes at 6 to 13 months among the controls versus users of either pill.

The class of gestational diabetes appeared to have the most profound impact on deterioration in glucose tolerance. The authors state, "In this study, only 7% of patients with class A_1 diabetes [antepartum fasting serum glucose levels <105 mg/dl] were seen to have diabetes mellitus compared with 29% of patients with class A_2 diabetes [antepartum fasting serum glucose levels ≥105 mg/dl]. The deterioration in glucose tolerance was closely related to the inherent disease process of gestational diabetes mellitus, rather than use of oral contraceptives."

Use of OCs in Women with Diabetes Mellitus

Early, small studies of insulin-dependent diabetic women using high-dose OCs yielded varying results. Two recent studies suggest, however, that OCs do not appear to enhance the progression of the illness. Klein et al assessed data from the population-based Wisconsin Epidemiologic Study of Diabetic Retinopathy.[11] Among approximately 1,000 women, 384 reported a history of OC use. The researchers found that "Neither current or past use nor number of years of use of oral contraceptives was associated with severity of retinopathy, hypertension or current glycosylated hemoglobin." The researchers caution that one limitation of the study is that it was not designed to assess whether or not OCs influence diabetic complications. They warn that selection bias may be influencing the results—physicians may have been more reluctant to prescribe the pill to women with diabetic complications.

Another study also suggests that OCs do not appear to influence the progression of diabetic renal and retinal complications.[12] Garg et al followed almost 300 young women with diabetes mellitus. In this retrospective, cohort study at a university hospital diabetes clinic, 43 diabetic women who had used OCs for 1 year or longer were compared with a control group of 43 diabetic women who had never used OCs. The outcomes measures were hemoglobin A_{1c} levels, albumin excretion rates and mean retinopathy scores. The investigators found that "The final mean albumin excretion rates, reflecting diabetic renal damage, and the mean eye grades were not significantly different between the groups." They concluded, "The use of OCs among young women with insulin-dependent diabetes mellitus does not pose an additional risk for the development of early diabetic retinopathy or nephropathy. ...The reasons for not seeing a harmful effect from OCs are unknown, but may be related to many other factors (eg, insulin dosage, diet, stress or exercise) having a much greater influence. ...[In addition,] with the knowledge that pregnancy hastens retinal damage, it is possible that OCs help to reduce retinal complications by preventing pregnancy. The additional benefit of allowing planned pregnancy during periods of excellent glucose control (to prevent birth defects) makes the use of OCs an important part of diabetes management."

OCs also have not been shown to accelerate progression of diabetic cardiovascular complications through glucose and/or lipid changes. One review of the literature states, "Despite occasional small changes in carbohydrate metabolism [and lipids] in OC users with previous gestational diabetes or with insulin-dependent diabetes, no prospective study has shown a significant dose-related increase in adverse cardiovascular or cerebrovascular events. In addition, much of the data that reported metabolic changes are from studies with OC formulations containing doses of estrogen and progestin that were higher than those of OCs in current use."[13]

OC Formulations

The differences among low-dose OC formulations also appear to be minimal.[14,15] Van der Vange and colleagues performed a comparative study of seven currently used low-dose combination OCs. They examined OCs containing 30 to 40 mcg EE and various progestins, including norethindrone, desogestrel, levonorgestrel, cyproterone acetate (not available in the United States) and gestodene (also not available). The area under the curve (AUC) for insulin and glucose did not change during treatment with any of the preparations, and the researchers inferred that none of these OCs had any adverse effect on glucose metabolism after 6 months. According to Joseph Goldzieher, MD, Associate Editor of *The Contraception Report*, "The vast majority of the studies find no change in fasting glucose and insulin, AUC of glucose and insulin and glycosylated proteins by monophasic or multiphasic formulations containing 35 mcg of ethinyl estradiol or less, and the progestins levonorgestrel, norethindrone, desogestrel, gestodene or norgestimate. Instead of focusing on minute differences between formulations, we should be carefully weighing the benefits versus the risks of OC use for diabetic women, in whom pregnancy carries such a high risk of progression of retinopathy, nephropathy, coronary heart disease and congenital malformations."

Weighing the Risk-to-Benefit Ratio

For healthy women, OCs pose no additional risk of diabetes; this also appears to be true for women with previous gestational diabetes. For the insulin-dependent diabetic woman, OCs may be used when the patient has made an informed decision

OCs and Diabetes: Summary Points

- Large epidemiologic studies show no increased risk of diabetes among women using OCs, even those using high-dose OCs (50+ mcg) for long periods.

- Women with prior gestational diabetes do not appear at increased risk of future diabetes due to OC use.

- Some evidence suggests OC use does not enhance the progression of either diabetic retinopathy or nephropathy among women with insulin-dependent diabetes.

- OCs have not been shown to accelerate the progression of diabetic cardiovascular complications.

- No significant difference in carbohydrate metabolism exists among various OC formulations.

- Risk-to-benefit ratio of OC use in diabetic women needs to be carefully assessed, as pregnancy carries potentially serious consequences for mother and fetus.

based on her current diabetic status and her willingness to use other methods. Jones and Wild suggest that a careful assessment needs to be made of the risk-to-benefit ratio for various contraceptives when considering their use among women with medical disorders.[3]

Among diabetics, the use of a highly effective birth control method should be encouraged. Pregnancy may then be planned during a time of optimal glycemic control. Although there is no evidence that OCs hasten the progression of cardiovascular complications in diabetic women, many clinicians recommend the intrauterine device (IUD) or progestin-only methods for diabetic women with peripheral vascular disease and/or coronary artery disease.

Alterations in the Lipid Profile

Are changes in the lipid profile induced by OCs relevant to clinical practice? The overall evidence suggests they are not. First, cardiovascular disease in women taking OCs is thought to be primarily thrombotic, rather than atherogenic, and has been attributed to the estrogen component. A reevaluation of early data linking OCs to serious cardiovascular events found that cigarette smoking largely confounded the results. The cardiovascular disease-OC link, however, led many to question whether there might be an atherogenic mechanism involved, as well. Although researchers have performed numerous studies comparing lipoprotein subfraction changes among various OC formulations, the differences are minor and their relevance to clinical practice is questionable.[2]

Second, large prospective studies have not found any increased risk of coronary heart disease among past users of OCs. If OC-induced lipid changes resulted in atherosclerosis, then one would expect a residual effect among past users, especially those who used the pill for long periods. No such increase in the risk of coronary heart disease has been found. On the contrary, the latest data from the Nurses' Health Study indicates no increased risk of coronary heart disease, stroke or other heart disease for past users of OCs.[16]

In one study of premenopausal women who had had a myocardial infarction (MI), typical diffuse coronary atherogenesis was found less frequently in OC users.[17] Among 76 women under the age of 50 years who experienced an MI, angiographic findings revealed that 45% did not have typical coronary atherosclerosis. Of these women, 79% were current users of OCs. What this suggests is that atherogenesis was not the etiology of their MIs.

Cigarette smoking was the only risk factor that appeared to be common to those women who did not have typical atherogenesis. Among the 27 women who used OCs and had no evidence of coronary atherogenesis, 20 had a positive smoking history while the presence of other risk factors, such as hypertension and hypercholesterolemia, was low. According to Engel et al, "If the adverse side effects of oral contraceptives on blood pressure and on carbohydrate and lipid metabolism had been responsible for these myocardial infarctions, then it should have been expected that these atherogenic risk factors had been more prevalent in group I patients [users of OCs without coronary atherosclerosis] than they actually were. Data from group I suggest that the analysis of atherogenic risk factors does not produce information about the propensity for cardiovascular side effects of oral contraceptives."

Data from cynomolgus macaque monkeys also do not support the notion that OCs increase the risk of atherogenic plaque formation.[18-21] Why are results from monkey studies relevant to women using OCs? This monkey serves as an important atherogenesis research model for several reasons:

1. The animals display a high susceptibility to diet-induced atherosclerosis.
2. The histology of macaque coronary atheromas is identical to that of humans.
3. The female monkey's reproductive physiology is similar to human females.
4. The species shows a gender difference in the development of coronary atherosclerosis similar to humans in Western societies. Specifically, male and premenopausal female monkeys develop comparable total plasma cholesterol concentrations, but the females, like human females, exhibit higher HDL (high-density lipoprotein) cholesterol concentrations than do males. In addition, coronary artery atherosclerosis is a little more than twice as extensive among male monkeys as females.

Work with this animal model suggests that the estrogenic effect of OCs may help to prevent atherosclerosis, especially among those at high risk.[20] Researchers compared the effects of two contraceptive preparations on diet-induced atherosclerosis in female macaques. One formulation contained EE plus norgestrel, the other contained EE plus ethynodiol diacetate (which metabolizes to norethindrone). The dose given to the animals was adjusted to be comparable to that given to women during high-dose OC treatment.

The effects of the atherogenic diet were evaluated in the control group and the two OC-treated groups via plasma lipid concentrations. The plasma lipid profiles were much more atherogenic in those treated with OCs: plasma HDL-cholesterol concentrations were lower, total plasma cholesterol concentrations tended to be higher and ratios of total cholesterol to HDL were higher. HDL concentrations were significantly lower in the OC treatment groups compared with the control group (p<0.05). Despite this, actual plaque formation was less than controls in both OC groups. Thus, the OCs *protected* against coronary plaque development, especially among those at high risk— for example, in high-risk animals, controls had a mean coronary artery plaque extent that was up to 10 times that of those treated with OCs.

Furthermore, the OCs prevented plaque formation in the face of adverse lipoprotein profiles. The researchers used a multiple regression model to calculate the expected amount of plaque among those monkeys treated with OCs. They then compared the expected amount of plaque with the amount that actually occurred (Figure 3). Based on plasma lipoprotein measurements, the predicted amount of coronary artery atherosclerosis among the OC groups should have been 1.3 to 2.7 times greater than that seen in the control animals. Instead, coronary atherosclerosis among the OC groups was reduced by 55% to 83%. The researchers concluded, "Considering either all of the animals or the high-risk subset, [the] OC treatment, while changing the plasma lipid profile in an atherogenic direction, actually resulted in less extensive coronary artery atherosclerosis than would be expected based upon the plasma lipid concentrations of the treated groups. This [apparent paradox] indicated that there must be a large positive or protective effect of OC treatment with respect to coronary artery atherosclerosis."

The following factors argue against the idea that OCs and specific progestins promote the development of atherogenic cardiovascular complications. One: large

Figure 3

Expected vs Actual Extent of Coronary Atherosclerosis in Cynomolgus Macaques Treated with Two Different High-Dose Oral Contraceptives

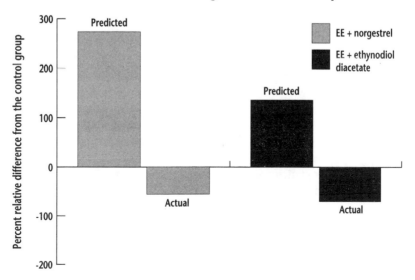

Source: Clarkson TB, et al, 1990 (see reference 20).

OCs and Lipids: Summary Points

- Cardiovascular complications in women using OCs are not atherogenic in origin.

- Latest data from the Nurses' Health Study indicate no increased risk of coronary heart disease, stroke or other heart disease among former OC users.

- Data from cynomolgus macaque monkeys, an accepted animal model for atherogenesis, suggest that the estrogen in OCs may protect against the development of atherosclerosis.

- Lipid values among OC users tend to vary only within the normal range and also to return to pretreatment values during the pill-free week.

- The androgenic properties of progestins used in low-dose combination OCs and their effect on lipids appear irrelevant for the later development of coronary atherogenesis.

---

prospective studies have shown that women using OCs are not at an increased risk of atherogenic cardiovascular disease. Two: angiographic data from young women who had an MI suggest that among OC users, the MIs resulted from some mechanism other than atherogenesis. Three: data from animal experiments suggest OCs may protect against coronary atherosclerosis, particularly among those who have unfavorable lipid profiles and are considered high risk. Four: studies of lipid profiles among OC users demonstrate lipid values that vary within the normal range, values that tend to return to pretreatment levels during the pill-free week.[22]

The relative androgenicity of the progestin given in low-dose combination OCs also appears to be unrelated to the later development of atherogenic cardiovascular disease. Both levonorgestrel and norethindrone [generally considered more androgenic than third-generation progestins (desogestrel, norgestimate and gestodene)] have been shown to have a similar minimal impact on lipids.[23,24] Moreover, in experimental animals, combination OCs containing either progestin protected against the development of atherosclerotic lesions.

Do newer, less "androgenic" progestins offer greater benefit in terms of the lipid profile? According to Luigi Mastroianni, Jr., MD, Associate Editor of *The Contraception Report*, "One of the goals in developing the third-generation progestins was to modify the molecule (levonorgestrel) to have less androgenicity, which would result in a more 'favorable' lipid profile. The developers accomplished their aim, but the clinical significance of reduced androgenicity remains obscure. Older progestins induce minimal lipid changes, which, in any case, appear to be irrelevant for the later development of cardiovascular disease in women using OCs."

Androgenicity of the Progestin Component

Recently, attention has centered on the relative androgenicity of the progestin component of OCs. Investigators have hypothesized that the androgenic effect of the progestin may aggravate or induce androgenic side effects, such as acne and hirsutism.

Some suggest that the androgenic effect on the lipid profile may interact with insulin resistance to increase a woman's risk of cardiovascular disease.

Is androgenicity of the progestin clinically relevant? In order to answer this question, it is important to understand the scope of the biological actions of progestational compounds, how the androgenic action of progestins is measured, the overall effect of a combination OC on the endogenous androgen environment and the workings of the sex hormone-binding globulin (SHBG) system.

First, androgenicity constitutes only one property of progestational agents. Progestational agents have at least 27 different biological actions.[2] For example, they have progestational, estrogenic, antiestrogenic, androgenic, antiandrogenic and corticoid properties, among many others. Each of these properties can be used as the basis of a bioassay.

A progestational agent is tested preclinically to determine its properties at various doses, which are often very high. These preclinical assays help ascertain other properties the compound may exhibit aside from its desired effect(s); eg, endometrial transformation and ovulation blockade. Researchers administer high doses to animals in order to determine what is known as a "dose separation." The dose separation is the difference between the amount needed to achieve the desired effect (eg, ovulation inhibition) and that amount needed to express other properties that may be undesirable.

One classic, preclinical assay to determine the androgenic properties of a progestin utilizes immature, castrated male rats. After giving the progestin at various doses, the growth in the sizes of the ventral prostate, seminal vesicle and levator ani are measured by weight. These measurements are then compared to that growth induced by the "standard" androgen, testosterone. Increased weight of the ventral prostate and seminal vesicle indicate androgenic activity, while increased weight of the levator ani can indicate anabolic activity.

Ventral prostate assays are useful preclinically, but have little relevance in terms of the clinical effects of combination OCs in women. One major factor that is often overlooked is that the effect of the combination of estrogen and progestin on androgen function far outweighs any androgenic potential of the progestin. As Dr. Goldzieher explained, "If you take the pure progestin and do a ventral prostate assay in mice, some progestins are more androgenic than others. But, that's got nothing to do with the clinical use of a combination of estrogen and a progestin for birth control in women. The concept of a combination OC being more androgenic completely ignores the fact that all OCs work to suppress androgen production by shutting down gonadotropins and, subsequently, ovarian production of androgen. And, to a certain extent, the pill also suppresses androgen production from the adrenals. The combination of suppression of the ovaries and the adrenals makes such an impact on the endogenous androgen environment that any androgenic action that the progestin would have on its own is *trivial* compared to the overall effect on the body." David A. Grimes, MD, Executive Editor of *The Contraception Report*, agrees. "The androgenic property of the progestin is unlikely to overwhelm the estrogen effect. The hypothesis that the androgenicity of the progestin matters in terms of the metabolic side effects of OCs remains unproved."

The progestin's potency also influences whether its androgenic property could manifest clinically.[2] For example, how much of the progestin is needed to achieve the desired antiovulatory effect? Is this amount high enough to exhibit the androgenic property? According to Dr. Goldzieher, the answer is no. "In considering the pharmacologic effects of a progestin, androgenic activity must be expressed in proportion to the progestational potency; thus, vastly larger quantities of the progestin must be used to produce an androgenic response than are required for expression of progestational activity. In clinical terms, the quantity of a progestin (combined with the augmentative effect of the estrogen) needed to inhibit ovulation is so small that androgenic action is simply not expressed."[2]

The purported androgenicity of first- and second-generation progestins, norethindrone and levonorgestrel, respectively, has been the subject of much debate. This is, perhaps, because they are, remotely, derivatives of 19-nortestosterone (as are the third-generation progestins desogestrel, gestodene and norgestimate). Levonorgestrel is generally considered the more androgenic of the two. When used at doses found in combination OCs, however, data suggest its androgenic properties are not expressed.

An evaluation of levonorgestrel found that the dose needed for its antiovulatory effect was much less than that needed to express androgenicity (Figure 4).[25] Researchers compared the effects of levonorgestrel, testosterone propionate and no treatment on the ventral prostate, seminal vesicles and levator ani of immature, castrated rats. Levonorgestrel produced a dose-dependent increase in the weights of the ventral prostate and seminal vesicles (indicating androgenic activity). The response paralleled, but was considerably less than that observed with testosterone

Figure 4

The Dose Separation between Antiovulatory Activity and Androgenic Activity of Levonorgestrel

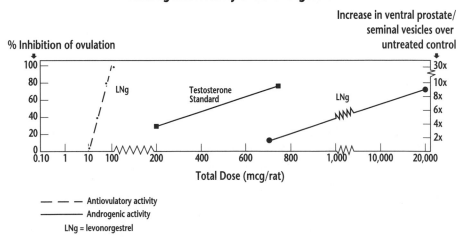

Antiovulatory activity

Androgenic activity

LNg = levonorgestrel

Source: Upton GV, Corbin A. The relevance of the pharmacologic properties of a progestational agent to its clinical effects as a combination oral contraceptive. Yale J Biol Med 1989;62:445-457. Reproduced with permission of the publisher, The Yale Journal of Biology and Medicine.

Androgenicity of the OC Progestin: Summary Points

• All combination OCs work to suppress gonadotropins and subsequent ovarian androgen production.

• OCs also partly suppress androgen production by the adrenals.

• The combination of suppression of the ovaries and adrenals far outweighs any androgenic action of the progestin alone.

• Any androgenic action of the progestin is unlikely to overwhelm the estrogen effect.

• The progestin's potency influences whether the androgenic action could be expressed at doses needed to suppress ovulation.

• An evaluation of levonorgestrel, generally classified as "androgenic," found that the dose used in OCs is insufficient to express androgenic effects.

---

propionate. Additionally, the effects on the levator ani resembled the anabolic effect of testosterone more than the androgenic property (data not shown).[25]

The dose separation between the amount of levonorgestrel needed to inhibit ovulation and the amount needed to exhibit androgenicity was very large. An estimated effective dose of 50 mcg to 100 mcg of the progestin was needed to suppress ovulation, whereas androgenic response (weight gain of ventral prostate and seminal vesicles) only occurred at doses of 700 mcg to 21,000 mcg. This dose separation is so wide that the amount of levonorgestrel used in current low-dose OCs would be predicted to be insufficient to express an inherent androgenic property, particularly in combination with an estrogen.

Androgenic Progestins and Acne

OCs have traditionally been used to treat hirsutism and acne, conditions often associated with a hyperandrogenic state. According to Dr. Goldzieher, "I use OCs to treat acne. I don't think the androgenicity or 'selectivity' of the progestin has much to do with a particular pill's overall impact on acne. In fact, the term 'androgenicity' carries a negative connotation by itself, conjuring up images of excessively hairy women with terrible skin problems. Pills don't cause these types of severe problems. The cause is usually some combination of factors, including a hyperandrogenic state and genetics. Remember, the net effect of prescribing an OC is to reduce endogenous androgen production, an effect far more substantial and important than the androgenicity of the synthetic progestin. Moreover, estrogens increase plasma levels of sex hormone-binding globulin, thereby lowering the bioavailability of circulating androgens, as measured by plasma free testosterone, for example."

The effects of various progestins on SHBG have been studied in an attempt to determine whether certain OC formulations have a more or less favorable effect on acne. Are some formulations better than others? Do those formulations with greater androgenicity worsen acne?

At this time, data are too scant to draw definitive conclusions about whether some OC formulations provide greater improvement in acne than others. Some data exist, however, which suggest that low-dose OCs (both monophasic and triphasic) containing androgenic progestins help improve, not worsen, acne.

Understanding how SHBG works to regulate levels of circulating androgens may help to explain this apparent paradox. The steroid-binding system is complex.[26,27] SHBG is a steroid-binding protein that circulates in plasma and regulates the concentration of free testosterone, dihydrotestosterone and, to a lesser extent, estradiol. Estrogen raises the amount of SHBG, while androgen lowers it. Progestins tend to counter the effect of estrogen. An equilibrium exists between the amounts of testosterone and estradiol that are bound to SHBG and essentially inactive, and the amounts of "free" circulating testosterone and estradiol, which remain biologically active. The small free fraction affects hormone action.

"Ideally," Dr. Goldzieher continued, "if you want to measure androgens, you want to measure the fraction of free circulating testosterone. It was not until quite recently that a good SHBG assay was available. If you wanted to measure bound versus free androgens accurately, you had to use an equilibrium dialysis—a lengthy, expensive test that was simply not practical for routine laboratory use. Clinicians have traditionally measured total SHBG levels and it's perfectly okay for most purposes, but when looking at sophisticated concepts, such as what an OC formulation does to the endogenous androgenic environment, then you have to scrutinize the levels of bound versus free androgens. Even in the condition of hirsutism, where half the time the total plasma testosterone is normal, if you look at the free testosterone, it's elevated. What's important clinically is not the total SHBG level, but the levels of free hormone (free testosterone) that remain biologically active."

A study by Palatsi et al found that SHBG levels were higher in women taking a desogestrel- as compared to a levonorgestrel-containing pill, but improvement in acne was similar.[28] The study divided 54 women with preexisting acne into two treatment groups given two different kinds of OCs: one contained 150 mcg desogestrel plus 30 mcg EE, the other contained 150 mcg levonorgestrel plus 30 mcg EE. Both OCs significantly improved acne. Importantly, although SHBG levels were much higher in the desogestrel group, both groups were found to have a 60% decrease in serum free testosterone, a fact the investigators credit for the improvement in acne.

Combination OCs decrease free testosterone levels, regardless of the pill's specific progestin. Fotherby and Caldwell examined over 40 studies of the effect of various OC formulations on serum proteins and adrenal steroids.[29] All studies indicated OCs produced a drop in free testosterone levels, whether the pills contained EE plus levonorgestrel, norethindrone, gestodene, desogestrel or norgestimate.

Combination OCs increase SHBG through the estrogen component, but to different degrees. Fotherby and Caldwell note, for example, that estrogen/progestin preparations containing either norethindrone or triphasic levonorgestrel increase SHBG, but to a lesser degree than those containing desogestrel and gestodene.[29] Nonetheless, comparative trials found no difference in effect on acne between low-

---

OCs, SHBG and Acne: Summary Points

• All OCs tend to improve acne by suppressing endogenous androgen production.

• Combination OCs decrease free testosterone while raising SHBG levels to varying degrees.

• An OC's effect on acne depends upon the combined effect of the estrogen and progestin, and the overall effect on ovarian, adrenal and peripheral metabolism.

• Combination OCs containing the progestins norgestimate, levonorgestrel, gestodene and desogestrel have been suggested to improve acne among women with preexisting acne.

• Few comparative clinical trials have been done comparing one formulation to another.

---

dose combination pills containing 150 mcg levonorgestrel and either 75 mcg gestodene[30] or 150 mcg desogestrel.[28]

At least one investigation has explored whether more androgenic progestins exacerbate acne.[31] Andre Lemay, MD, PhD, Professor of Obstetrics and Gynecology at Laval University in Quebec, Canada, and his colleagues used a triphasic OC containing levonorgestrel [as dl-norgestrel] in 41 postpubertal women with acne. Mean baseline levels of testosterone, 17-hydroxyprogesterone and dehydroepiandrosterone sulfate were in the upper third of the normal range, with elevated individual values in 19%, 37% and 27% of women, respectively. SHBG levels were below the normal range in 27% of the cases.

Just over two-thirds (69%) of patients had clinical improvement in their acne. At the end of the first OC cycle, the pill significantly decreased all androgen precursors (p<0.01) and resulted in a twofold increase in SHBG. Androstenedione and free testosterone dropped into the normal range during OC treatment. "These results [suggest] that the...OC has significantly improved acne in postpubertal women for whom acne was the main manifestation of mild hyperandrogenic activity. The improvement in acne corresponded to a decrease in adrenal/ovarian androgens and free T [testosterone], which led to a decreased metabolism to 3α-diol-G, presumably by the sebaceous glands. The increase in SHBG is considered an estrogenic effect, and the triphasic formulation containing low-dose levonorgestrel is not androgenic, but rather an estrogen-dominant formulation; as such, this product is recommended in women requiring contraception who also have idiopathic acne."[31]

Dr. Lemay emphasized that the overall effect of the OC is more important than the degree of androgenic expression of its progestational component. In an interview he said, "There has been some prejudice against compounds containing the progestins that are considered androgenic. It's essential to remember that the most important element is the compound effect of the estrogen and the progestin together, and the overall effect on ovarian, adrenal and peripheral metabolism. The effect on acne will depend on the balance of estrogen and progestin. Each pill formulation should be tested for its effect on acne because it is the overall effect of the combination that counts. There have been few comparative trials between pills, so far. Triphasic levonorgestrel has been shown to help improve acne.[31,32] Some of the newer pills containing desogestrel[33] or gestodene also have been tested and been found to improve acne."

Indeed, one OC has now been approved by the Food and Drug Administration for use in treating acne in women >15 years of age. The triphasic OC contains 35 mcg ethinyl estradiol and norgestimate.

References

1. Watanabe RM, Azen CG, Roy S, et al. Defects in carbohydrate metabolism in oral contraceptive users without apparent metabolic risk factors. *J Clin Endocrinol Metab* 1994;79:1277-1283.

2. Goldzieher JW. *Hormonal Contraception: Pills, Injections & Implants*. Third edition. London, Ontario, Canada: EMIS-Canada, 1994.

3. Jones KP, Wild RA. Contraception for patients with psychiatric or medical disorders. *Am J Obstet Gynecol* 1994;170:1575-1580.

4. Skouby SO, Molsted-Pedersen L, Petersen KR. Contraception for women with diabetes: an update. *Clin Obstet Gynecol* 1991;5:493-503.

5. Russell-Briefel R, Ezzati TM, Perlman JA, et al. Impaired glucose tolerance in women using oral contraceptives: United States, 1976-1980. *J Chron Dis* 1987;40:3-11.

6. Wingrave SJ, Kay CR, Vessey MP. Oral contraceptives and diabetes mellitus. *BMJ* 1979;1:23.

7. Hannaford PC, Kay CR. Oral contraceptives and diabetes mellitus. *BMJ* 1989;299:1315-1316.

8. Rimm EB, Manson JE, Stampfer MJ, et al. Oral contraceptive use and the risk of type 2 (non-insulin-dependent) diabetes mellitus in a large prospective study of women. *Diabetologia* 1992;35:967-972.

9. Duffy TJ, Ray R. Oral contraceptive use: prospective follow-up of women with suspected glucose intolerance. *Contraception* 1984;30:197-208.

10. Kjos SL, Shoupe D, Douyan S, et al. Effect of low-dose oral contraceptives on carbohydrate and lipid metabolism in women with recent gestational diabetes: results of a controlled, randomized, prospective study. *Am J Obstet Gynecol* 1990:163:1822-1827.

11. Klein BEK, Moss SE, Klein R. Oral contraceptives in women with diabetes. *Diabetes Care* 1990;13:895-898.

12. Garg SK, Chase HP, Marshall G, et al. Oral contraceptives and renal and retinal complications in young women with insulin-dependent diabetes mellitus. *JAMA* 1994;271:1099-1102.

13. Mestman JH, Schmidt-Sarosi C. Diabetes mellitus and fertility control: contraception management issues. *Am J Obstet Gynecol* 1993;168:2012-2020.

14. Van der Vange N, Kloosterboer HJ, Haspels AA. Effect of seven low-dose combined oral contraceptive preparations on carbohydrate metabolism. *Am J Obstet Gynecol* 1987;156:918-922.

15. Simon D, Senan C, Garnier P, et al. Effects of oral contraceptives on carbohydrate and lipid metabolism in a healthy population: The Telecom Study. *Am J Obstet Gynecol* 1990;163:382-387.

16. Colditz GA and The Nurses' Health Study Research Group. Oral contraceptive use and mortality during 12 years of follow-up: The Nurses' Health Study. *Ann Intern Med* 1994;120:821-826.

17. Engel HJ, Engel E, Lichtlen PR. Coronary atherosclcerosis and myocardial infarction in young women—role of oral contraceptives. *Eur Heart J* 1983;4:1-8.

18. Adams MR, Clarkson TB, Koritnik DR, et al. Contraceptive steroids and coronary artery atherosclerosis in cynomolgus macaques. *Fertil Steril* 1987;47:1010-1018.

19. Clarkson TB, Adams MR, Kaplan JR, et al. From menarche to menopause: coronary artery atherosclerosis and protection in cynomolgus monkeys. *Am J Obstet Gynecol* 1989;160:1280-1285.

20. Clarkson TB, Shively CA, Morgan TM, et al. Oral contraceptives and coronary artery atherosclerosis of cynomolgus monkeys. *Obstet Gynecol* 1990;75:217-222.

21. Adams MR, Kaplan JR, Manuck SB, et al. Inhibition of coronary artery atherosclerosis by 17-beta estradiol in ovariectomized monkeys. Lack of an effect of added progesterone. *Arteriosclerosis* 1990;10:1051-1057.

22. Marz W, Jung-Hoffmann C, Heidt F, et al. Changes in lipid metabolism during 12 months of treatment with two oral contraceptives containing 30 mcg ethinyl estradiol and 75 mcg gestodene or 150 mcg desogestrel. *Contraception* 1990;41:245-258.

23. Patsch W, Brown SA, Gotto AM, et al. The effect of triphasic oral contraceptives on plasma lipids and lipoproteins. *Am J Obstet Gynecol* 1989;161:1396-1401.

24. Notelovitz M, Feldman E, Gillespy M, et al. Lipid and lipoprotein changes in women taking low-dose, triphasic oral contraceptives: a controlled, comparative, 12-month clinical trial. *Am J Obstet Gynecol* 1989;160:1037-1048.

25. Upton GV, Corbin A. The relevance of the pharmacologic properties of a progestational agent to its clinical effects as a combination oral contraceptive. *Yale J Biol Med* 1989;62:445-457.

26. Rosner W. Plasma steroid-binding proteins. *Endocrinol Metab Clin North Am* 1991;20:697-720.

27. Rosner W, Hryb DJ, Khan MS, et al. Sex hormone-binding globulin: anatomy and physiology of a new regulatory system. *J Steroid Biochem Mol Biol* 1991;40:813-820.

28. Palatsi R, Hirvensalo E, Liukko P, et al. Serum total and unbound testosterone and sex hormone-binding globulin (SHBG) in female acne patients treated with two different oral contraceptives. *Acta Derm Venereol* 1984;64:517-523.

29. Fotherby K, Caldwell ADS. New progestogens in oral contraception. *Contraception* 1994;49:1-32.

30. Loudon NB, Kirkman RJE, Dewsbury JA. Double-blind comparison of Femodene and Microgynon. *Eur J Obstet Gynecol Reprod Biol* 1990;34:257-266.

31. Lemay A, Dewailly SD, Grenier R, et al. Attenuation of mild hyperandrogenic activity in postpubertal acne by a triphasic oral contraceptive containing low doses of ethinyl estradiol and dl-norgestrel. *J Clin Endocrinol Metab* 1990;71:8-14.

32. Vermeulen A, Thiery M. Metabolic effects of the triphasic oral contraceptive Trigynon®. *Contraception* 1982;26:505-513.

33. Cullberg G, Hamberger L, Mattsson LA, et al. Effects of a low-dose desogestrel-ethinyl estradiol combination on hirsutism, androgens and sex hormone-binding globulin in women with a polycystic ovary syndrome. *Acta Obstet Gynecol Scand* 1985;64:195-202.

1.8: Trends in Development and Utilization

During the past 3 decades, oral contraceptives (OCs) have changed substantially. These changes have occurred in the dose and type of both the estrogen and progestin components, as well as in the sequencing or phasing of these steroids.

Prescribing has also changed. Clinicians now dispense pills with far less estrogen and progestin than used in early preparations. In addition, clinicians are more aware of the importance of compliance and use effectiveness.

What forces have shaped the development of today's birth control pills? The first part of this section examines how the birth control pill was developed, describes trends in use and prescribing, and presents data specifically for low-dose pills. The second part covers the current evidence concerning the lowest-dose pills—those with 20 mcg of ethinyl estradiol (EE). We look at their safety, efficacy, side effect profile and health benefits.

The Development of Oral Contraceptives

Serendipity played a role in the development of the combination oral contraceptive.[1] Furthermore, within this story lies the explanation for why birth control pills have evolved to the formulations available today.

Developers of the contraceptive pill were working with the progestational agents norethynodrel and norethindrone. Joseph Goldzieher, MD, one of the researchers involved in the early development of norethindrone preparations and Associate Editor of *The Contraception Report*, shared his perspective on this research. "In the 1950s, the quest began in earnest to use progestins as a contraceptive agent; ie, a progestin-only pill. The first investigators decided upon the original dose of 10 mg of norethynodrel after extrapolation from animal data. Importantly, the norethynodrel coming from the factory was contaminated with an estrogen, mestranol. This fact would greatly impact the later development of the pill.

"The norethynodrel contained 0.15% of mestranol. To a chemist, 0.15% contamination is minute. However, in pills containing 10 mg of norethynodrel, that 0.15% translated into 150 mcg of mestranol—a huge dose!

"The importance of mestranol was finally recognized because the norethynodrel coming from the factory became purer. As the mestranol was eliminated, the pill provided less effective cycle control, so the researchers decided to put it back in.

"No one recognized, however, that the mestranol also had powerful contraceptive effects of its own. At that time, it was known that estrogens of other kinds—conjugated equine estrogens, estradiol and others—do not inhibit the pituitary very well. I became curious about the 'contaminant' mestranol and began research with this compound. As it turned out, the 17-α-ethinyl group, which is present in mestranol and ethinyl estradiol, confers an extraordinary amount of pituitary inhibiting action, a property not shared by any other type of derivative.[2] This unique contraceptive property prompted further investigation into oral contraceptive preparations.

"I then became involved in developing the sequential pill. The idea was that if the ethinyl estrogen inhibits the pituitary so effectively, then we should be able to give less progestin. We developed a pill with mestranol and 10 days of a progestin. As estrogen doses got much below 80 mcg mestranol, however, the effectiveness dropped. Today, we don't have any sequential pills because we're using much lower doses of estrogen.

"When we started lowering the estrogen dose, we found out that the estrogen and progestin acted *synergistically* to inhibit the pituitary. Therefore, it required even less of each component for effective ovulation inhibition than might have been anticipated from their individual effects. This finding was the breakthrough that made possible the current generation of low-dose OCs."

Research Trends

Manufacturers continue to research and develop new birth control pill formulations. These efforts are focused on reducing the amount of estrogen to the lowest contraceptively effective dose and combining it with a type and dose of progestational agent that provides good cycle control and minimizes side effects.

Developers are concentrating their attention on pills with <35 mcg of EE. In the United States, several OC formulations with 30 mcg of EE and various progestins are available. As of press time, one 20 mcg formulation is available (20 mcg EE plus 1 mg norethindrone acetate); however, other 20 mcg formulations are being investigated. In Europe, three 20 mcg pills are available—20 mcg EE plus 1 mg norethindrone acetate, 20 mcg EE plus 100 mcg levonorgestrel and 20 mcg EE plus 150 mcg desogestrel.

Two lower-dose products should be available in the U.S. in 1997. The monophasic preparation with 20 mcg EE and 100 mcg levonorgestrel should come to market within the next few months.[3] Another low-dose product that uses phased doses of estrogen was approved by the Food and Drug Administration (FDA) in late 1996.[4] This pill phases the estrogen, using 20 mcg EE for the first 5 days, 30 mcg EE for the next 7 days and 35 mcg EE for the last 9 days, combined with a constant dose of 1 mg norethindrone acetate for 21 days. Some research is even under way on pills with less than 20 mcg of EE.

Trends in Utilization and Prescribing: 1964-1988

Gerstman et al used national audit data to analyze U.S. trends in OC formulation and prescribing between 1964 and 1988.[5] The researchers gathered information from two pharmaceutical marketing research databases produced by IMS America, Ltd. (Plymouth Meeting, Pennsylvania). The National Prescription Audit provided information on the number of OC prescriptions dispensed by retail pharmacies in the contiguous United States. The National Disease and Therapeutic Index (NDTI) provided age-related information from office-based physicians.

Several trends emerged. First, the use of low-dose pills, those with <50 mcg of estrogen, steadily rose (Figure 1). According to the authors, "In 1968, fewer than 1% of the estimated 54 million retail prescriptions for oral contraceptives were for formula-

Figure 1

Percentage of Retail Prescriptions Written for Oral Contraceptives by Estrogen Dose and Year

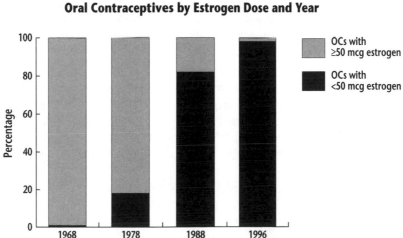

Source: Gerstman BB, et al, 1991 (see reference 5) and IMS America National Prescription Audit, November 1996.

tions containing less than 50 mcg of estrogen, whereas in 1988, approximately 82% of the approximately 57 million retail prescriptions were for formulations with less than 50 mcg of estrogen."[5] By about 1986, prescriptions for pills with <50 mcg estrogen outnumbered those for higher-dose pills. The mean dose of progestin in low-dose pills also declined steadily.

Second, multiphasic pills increased in popularity after they were introduced in 1982. By 1988, multiphasic pills, which included both triphasic and biphasic preparations, accounted for 37% of all retail OC prescriptions.

Trends in Utilization and Prescribing: 1991-1996

The editors of *The Contraception Report* performed a similar analysis of trends in OC use over the past 6 years. We used data from the National Prescription Audit of IMS America, but focused specifically on trends in use of low-dose pills. While the Gerstman et al report clearly indicated that prescribing pills containing <50 mcg of estrogen had become the norm, it did not differentiate among pills containing ≤35 mcg of estrogen.

We separated prescriptions containing 20 mcg, 30 mcg and 35 mcg of estrogen. Pills containing 50 mcg of mestranol were grouped with 35 mcg estrogen pills. Mestranol must be converted to the active estrogen, ethinyl estradiol. Data indicate that 30% of mestranol is lost in this conversion, making 50 mcg mestranol pills bioequivalent to 35 mcg EE formulations.[6,7]

We also looked at trends in use of monophasic or phasic preparations, again limiting the analysis to low-dose formulations. We included multiphasic pills with consistent use of 35 mcg EE throughout the cycle with 35 mcg estrogen products.

Those multiphasic pills using less than a mean of 35 mcg of estrogen were included with 30 mcg estrogen products. Doing so did not change the trend for 30 mcg pills, except perhaps to underestimate slightly the number of prescriptions being filled for 30 mcg pills. This was because the number of prescriptions for multiphasic pills declined over the 6-year period.

As of October 1996, low-dose pills accounted for virtually all retail OC prescriptions—98%. This represents about an 11% increase from 1988. Not surprisingly, use of pills with 50 mcg estrogen dropped 57% between 1991 and 1996. In 1991, almost 3 million prescriptions were written for products containing 50 mcg estrogen; in 1996, only 1.2 million prescriptions were written for high-dose products.

Among low-dose pills, use of 35 mcg pills declined, while use of 30 mcg and 20 mcg pills increased. Formulations containing 35 mcg estrogen, while still accounting for the majority of prescriptions until 1994, dropped steadily over the 6-year period. In 1995, prescriptions for 30 mcg pills outnumbered those for 35 mcg preparations for the first time (Figure 2).

The most rapid change occurred in pills with the lowest dosage of estrogen—20 mcg. Between 1991 and 1996, the number of retail prescriptions for these pills increased 10-fold. This increase occurred both among older women (≥40 years of age) and among younger women (20 to 39 years of age). Almost no use occurred among women 19 years old or younger.

Figure 2

Total Number of Retail Prescriptions for Low-Dose Oral Contraceptives by Estrogen Dose: United States, 1991-1996

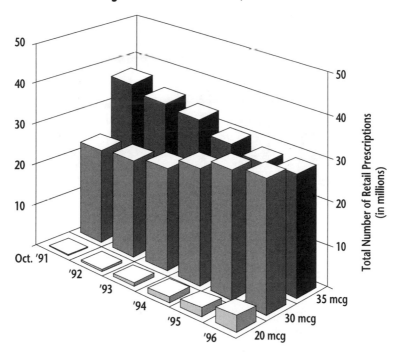

Source: IMS America, Ltd., National Prescription Audit, November 1991-1996.

Multiphasic preparations, however, declined in popularity. Between 1991 and 1996, retail prescriptions fell 14%. On the other hand, during the same time period, total retail prescriptions for low-dose monophasic formulations rose from 52% to 62% (Figure 3).

Implications of Further Reducing Steroid Dosage

What are the implications of continuing to reduce the steroid dosages in oral contraceptives? The following section examines data concerning pills containing the lowest dose of estrogen—20 mcg of EE—in terms of their safety, efficacy, side effects and health benefits.

Safety of Lower-Dose Pills

The FDA recommends that women use pills containing the lowest effective amount of estrogen. An October 1993 FDA debate about the safety of 50 mcg pills came about after the agency had considered removing all such products from the U.S. market. After reviewing the literature on the relationship between OC dose and myocardial infarction, venous thromboembolism and stroke, the committee concluded that the evidence against higher-dose pills was not definitive. In addition, they recognized the

Figure 3

**Total Number of Retail Prescriptions for Monophasic and Multiphasic
Low-Dose* Oral Contraceptives: United States, 1991-1996**

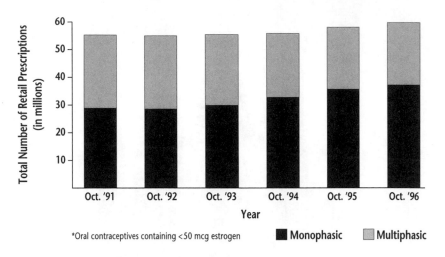

*Oral contraceptives containing <50 mcg estrogen   ■ **Monophasic**   ▨ **Multiphasic**

Source: IMS America, Ltd., National Prescription Audit, November 1991-1996.

need for high-dose products for some patients; for example, those taking anticonvulsants. The agency left higher-dose products on the market, but strongly recommended that women use the lowest estrogen dose necessary for contraceptive efficacy.

Most agree that sound medical practice warrants using the lowest effective dose possible. In an interview, Ian Thorneycroft, MD, PhD, Professor and Chairman of the Department of Obstetrics and Gynecology at the University of South Alabama, commented on this issue. "My feeling is that the lower the dose of estrogen, the better off you are. After the venous thromboembolism data came out in the 1960s and 1970s, we realized that we didn't need that much estrogen. Since we don't need the estrogen for efficacy and there's some question with regard to safety, I think it makes sense to reduce the estrogen dose. And, that's one reason why I think we'll see greater utilization of 20 mcg pills in the future as more of these preparations come on the market."

Efficacy of 20 mcg Pills

Should efficacy be a concern when using very low-dose pills? Most agree that it should not. Although the pharmacology of birth control pills is such that a wide inter- and intraindividual variability in steroid metabolism exists, the data are reassuring that low-dose pills are, nonetheless, highly effective. According to Dr. Goldzieher, "Marketed formulations are very much the result of clinical trial-and-error experience because of these inter- and intraindividual differences in steroid metabolism. In a given individual, the blood levels from the same dose will not be the same from day to day. Also, the bioavailability of both the estrogen and progestin do not change in parallel. A woman makes her own varying blend of contraceptive each day she takes an OC.

"Despite this, even very low-dose OCs are highly effective. The clinical trials of pills with 20 mcg EE show the pregnancy rate is no different than with 35 mcg pills. Clearly, the 20 mcg dose is enough for contraceptive control. Again, that's because of the synergistic effect of the estrogen and the progestin.

"There were two reports that suggested that lower-dose OCs were associated with higher failure rates. One, a retrospective investigation by Meade et al, found about twice as much risk of failure with lower-dose formulations (30 mcg EE).[8] In practical reality, however, the chance of failure was so small as to be inconsequential. The 50 mcg and 30 mcg preparations had failure rates between 0.1 and 0.2 per 100 women-years.

"The other study utilized data recorded from women obtaining an abortion in The Netherlands from 1982 to 1984.[9] In The Netherlands, over 1 million women use OCs. From detailed interviews, Ketting estimated that the true OC failure rate (ie, with correct use) was an extraordinary 0.02 pregnancies per 100 women-years for all types of OCs combined. The pregnancy rates were no different for monophasic OCs containing 50 mcg EE compared to those with <50 mcg EE; however, there was a small, but statistically significant, higher pregnancy rate with triphasics that could not be explained by gastrointestinal disorders or drug interactions.

"Despite this finding, overall, the efficacy data are reassuring. Of course, as with any OC, women should be counseled carefully to help improve compliance and be advised to take their pill at the same time every day to minimize the chance of failure."

Dr. Thorneycroft explained that concerns about efficacy with low-dose pills are most likely overstated. "I think clinicians really shouldn't worry about efficacy because the Food and Drug Administration must weigh the data very carefully before approving any new contraceptive pill—efficacy is not something that can be sacrificed.

"The concern is reminiscent of when we used 80 and 50 mcg pills. When the 35 mcg pills came out, some of us weren't really trusting of the lower-dose pills. Now, we think of 35s as the standard and have no concerns about using them. I think the same will be true of the 20 mcg pills, which are likely to be used more and more as first-line pills as newer agents come on the market. I have no major concerns about efficacy with the 20 mcg pills."

In May 1993, a group of European experts met to debate issues surrounding 20 mcg pills.[10] With regard to efficacy, the group stated, "On the evidence available, 20 mcg formulations in association with the new gonane progestogens appear to have the same level of effectiveness as 30 mcg formulations, providing they are taken as prescribed." Like Dr. Goldzieher, the group noted that individual variations in metabolism may narrow the margin of error with regard to pill omissions and emphasized that clinicians educate women to improve compliance with the pill-taking regimen.

Other mechanisms of action likely support the efficacy of 20 mcg (and higher-dose) combination pills.[7,11] For example, the progestational agent makes the cervical mucus more viscous, scanty and cellular. These effects are thought to impede the ascent of both sperm and organisms into the upper reproductive tract, helping to protect OC users from pregnancy and some sexually transmitted diseases. Other suspected and possible mechanisms of action include alterations in the endometrium and tubal transport processes.

61

In fact, most pill failures are due to user mistakes rather than method failure. According to Dr. Goldzieher, "The critical factor in efficacy, today, is not 'theoretical effectiveness,' but user compliance. Compliance is intimately related to side effects and the user's perceptions of risks and benefits, a factor heavily influenced by media-generated misinformation."

Importantly, side effects can cause women to stop using the pill.[12] Side effects formerly thought of as "nuisance" side effects—breakthrough bleeding, nausea, breast tenderness and weight gain—can have a major impact on compliance.[13,14]

Side Effects

Cycle Control

Cycle control greatly affects the pill's acceptability to women.[15] Breakthrough bleeding and amenorrhea can be confusing and frightening. A woman may be concerned about whether the bleeding or spotting is her "real" period, if she should stop taking the pills and/or if something is wrong with her (a fear of cancer or sexually transmitted disease). If a woman experiences amenorrhea, she may fear she is pregnant. Unless thoroughly counseled as to the nature of breakthrough bleeding, women may stop taking the pill on their own—and often fail to use a substitute contraceptive.

Breakthrough bleeding is also a common cause for phone calls to the clinician's office. According to S. Jean Emans, MD, Associate Editor of *The Contraception Report*, "Breakthrough bleeding causes the most concern and phone calls to the office. I use the current 20 mcg pill (20 mcg EE, 1 mg norethindrone acetate) primarily as a 'step-down' pill if patients have side effects using 30 or 35 mcg pills. If the patient has had a lot of nausea or headaches or a mild elevation of blood pressure, stepping down to 20 mcg formulation is well tolerated. Additionally, the patient has already gotten through the first 3 or 4 months of use, which is when breakthrough bleeding is most common. My feeling is that if a 20 mcg pill can be developed that provides improved cycle control, this would be beneficial. I would use such a formulation for new starts."

Whether some progestational agents provide better cycle control than others has been the subject of debate. Paula J. A. Hillard, MD, Associate Editor of *The Contraception Report*, commented, "Thus far, some clinicians have shied away from 20 mcg pills

---

Mechanisms of Action of Combination Oral Contraceptives

CONFIRMED

• Suppression of ovulation via hypothalamic and pituitary effects
  – Suppression of luteinizing and follicle-stimulating hormones (LH and FSH)
  – Absence of LH surge
  – Diminished frequency of gonadotropin-releasing hormone (GnRH) pulses
  – Decreased pituitary responsiveness to GnRH

• Progestin-mediated alterations in the consistency and properties of cervical mucus

SUSPECTED

• Alterations in the endometrial lining

POSSIBLE

• Alterations of tubal transport mechanisms

Source: Goldzieher J, 1994 and Goodman & Gilman's The Pharmacological Basis of Therapeutics — 9th Edition, 1996 (see references 7 and 11).

because of a concern about a greater risk of breakthrough bleeding; however, differences in breakthrough bleeding among various formulations are difficult to measure and few head-to-head comparisons have been done. I don't think any have been done comparing 20 mcg pills to 30 or 35 mcg pills. One of the big problems with the studies we do have is that the definitions of bleeding and spotting, as well as the patient populations, vary, so it's really very hard to compare them."

A 1992 review of the literature by Rosenberg et al evaluated 25 studies of cycle control with various OCs.[16] These authors concluded that, in general, products containing norgestrel and levonorgestrel have a lower incidence of spotting and breakthrough bleeding compared with norethindrone acetate and norethindrone, whether triphasic or monophasic.[17-22] They emphasized, however, that cycle control problems tend to disappear within a few months of OC use, regardless of formulation. In terms of 20 mcg pills, data suggest desogestrel plus 20 mcg EE has as good cycle control as desogestrel plus 30 mcg EE.[23]

Dr. Goldzieher provided some insight as to how cycle control is impacted by estrogen and progestin. "When the pill was originally developed, it was the estrogen component, the mestranol, that was found to help cycle control. But, in addition to the cycle control mediated by the estrogen, the progestin also provides endometrial support."

The half-life of different progestational agents may explain why they provide poorer or better endometrial support. For example, the mean elimination half-life of norethindrone is 7.5 hours compared to 11.4 hours for levonorgestrel.[7] "The longer the half-life of the progestin," Dr. Goldzieher explained, "the better you protect the endometrium from collapsing. The bottom line is that you can lower the estrogen dose quite far and keep cycle control when the progestational agent is providing an additive endometrial support function.

"One area where lower-dose preparations are not as effective as 50 mcg preparations is early cycle control. The data on breakthrough bleeding suggest that there is about 30% breakthrough bleeding in the first cycle, which drops within about 3 months. But, with the 50 mcg pills, cycle control was better."

One trial that investigated bioavailability of steroids and bleeding patterns found decreasing cycle control with decreasing doses of both estrogen and progestin.[24] This study looked at three different preparations, all containing EE plus norethindrone, but in different dosages. The pills contained either 50 mcg EE plus 1 mg norethindrone, 35 mcg EE plus 1 mg norethindrone or 35 mcg EE and 0.5 mg norethindrone. The number of intermenstrual bleeding days was significantly higher (p=0.01) among women taking the lowest-dose pill compared to the highest.

David Archer, MD, provided another perspective on cycle control with 20 mcg formulations. Dr. Archer is Professor of Obstetrics and Gynecology at Eastern Virginia Medical School and Director of the Clinical Research Unit at the Jones Institute for Reproductive Medicine in Norfolk, Virginia. In an interview he said, "I was involved in a study that looked at 20 mcg EE combined with 100 mcg levonorgestrel.[3] What we found was that this combination provided pregnancy protection and good cycle control with no greater incidence of side effects, such as nausea, breast tenderness and weight gain.

"It is hypothesized that the cycle control provided by this combination is related to the ratio of estrogen to progestin. If you take a 30 mcg EE pill with 150 mcg of a progestin, that's a 1:5 ratio between the two steroids. This pill—20 mcg EE and 100 mcg levonorgestrel—keeps the same ratio. Of course, whether this balance of the steroids is the reason this formulation provided effective cycle control remains unproven, but that is the hypothesis."

Nausea, Breast Tenderness and Weight Gain

The incidence of other side effects has also diminished with lower-dose preparations. Dr. Goldzieher stated, "Side effects related to estrogen, such as nausea, headaches, bloating and sodium retention, have definitely diminished. Some women get progestational side effects and these have diminished, as well. It's possible that since estrogen side effects are dose-related, we might see a further decrease with 20 mcg pills, but that remains to be seen."

Increased Blood Pressure

Elevated blood pressure with OC use is uncommon, but does occur in a small minority of women. A recent analysis from the Nurses' Health Study II suggested that only about 42 cases of elevated blood pressure occurred per 10,000 person-years in women using current low-dose pill formulations.[25] Whether reducing the estrogen dosage even further may help to decrease the incidence of elevated blood pressure is unknown.

Lipids

Should clinicians worry about alterations in the lipid profile when choosing an OC? Do some formulations have advantages over others because they have a more "favorable" impact on lipids? The scientific evidence suggests the answer is no. Lipid profiles, including the measurement of high-density lipoproteins (HDL), low-density lipoproteins (LDL), triglycerides and other lipid subfractions, are risk markers of cardiovascular disease in men and in postmenopausal women not taking estrogen. What many clinicians may not realize, however, is that this relationship does not appear to hold true in women with adequate levels of estrogen. Experts hypothesize that estrogen exerts a cardioprotective effect in several ways other than by its favorable impact on lipids.[26]

Premenopausal women may experience OC-induced alterations in lipid profiles, but the clinical relevance of these alterations is unsubstantiated. In fact, data from cynomolgus monkeys, an accepted animal model for studying atherosclerosis in the human, dispute the idea that OC-induced lipid changes accelerate the development of atherosclerotic cardiovascular disease.[27-29]

"I would ignore lipid data when prescribing OCs," advised Dr. Thorneycroft. "I don't believe they have any relevance for the usage of birth control pills because the primate studies clearly show that atherosclerosis was decreased, not increased, while using the pill. Of course, if a woman comes in and she already has a hyperlipidemia, then it's important to treat that disorder. But, in choosing a birth control pill, the lipid data have no relevance as to which pill to use." (For further discussion of OCs and lipids, see section on metabolic effects in this chapter.)

Androgenicity and Acne

Should worries about the "androgenicity" of the progestin and subsequent acne influence the choice of pill? Again, the weight of the scientific evidence suggests no. Although it is true that some progestational agents are more "androgenic" when measured alone at high doses by specific assays in animals, these measurements are not necessarily clinically relevant.[30]

The data are scant with regard to direct comparisons of various preparations, but at least some evidence exists which contradicts the suggestion that OCs containing "androgenic" progestins worsen or cause acne.[31-34]

Dr. Thorneycroft commented on where the idea that the androgenicity of the progestin mattered originated. He said, "As far as I'm concerned, no birth control pill is androgenic. Androgenicity dates back to the lipid issue. When lipids were becoming the focus of attention, the progestin's effect on lipids became a point of concern. Androgenic pills were said to have the worst lipid profile. Since lipids are irrelevant, androgenicity is irrelevant.

"There are too few data to say that one pill has an advantage over another with regard to androgenicity and acne. In fact, some data suggest that pills with progestins considered androgenic help improve acne. In my opinion, what data do exist suggest all low-dose birth control pills reduce acne and hirsutism, and do so to a comparable degree. My advice to clinicians is to choose the pill they feel most comfortable prescribing without worrying about androgenicity or lipids." (For further discussion of OCs and androgenicity, see section on metabolic effects in this chapter.)

Health Benefits

Will the health benefits of the pill be lost with 20 mcg preparations? This concern has been raised by some clinicians. Health benefits of the pill include protection from ovarian and endometrial (and possibly colon) cancers, suppression of ovarian cyst development (with high-dose pills), relief of dysmenorrhea and irregular menstrual cycles, and prevention of benign breast disease, iron deficiency anemia and premenopausal loss of bone mineral density.

Little evidence exists regarding the effect of low-dose pills (35 mcg or less) on the maintenance of health benefits. This is because data on health benefits were derived from older studies conducted in the 1970s, when higher-dose formulations were used. What data do exist suggest that the only health benefit that may be appreciably attenuated is the effect of OCs on ovarian cyst development.

Ovarian Function

What is the effect of lowering the dose of EE to 20 mcg on ovarian function? Is escape ovulation more likely to occur? Will women using 20 mcg pills be more likely to develop ovarian cysts? The weight of the evidence suggests that ovulation is effectively inhibited with 20 mcg pills. It also suggests that, although follicular development occurs more frequently with 20 mcg than with 30 mcg and 35 mcg pills, this follicular activity is not necessarily indicative of more ovarian cysts.

For example, three studies of 20 mcg EE in combination with desogestrel, gestodene or levonorgestrel found some follicular development, but no ovulation, among women taking these preparations.[35-37] The first study compared two 20 mcg pills containing either desogestrel or gestodene to a new triphasic OC.[35] Among 51 women having 86 cycles monitored by ultrasonography, follicular-like structures were observed in nine women. The frequency of follicular growth was similar with all three OC preparations. No follicle progressed to more than 19 mm in diameter. The authors concluded, "The results of this study suggest that during OC use (even with a low dose of ethinyl estradiol), a little ovarian activity may be present without ovulation."

The second investigation looked at ovarian activity during use of 20 mcg EE in combination with 100 mcg levonorgestrel.[36] Again, although some follicular activity was present, no escape ovulation occurred. The third study, comparing 20 mcg EE preparations containing either desogestrel or gestodene, found similar results.[37]

Dr. Archer believes that even if follicular development is not completely suppressed, the residual ovarian activity is not clinically important. He said, "There may well be more follicular development with newer 20 mcg pills coming to the market, but that remains to be seen. It has been shown that there is always a small percentage of women who, upon ultrasound examination, appear to be ovulatory when using OCs. However, whether or not they will become pregnant is questionable. They probably will not become pregnant because of other OC mechanisms of action, such as changes in the cervical mucus and endometrial lining."

Ovarian Cyst Development

Early data indicated that OCs protect against the development of ovarian cysts.[38] Newer data suggest that the strength of the inhibition of ovarian cysts is attenuated with lower-dose pills.[39] Importantly, ovarian follicles must not be confused with cysts. According to experts in the field, follicles that develop during OC use "generally disappear spontaneously with continued use of the OC and very rarely give [rise] to symptoms, nor do they need treatment. ...follicles with a homogenous appearance on ultrasound and a diameter less than 35 mm should not be called ovarian cysts...[In addition,] medical interference or the discontinuation of OC use in women with... follicle activity without symptoms is unwanted."[40]

A study by Egarter et al found that a 20 mcg preparation did not lead to more ovarian follicles or cysts compared with a 35 mcg preparation.[41] Using vaginal ultrasonography, the researchers measured the size of ovarian follicles at baseline and during two treatment cycles in 63 women. The investigators found that only one woman had a follicle progress to an ovarian cyst of 35 mm in diameter. This woman took the higher-dose OC. No significant difference occurred in the number of women with follicles 10 mm in diameter between those taking 20 mcg EE plus 150 mcg desogestrel compared to those taking 35 mcg EE plus 250 mcg norgestimate. After 2 months of treatment, there were significantly fewer follicles after two cycles compared to baseline ($p<0.05$).

According to Dr. Thorneycroft, "We are not sure what the effect of reducing the dose of EE to 20 mcg will be on functional ovarian cysts. With the 35 mcg pills, women certainly have more cysts than in the past when we used 50 mcg pills, but it is still less than if women are not on the pill. There's a 90% reduction of corpus luteum cysts and a 50% reduction in cysts with 35 mcg pills, whereas there is almost complete suppression with high-dose pills."

Other clinicians agree that the suppression of follicular development with 20 mcg pills may not be as complete as with higher doses. Dr. Hillard commented, "It does look like there's a stepwise ability to suppress cysts with higher doses being more effective. If ovarian cyst suppression were my primary indication for a patient, then I probably wouldn't prescribe a 20 mcg pill, I'd use a higher-dose pill."

Ovarian and Endometrial Cancers

Will the reduction in estrogen dose to 20 mcg affect the protection seen against ovarian and endometrial cancers? Few data are available on new lower-dose preparations (≤35 mcg EE) and risk of ovarian cancer; however, if prevention of "incessant" ovulation is the cause, then lower-dose pills likely result in similar protection.[10]

Data from the World Health Organization's Collaborative Study of Neoplasia and Steroid Contraceptives suggest that low-dose preparations do protect against ovarian cancer, but perhaps to a slightly smaller degree.[42] The international case-control study found an odds ratio (OR) slightly lower for women who used higher-dose (OR=0.7; 95% confidence interval [CI], 0.4-1.1) as compared to lower-dose preparations (OR=0.8; 95% CI, 0.5-1.3). The authors conclude, "both high-dose and low-dose oral contraceptives protect against ovarian cancer, but the degree of protection may be slightly weaker for the newer, low-dose products."

Similar results were found by the Case-Control Surveillance Study.[43] Researchers performed a case-control study of patients with ovarian cancer between 1977 and 1991 in Boston, New York, Philadelphia and Baltimore. As in previous studies, these researchers found about a 40% reduction in risk with 3 years of OC use. Available data, though scant, suggested that 3 years of use conferred similar protection for users of pills with <50 mcg EE (RR=0.6; 95% CI, 0.2-2.2) compared to those using 50 mcg EE (RR=0.4; 95% CI, 0.1-1.0). The relative risk (RR) was similar for products containing 50 mcg mestranol (RR=0.7; 95% CI, 0.2-2.0).

Use of OCs reduces the occurrence of endometrial cancer, a protection that increases with longer duration of use. Some data on the protection with various formulations are available from the Cancer and Steroid Hormone Study, conducted at eight U.S. centers.[44] This investigation found no significant difference between users of low- and high-dose OCs with regard to protection against this cancer.

In fact, because unopposed estrogen causes endometrial cancer, using lower doses might actually help improve the protection. According to Dr. Thorneycroft, "With regard to protection against endometrial cancer, I think this health benefit will certainly hold up. The progestin acts to create an atrophic endometrium, decreasing mitosis. Decreasing the estrogen might actually increase the efficacy."

Dysmenorrhea, Menorrhagia and Iron Deficiency Anemia

Quality-of-life health benefits, such as alleviation of dysmenorrhea, menorrhagia and iron deficiency anemia, will likely remain, as well. "Protection against dysmenorrhea and menorrhagia probably will be maintained," said Dr. Hillard. "I've never seen any data to indicate that the 20 mcg pill now on the market isn't as good as other pills at providing relief of dysmenorrhea. One study comparing two 20 mcg pills containing either gestodene or desogestrel found that gestodene had a more favorable effect on dysmenorrhea.[45] But, we're going to have to see data for individual formulations as they come to the U.S. market. Of course, if the pills relieve menorrhagia, they should help prevent iron deficiency anemia. In any case, I wouldn't let a concern about a possible lessening of these benefits deter me from using 20 mcg pills."

Benign Breast Disease

The decrease in benign breast disease with OCs is mediated by progestin. The Royal College of General Practitioners' Oral Contraception Study found more protection with higher doses of progestin.[46] The Oxford Family Planning Association study also found decreasing risk of benign breast disease with increasing years of OC use.[47] How lowering the dose of both estrogen and progestin in OCs will affect this outcome is unknown.

Bone Mineral Density

A growing body of evidence suggests that premenopausal use of OCs preserves bone mineral density. A 1996 review of the literature concluded that preparations containing 20 mcg of estrogen should be satisfactory.[48] At least one investigation found that use of a 20 mcg EE pill with desogestrel significantly increased vertebral bone density ($p<0.001$) in oligomenorrheic, perimenopausal women.[49]

In fact, 20 mcg of EE should be more than enough, as postmenopausal doses of estrogen used to prevent osteoporosis are well below that dose.[50] "Many researchers estimate that 0.625 mg of conjugated equine estrogen is equivalent to about 5 or 6 mcg of EE," Dr. Thorneycroft explained. "We know that dose in most postmenopausal women is sufficient to prevent osteoporosis, so there's no reason why we should lose that protection with 20 mcg pills."

Patient Populations

Several patient populations may particularly benefit from using 20 mcg pill preparations. For example, Dr. Goldzieher believes it's quite advantageous to use 20 mcg pills for "adolescents who are very sensitive to estrogen and may have more nausea, for the underweight and for perimenopausal women. Perimenopausal women who are not infertile still need effective contraception, but do not need the higher doses. Yet, they still receive the advantages of cycle regularity and reduction of hormonal instability."

Dr. Hillard agrees that 20 mcg preparations are quite beneficial for perimenopausal women and adolescents, but thinks they will be good for all women. "As more 20 mcg products become available, especially ones that provide acceptable cycle control, I don't see why these products should be used in 'special' patient populations. I believe that using the lowest effective dose of estrogen is wise. My feeling is that lower estrogen dose pills represent an advance in contraception. Thus, I see newer 20 mcg pills as first-line choices for most women. The only exception I can think of is the situation in which I was aiming for more complete ovarian shutdown. Then, I would likely go with a higher-dose pill."

Are smokers good candidates for 20 mcg pills? Perhaps. Women under age 35 years who smoke are at no increased risk of cardiovascular complications when using OCs. Dr. Hillard comments, "In women under age 35, I see no reason not to use a low-dose pill. Among adolescents, I am concerned about their smoking, not because they're using OCs, but because of the substantial health dangers of smoking alone."

Should women over age 35 years who smoke but want to use OCs be put on a lower-dose pill? Dr. Archer commented, "Although it makes intuitive sense that less estrogen might be better in smokers, there are no data that actually show that use of a 20 mcg EE pill is safer than a 30 or 35 mcg pill in smokers. I'd recommend they quit smoking."

Future Directions

Are 20 mcg pills the wave of the future? Actually, the idea of a 20 mcg pill is not new. The 20 mcg formulation containing 1 mg norethindrone acetate was introduced to the U.S. market in 1973.

Dr. Archer shared his perspective on the future of oral contraception. "I think the FDA mandates that we continue to look at the safety and efficacy of lower-dose pills. Some evidence in the literature is suggestive of a reduction in cardiovascular risk with lower doses of estrogen. While it's not certain that this is the case, without a clear-cut epidemiologic answer, I maintain that based on what we know, utilizing a lower-dose OC is beneficial for the patient.

"I believe 20 mcg pills are not only here to stay, but they will be picked up and utilized to a greater degree in the future as we get more of them on the market. To my knowledge, in the next 12 months, we'll see at least one, and maybe more than one, 20 mcg pill come on the U.S. market.

"I think 20 mcg pills can represent an improved product. Not improved necessarily in terms of side effects, although it's possible we could see even further reduction of estrogen-related side effects, but in terms of a total reduction in estrogen dose. Still, the ideal pill will need to provide comparable efficacy and acceptable cycle control to what we have now. These attributes cannot be sacrificed; otherwise, there's no sense in continuing to drop the estrogen dose."

Pills with Less Than 20 mcg Estrogen?

Is it possible we will see pills with even less than 20 mcg estrogen? It's possible, although at some point, the lowest dose of estrogen must be reached. Dr. Thorneycroft said, "I think we could see even lower-dose pills than 20 mcg EE. Of course, at some point, it will be too low. There's got to be a stopping point for the combination birth control pill; otherwise, it will be a progestin-only pill. I think that starting patients on 20 mcg pills and seeing how they do is a reasonable option, and I think as we get more of these pills on the market over the next several years, clinicians will be doing more of that."

References

1.   Perone N. The progestins. In: Goldzieher JW, Fotherby K, eds. *Pharmacology of the Contraceptive Steroids*. New York: Raven Press, 1994:5-25.

2. Goldzieher JW, de la Pena A, Chenault CB. Ovulation-inhibiting action of ethinyl estrogen. *Fertil Steril* 1974;25:299-300.

3. Archer DF, DelConte A. The efficacy and safety of a new monophasic, low-dose, 21-day oral contraceptive containing levonorgestrel 100 mcg and ethinyl estradiol 20 mcg. Poster presentation #354. American Society for Reproductive Medicine Annual Meeting, November 2-6, 1996, Boston, MA.

4. *F-D-C Reports*. October 14, 1996; T&G 2.

5. Gerstman BB, Gross TP, Kennedy DL, et al. Trends in the content and use of oral contraceptives in the United States, 1964-1988. *Am J Public Health* 1991;81:90-98.

6. Brody SA, Turkes A, Goldzieher JW. Pharmacokinetics of three bioequivalent norethindrone/mestranol-50 mcg and three norethindrone/ethinyl estradiol-35 mcg OC formulations: are "low-dose" pills really lower? *Contraception* 1989;40:269-284.

7. Goldzieher JW. *Hormonal Contraception: Pills, Injections & Implants*. Third edition. London, Ontario, Canada: EMIS-Canada, 1994.

8. Meade TW, Greenberg G, Thompson SG. Progestogens and cardiovascular reactions associated with oral contraceptives, and a comparison of the safety of 50- and 30-mcg oestrogen preparations. *BMJ* 1980;1157-1161.

9. Ketting E. The relative reliability of oral contraceptives; findings of an epidemiological study. *Contraception* 1988;37:343-348.

10. Elstein M. Consensus paper. Low-dose contraceptive formulations: is further reduction in steroid dosage justified? *Adv Contraception* 1994;10:1-4.

11. Hardman JG, Limbird LE, editors-in-chief. *Goodman & Gilman's The Pharmacological Basis of Therapeutics—9th Edition*. Section XIII: Hormones and hormone synthesis. The McGraw-Hill Companies, Inc., New York:1996.

12. Hillard PJA. Oral contraception noncompliance: the extent of the problem. *Adv Contraception* 1992;8(suppl 1):13-20.

13. Rosenberg MJ, Burnhill MS, Waugh MS, et al. Compliance and oral contraceptives: a review. *Contraception* 1995;52:137-141.

14. Emans SJ, Grace E, Woods ER, et al. Adolescents' compliance with the use of oral contraceptives. *JAMA* 1987;257:3377-3381.

15. Hillard PJA. The patient's reaction to side effects of oral contraceptives. *Am J Obstet Gynecol* 1989;161:1412-1415.

16. Rosenberg MJ, Long SC. Oral contraceptives and cycle control: a critical review of the literature. *Adv Contraception* 1992;8(suppl 1):35-45.

17. Droegemueller W, Katta LR, Bright TG, et al. Triphasic Randomized Clinical Trial: comparative frequency of intermenstrual bleeding. *Am J Obstet Gynecol* 1989;161:1407-1411.

18. Schilling LH, Bolding OT, Chenault CB, et al. Evaluation of the clinical performance of three triphasic oral contraceptives: a multicenter, randomized comparative trial. *Am J Obstet Gynecol* 1989;160:1264-1268.

19. Dunson TR, McLaurin VL, Israngkura B, et al. A comparative study of two low-dose combined oral contraceptives: results from a multicenter trial. *Contraception* 1993;48:109-119.

20. Anstee P, Kovacs GT. A prospective, randomized study comparing the clinical effects of a norethisterone and a levonorgestrel containing low-dose oestrogen oral contraceptive pills. *Aust NZ J Obstet Gynaecol* 1993;33:81-83.

21. Edgren RA, Nelson JH, Gordon RT, et al. Bleeding patterns with low-dose monophasic oral contraceptives. *Contraception* 1989;40:285-297.

22. Ramos R, Apelo R, Osteria T, et al. A comparative analysis of three different dose combinations of oral contraceptives. *Contraception* 1989;39:165-177.

23. Akerlund M, Rode A, Westergaard J. Comparative profiles of reliability, cycle control and side effects of two oral contraceptive formulations containing 150 mcg desogestrel and either 30 mcg or 20 mcg ethinyl estradiol. *Br J Obstet Gynaecol* 1993;100:832-838.

24. Saleh WA, Burkman RT, Zacur HA, et al. A randomized trial of three oral contraceptives: comparison of bleeding patterns by contraceptive types and steroid levels. *Am J Obstet Gynecol* 1993;168:1740-1747.

25. Chasan-Taber L, Willett WC, Manson JE, et al. Prospective study of oral contraceptives and hypertension among women in the United States. *Circulation* 1996;94:483-489.

26. Sarrel PM. Ovarian hormones and circulation. *Maturitas* 1990;11:287-298.

27. Adams MR, Clarkson TB, Koritnik DR, et al. Contraceptive steroids and coronary artery atherosclerosis in cynomolgus macaques. *Fertil Steril* 1987;47:1010-1018.

28. Clarkson TB, Adams MR, Kaplan JR, et al. From menarche to menopause: coronary artery atherosclerosis and protection in cynomolgus monkeys. *Am J Obstet Gynecol* 1989;160:1280-1285.

29. Clarkson TB, Shively CA, Morgan TM, et al. Oral contraceptives and coronary artery atherosclerosis of cynomolgus monkeys. *Obstet Gynecol* 1990;75:217-222.

30. Upton GV, Corbin A. The relevance of the pharmacologic properties of a progestational agent to its clinical effects as a combination oral contraceptive. *Yale J Biol Med* 1989;62:445-457.

31. Lemay A, Dewailly SD, Grenier R, et al. Attenuation of mild hyperandrogenic activity in postpubertal acne by a triphasic oral contraceptive containing low doses of ethinyl estradiol and dl-norgestrel. *J Clin Endocrinol Metab* 1990;71:8-14.

32. Palatsi R, Hirvensalo E, Liukko P, et al. Serum total and unbound testosterone and sex hormone-binding globulin (SHBG) in female acne patients treated with two different oral contraceptives. *Acta Derm Venereol* 1984;64:517-523.

33. Loudon N, Biddell S. The effect of the triphasic oral contraceptive on acne vulgaris: an interim report of an open multicenter study. In: Elstein M (ed.). *Update on Triphasic Oral Contraception.* Princeton, NJ: Excerpta Medica, 1982:75-81.

34. van der Vange N, Blankenstein MA, Kloosterboer HJ, et al. Effects of seven low-dose oral contraceptives on sex hormone-binding globulin, corticosteroid-binding globulin, and total and free testosterone. *Contraception* 1990;41:345-352.

35. Crosignani PG, Testa G, Vegetti W, et al. Ovarian activity during regular oral contraceptive use. *Contraception* 1996;54:271-273.

36. Spona J, Feichtinger W, Kindermann Ch, et al. Inhibition of ovulation by an oral contraceptive containing 100 mcg levonorgestrel in combination with 20 mcg ethinyl estradiol. *Contraception* 1996;54:299-304.

37. Fitzgerald C, Feichtinger W, Spona J, et al. A comparison of the effects of two monophasic, low-dose oral contraceptives on the inhibition of ovulation. *Adv Contraception* 1994;10:5-18.

38. Vessey M, Metcalfe A, Wells C, et al. Ovarian neoplasms, functional ovarian cysts, and oral contraceptives. *BMJ* 1987;294:1518-1520.

39. Lanes SF, Birmann B, Walker AM, et al. Oral contraceptive type and functional ovarian cysts. *Am J Obstet Gynecol* 1992;166:956-961.

40. Leroy F, Petersen K, Breckwoldt W, et al. Letter to the editor. *Contraception* 1992;45:519-521.

41. Egarter Ch, Putz M, Strohmer H, et al. Ovarian function during low-dose oral contraceptive use. *Contraception* 1995;51:329-333.

42. Rosenblatt KA, Thomas DB, Noonan EA, and the WHO Collaborative Study of Neoplasia and Steroid Contraceptives. High-dose and low-dose combined oral contraceptives: protection against epithelial ovarian cancer and the length of the protective effect. *Eur J Cancer* 1992;28A:1872-1876.

43. Rosenberg L, Palmer JR, Zauber AG, et al. A case-control study of oral contraceptive use and invasive epithelial ovarian cancer. *Am J Epidemiol* 1994;139:654-661.

44. The Cancer and Steroid Hormone Study of the Centers for Disease Control and the National Institute of Child Health and Human Development. Combination oral contraceptive use and the risk of endometrial cancer. *JAMA* 1987;257:796-800.

45. Endrikat J, Jaques M-A, Mayerhofer M, et al. A 12-month comparative clinical investigation of two low-dose oral contraceptives containing 20 mcg ethinyl estradiol/75 mcg gestodene and 20 mcg ethinyl estradiol/150 mcg desogestrel, with respect to efficacy, cycle control and tolerance. *Contraception* 1995;52:229-235.

46. Royal College of General Practitioners' Oral Contraception Study. Effect on hypertension and benign breast disease of progestagen component in combined oral contraceptives. *Lancet* 1977;1:624.

47. Brinton LA, Vessey MP, Flavel R, et al. Risk factors for benign breast disease. *Am J Epidemiol* 1981;113:203-214.

48. DeCherney A. Bone-sparing properties of oral contraceptives. *Am J Obstet Gynecol* 1996;174:15-20.

49. Gambacciani M, Spinetti A, Taponeco F, et al. Longitudinal evaluation of perimenopausal vertebral bone loss: effects of a low-dose oral contraceptive preparation on bone mineral density and metabolism. *Obstet Gynecol* 1994;83:392-396.

50. The Writing Group for the PEPI Trial. Effects of hormone therapy on bone mineral density. Results from the Postmenopausal Estrogen/Progestin Interventions (PEPI) Trial. *JAMA* 1996;276:1389-1396.

1.9: Myths

Both patients and clinicians may harbor unwarranted fears about oral contraceptives (OCs). This section takes a look at various misperceptions and the current facts regarding each.

i. Weight Gain

In a nation obsessed with appearance and body image, the prospect of gaining weight because one uses a birth control method is worrisome. Women are particularly vulnerable to media images that clearly present a slender body as the ideal. With societal pressures so strong, many women, if they believe the pill can make them gain weight, will reject the method without knowing the truth.

A study by Emans et al confirmed that 45% of adolescents were very concerned about the possibility of weight gain on the pill. Teens seen in a suburban private practice were significantly more concerned about weight gain than those seen in a hospital-based adolescent clinic (86% vs 32%, p=0.001). Although there was no statistically significant difference in weight gain between the noncompliant and compliant patients, noncompliant patients were more likely to have *perceived* that they had gained weight while taking OCs even though actual weight was often unchanged.[1] Carpenter and Neinstein found that sexually active adolescents using OCs for 12 months were no more likely to gain weight than those using intrauterine devices (IUDs) or barrier contraception.[2]

Thus, young women should be reassured that studies show that as many young women lose as gain weight while on the pill. They should be counseled about healthy eating habits and told that their weight will be checked during each visit. Importantly, addressing patient concerns will improve compliance with contraceptive use.

References

1. Emans SJ, Grace E, Woods ER, et al. Adolescents' compliance with the use of oral contraceptives. *JAMA* 1987;257:3377-3381.

2. Carpenter S, Neinstein LS. Weight gain in adolescent and young adult oral contraceptive users. *J Adol Health Care* 1986;7:342-344.

ii. Taking a Rest

One of the myths that has surrounded the use of oral contraceptives has been the idea that a woman should periodically take a "rest" from pill use. The origin of this myth has been attributed to a British family planning practitioner who wrote a letter to a prominent British medical journal suggesting that it would be a good idea for women to get off the pill once a year, although no scientific evidence was offered to support this suggestion.

Perhaps some practitioners have suggested a rest from the pill to allow the ovary to recover its function before an attempt at pregnancy. At this time, however, there is no evidence to suggest that taking a rest from the pill is medically necessary or beneficial.

Importantly, taking a rest from the pill may lead to negative consequences for the patient. These consequences include unintended pregnancy and abortion. Studies have suggested that a woman who stops taking the pill may not use another form of birth control or may switch to a less effective method, thus increasing her risk of unintended pregnancy.[1]

In addition, taking a rest from the pill can perpetuate compliance problems. Side effects such as breakthrough bleeding and amenorrhea, which can initiate compliance problems, are common during the first few months of OC use. Discontinuing and restarting the pill may cause another few months of these unpleasant side effects. Such side effects are frequently perceived negatively by women. Compliance problems may result, causing discontinuation and possibly leading to unintended pregnancy or abortion.

Given the fact that there is no scientific evidence to suggest a woman should take a rest from the pill, important advice for the patient is: "There's no need to take a 'rest' from the pill. Please don't stop taking it without calling me."

References
1. Pratt WF, Bachrach CA. What do women use when they stop using the pill? *Fam Plann Perspect* 1987;19:257-266.

iii. Birth Defects

Many women are concerned about the possibility of birth defects with oral contraceptive use. For example, a study by Emans et al has shown that 11% of teens seen in an adolescent clinic were concerned that the pill would cause birth defects.[1] A classic review article by Wilson and Brent[2] and a more recent meta-analysis by Bracken[3] have shown that there is no proven association between oral contraceptives and birth defects. Some earlier reports suggested an association between OCs and such defects as anencephaly, transposition of the great vessels, limb reductions and other gross malformations. The 1981 overview by Wilson and Brent found that the use of exogenous hormones during pregnancy was not proven to cause abnormality in nongenital organs and tissues.

Wilson and Brent based their conclusions on several important findings. First, many of the older studies had serious flaws, such as small sample size. Second, as the use of OCs increased, the incidence of the suspected birth defects would be expected to rise if there was an association; however, surveillance data have shown that this is not the case. Third, more reports in the literature show no association than suggest a relationship. Fourth, no animal model has been able to demonstrate a causal relationship between administration of exogenous hormones in normal therapeutic doses, period of gestational development and teratogenic effects. Furthermore, because hormones act specifically on target tissues, there seems to be no reasonable biologic mechanism whereby exogenous sex hormones could act to damage nongenital fetal tissue.

In a meta-analysis by Bracken, the relative risks of specific types of fetal malformations were calculated. The relative risk from 12 prospective studies analyzed was 1.0 (95% confidence interval [CI], 0.8-1.2) for all malformations. Thus, no increased risk was found for birth defects. When congenital heart defects were analyzed, the relative risk was 1.1 (95% CI, 0.7-1.6); for limb reduction defects, the relative risk was 1.0 (95% CI, 0.3-3.6), again demonstrating no increased risk. These data provide very strong evidence that exposure to OCs in early pregnancy does not have a teratogenic effect. It is unlikely in a group this large that a single source of bias would have influenced all these studies. Therefore, a woman who inadvertently takes OCs prior to or at the time of conception, or in early pregnancy, should be reassured that OCs do not cause birth defects.

References

1. Emans SJ, Grace E, Woods ER, et al. Adolescents' compliance with the use of oral contraceptives. *JAMA* 1987;257:3377-3381.

2. Wilson JG, Brent RL. Are female sex hormones teratogenic? *Am J Obstet Gynecol* 1981;141:567-580.

3. Bracken MB. Oral contraception and congenital malformations in offspring: a review and meta-analysis of the prospective studies. *Obstet Gynecol* 1990;76:552-557.

iv. Infertility

Infertility after pill use is a concern of many women. The fear of permanent damage may cause a woman to choose a less effective contraceptive. In a review of the literature, Fraser and Weisberg found no evidence to suggest that oral contraceptive use causes permanent infertility.[1] However, many studies have found a temporary delay in conception after use of OCs.

A retrospective analysis of women stopping the pill in order to conceive compared with women stopping other methods was done by Harlap and Baras.[2] They found that women who had used oral contraceptives were 30% less likely to conceive in the first month after stopping the pill than women who had stopped other methods. This discrepancy disappeared, however, by the third month.

A recent study by Bracken et al suggests that delayed conception occurs in pill users more frequently than in nonusers and that high-dose OCs delay conception more than low-dose OCs.[3] The study was conducted over 25 months and evaluated 248 former OC users and 1,365 women who discontinued using other methods, such as diaphragms, spermicides or intrauterine devices. The mean time for nonusers to conceive was 3.6 cycles; low-dose pill users took a mean 4.0 cycles to conceive; high-dose pill users took a mean of 4.8 cycles to conceive. Because a dose-related effect appeared to be taking place, the investigators believed the fertility delays were caused by the OC use rather than by naturally occurring ovulatory disturbances.

Women need to understand that a delay in conception may be experienced after discontinuing the pill. They should be reassured, however, that the delay is temporary and that previous fertility levels usually return within 3 months.

References

1. Fraser IS, Weisberg E. Fertility following discontinuation of different methods of fertility control. *Contraception* 1982;26:389-415.

2. Harlap S, Baras M. Conception-waits in fertile women after stopping oral contraceptives. *Int J Fertil* 1984;29:73-80.

3. Bracken MB, Hellenbrand KG, Holford TR. Conception delay after oral contraceptive use: the effect of estrogen dose. *Fertil Steril* 1990;53:21-27.

v. Stunted Growth

Some young women may be concerned about whether taking oral contraceptives will stunt their growth. The origin of this myth may stem from the known effect of estrogen on bone epiphyses. Young women predicted to have excessively tall stature are treated with high doses of estrogen for several years in order to accelerate bone maturation and limit final height. This practice may explain why an association has been suggested between OCs and stunting one's growth.

Several factors make it unlikely that oral contraceptives could limit growth. Most young women are substantially past the age of menarche when OCs are prescribed. Therefore, an extremely limited percentage of further growth could be potentially influenced. Skeletal maturation or "bone age" is often determined by comparing a radiograph of the wrist and hand with established standards. For example, a young woman found to have a bone age of 12.5 to 13 (the typical age for menarche) has reached nearly 96% of final height. A girl with a bone age of 14 years has reached 98% of her final height. Most importantly, current OCs have three to 10 times less estrogen than the typical doses that are used daily (not in cycles) to treat tall stature, a process that takes several years to achieve only 3 cm to 7 cm of height reduction in girls with bone age measurements typically less than 12.5 years.[1] Additionally, a German study of 80 mcg mestranol given in cycles with progestin found a satisfactory reduction in predicted height only in girls with a bone age of 9 to 10 years.[2] Thus, current low-dose oral contraceptives given after menarche are unlikely to affect final height.

References

1. Prader A, Zachmann M. Treatment of excessively tall girls and boys with sex hormones. *Pediatrics* 1978;62(suppl):1202-1210.

2. Schambach H, Nitschke U. Treatment of constitutionally tall girls with physiological estrogen doses in the prepuberty period. An alternative to high-dose estrogen therapy. *Monatsschr-Kinderheilkd* 1985;133:32-37.

vi. Treatment of Functional Ovarian Cysts

Older oral contraceptives were known to help prevent the *development* of functional ovarian cysts,[1] though there is little evidence that they hasten the resolution of such cysts once they have formed.

The descriptive study by Spanos documented the regression of functional ovarian cysts after treatment with high-dose OCs in 286 patients who presented with a cystic adnexal mass.[2] He hypothesized that a trial of 6 weeks of OC therapy would make the differential diagnosis between functional ovarian cysts and ovarian neoplasms an easier task. It was thought that pituitary suppression would cause ovarian cysts to regress, while not affecting the course of an ovarian neoplasm.

In Spanos' study, 81 of 286 patients treated with estrogen/progestin therapy had a persistent mass on reexamination. These 81 patients had laparotomies; none had functional cysts. Spanos concluded that a trial of 6 weeks of OC therapy was desirable to hasten the regression of functional ovarian cysts before a patient had exploratory surgery.[2]

In 1990, however, a randomized, prospective trial of the effect of OC therapy on adnexal cysts in women of reproductive age found no evidence to support this practice.[3] The study involved 48 infertility patients enrolled in a program of ovulation induction. The majority had been treated with clomiphene citrate and/or human menopausal gonadotropin. Researchers identified cysts by transvaginal sonography. The patients were randomized to either receive norethindrone 1 mg/mestranol 0.05 mg/day or no treatment for up to 6 weeks. At 6 weeks, the cysts had resolved in all but one patient in each group. By 9 weeks, both groups had complete resolution of their cystic adnexal masses.

Two possible explanations may account for the lack of benefit observed. This may be due to the low power of the study (a small sample size) or to use of an inadequate dose of steroids to suppress the cysts. Also, the majority of women had cysts that were hormonally induced; therefore, according to the investigators, the "findings can be generalized only with caution to spontaneously ovulating women."[3]

Regardless of these limitations, the authors concluded that "there remains little evidence that these medications are effective in hastening the disappearance of these cysts once they are formed."[3] A similar, but larger, study of women with spontaneously occurring cysts will be required to settle this issue.

References

1.   Vessey M, Metcalfe A, Wells C, et al. Ovarian neoplasms, functional ovarian cysts, and oral contraceptives. *BMJ* 1987;294:1518-1520.

2.   Spanos WJ. Preoperative hormonal therapy of cystic adnexal masses. *Am J Obstet Gynecol* 1973;116:551-556.

3.   Steinkampf MP, Hammond KR, Blackwell RE. Hormonal treatment of functional ovarian cysts: a randomized, prospective study. *Fertil Steril* 1990;54:775-777.

vii. Increased Sexual Activity among Teens

The rise in teenage pregnancy and the increase in sexually transmitted diseases (STDs) among the young has generated much concern.[1] Some say the increased availability and acceptance of oral contraceptives are directly related to an increase in sexual activity among teens.

Statistics characterizing adolescent first intercourse do not bear out this assumption.[2,3] In 1982, less than 50% of women ages 15 to 19 years used a contraceptive method at first intercourse. This rose to 65% by 1988. According to the National Survey of Family Growth, teens engaging in sexual intercourse for the first time who are inclined to use a contraceptive method typically choose the condom (Table 1).[3] In fact, the use of a condom more than doubled during the period from 1982 to 1988.

With teens, little indication exists that the availability of oral contraceptives or, for that matter, any type of contraceptive leads to an increase in sexual activity. The increase in teen sexual activity over the years does not coincide with an increase in pill use at first intercourse. The availability of oral contraceptives does not sanction, condone, encourage or influence early sexual practice patterns of adolescents.

Education will have the most profound effect on reversing the trend toward early, unprotected intercourse. Abstinence should be encouraged. Prevention efforts are best targeted to the very young adolescent, which means that education must begin in elementary school. Education should stress abstinence, but also include facts about sex, contraception and disease prevention. This is essential because 37% of teens are sexually active by ninth grade.[1]

In addition to presenting facts about sex, children need to learn skills to cope with the pressures of sexual performance. Skills can focus on changing behavior, such as learning to delay intercourse, building self-esteem as well as proper use of contraceptives. Helping teens learn the interpersonal skills necessary to postpone sexual involvement can help them cope with the peer structure and media images that frequently approve of and encourage teen sex. Easy, confidential and nonthreatening access to medical care may also help prevent many unintended pregnancies and the spread of STDs.

Frank discussion and education about sex and birth control in The Netherlands has resulted in high contraceptive use at first intercourse and a low abortion rate among teens.[4] In 1995, the Youth and Sex Survey of Dutch adolescents reported that 85% of teens used a contraceptive method at first intercourse. In addition, the use of two methods at first intercourse—the pill and the condom—for pregnancy and STD prevention rose from 9% in 1990 to 24% in 1995.

Table 1

Contraceptive Methods Chosen at First Intercourse by Women Ages 15 to 19 Years

Method	Percent Use	
	1982	1988
Total using any method	48%	65%
Condom	23%	47%
Oral contraceptives	8%	8%
Withdrawal	13%	8%
Other	4%	1%

Source: Forrest JD, et al, 1990 (see reference 3).

References
1. Centers for Disease Control and Prevention. Youth Risk Behavior Surveillance—United States, 1995. *MMWR* 1996;45:i-85.
2. Mosher WD, Bachrach CA. First premarital contraceptive use: United States, 1960-1982. *Stud Fam Plann* 1987;18:83-95.
3. Forrest JD, Singh S. The sexual and reproductive behavior of American women, 1982-1988. *Fam Plann Perspect* 1990;22:206-214.
4. David HP, Rademakers J. Lessons from the Dutch abortion experience. *Stud Fam Plann* 1996;27:341-343.

1.10: Compliance

Used absolutely consistently and correctly, oral contraceptives (OCs) have an annual failure rate of 0.1%, making them one of the most effective contraceptive methods available. Oral contraceptive failure rates during typical use, however, average 3% per year among married women studied in clinical trials.[1] The true failure rate is estimated to escalate in certain populations; eg, up to 18% in unmarried black adolescents and up to 20% in women in developing countries.[2] The main reason for this wide discrepancy is lack of compliance with the prescribed regimen—inconsistent use, missed pills or incorrect transition between pill packs. Studies of how women take the pill have found that many use it incorrectly.[3-6]

i. Overview

Another concern that falls under the category of noncompliance and contributes to unintended pregnancy is discontinuation; approximately 25% of oral contraceptive users in the United States discontinue use of the method during the first year, many without adopting an alternate means of birth control.[1]

Improving patient compliance with oral contraceptives could help reduce the number of unintended pregnancies that occur each year. Reducing the user failure rate by just one percentage point (eg, from 3% to 2%) *would prevent at least 630,000 accidental pregnancies each year worldwide*[7]—nearly 170,000 in the U.S. alone.

Pill Taking: Selected Study Results

- Only 28% of patients took the pill correctly.[3]

- Only 42% took a pill every day.[4]

- 16% had pills left at the end of the month.[4]

- Approximately 33% of adolescents missed a pill in the previous 3 months.[5]

- 17% did not know they needed a 7-day break with 21-day pill packs.[6]

Managing noncompliance is a challenging proposition for clinicians. One factor that greatly complicates such efforts is that noncompliance with OCs may not be a willful, conscious act; often, it is due to human error or misunderstanding. Failure to understand pill instructions, uncertainty over how to deal with missed pills and fear and misunderstanding of side effects all contribute to the problem.

Adequate counseling is crucial. Reproductive health practitioners need to provide a thorough explanation of how pills should be taken, when to start a new package and what to do if pills are missed. They also need to explain possible side effects and the overall risks and benefits of using OCs.

Unrealistic Fears

Two Gallup polls confirm that women hold an exaggerated view of the risks associated with the pill.[8,9] Educated women also harbor unrealistic fears about OCs (Figure 1). Researchers surveyed women faculty, students and employees (and their families) of Yale University about the pill.[10] Almost half (47%) reported that the pill

Figure 1

Risks of Oral Contraceptives Cited by Women Faculty, Students and Employees of Yale University*

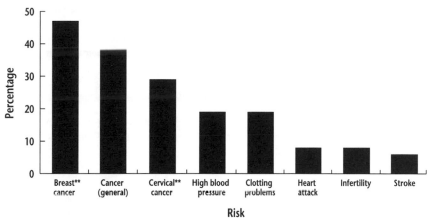

*Response to an open-ended question. **Response to a specific, multiple-choice question.

Source: Peipert JF, et al, 1993 (see reference 10).

caused breast cancer, 29% thought it caused cervical cancer, and 38% believed that cancer in general was the main risk of the pill. Other risks cited include high blood pressure, clotting problems, heart attack and infertility. Importantly, this survey suggests education *per se* does not predict a more accurate view of OCs—over 90% of the respondents had at least 1 year of college education.

Adolescents also report fears concerning the pill. In one study of teens attending either a suburban private practice or an urban clinic, fear of side effects was common.[11] Almost all (85%) of the teenage women in the private practice were very concerned about weight gain. Other concerns reported by clinic patients include fears of infertility, blood clots and birth defects. Another study found that the fear that contraception is dangerous caused teens to delay accessing services at a contraceptive clinic.[12] This fear was cited by 40% of teens who never visited the clinic. Other researchers have found that teens who perceived substantial health-related problems with the pill were least likely to continue to use it.[13]

Side Effects and Noncompliance

Possible side effects require considerable provider-patient discussion. Even the *perception* of side effects can lead to noncompliance.[14] Breakthrough bleeding, amenorrhea, actual or perceived weight gain, nausea, headaches and mood changes are among the usually transient side effects that may affect compliance. In addition, misinformation and fear of cancer may cause women to stop taking the pill and result in an unintended pregnancy (Figure 2).

Among women who stop using oral contraceptives, side effects or fear of potential side effects are cited as the most frequent reasons for method discontinuation.[15] This

79

suggests the need for anticipatory guidance—that is, careful education of patients about "nuisance" side effects, such as breakthrough bleeding and lack of withdrawal bleeding. Practitioners must identify and address a patient's initial and ongoing concerns about side effects, clarify any misperceptions, and provide advice on management of side effects and reassurance of their probable temporary nature.

Patient counseling to counteract exaggerated perceptions of the risks of OCs is essential. Clinicians need to uncover patient fears about the pill as an initial step. No matter what other counseling steps are taken, if the patient has unexpressed reservations about taking the pill, she may eventually stop taking it without informing her health care provider.

Figure 2

Side Effects and Noncompliance: "Minor" Side Effects May Lead to Major Consequences

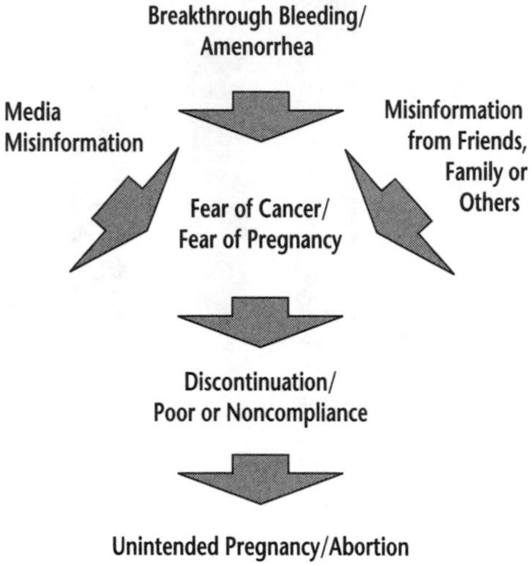

Breakthrough Bleeding/ Amenorrhea

Media Misinformation

Misinformation from Friends, Family or Others

Fear of Cancer/ Fear of Pregnancy

Discontinuation/ Poor or Noncompliance

Unintended Pregnancy/Abortion

Information on Risks

Clinicians may want to include several steps when counseling patients about the risks and benefits of OCs. First, ask the patient what negative stories she's heard about OCs. Don't wait for patients to volunteer that information, as many of them may not be consciously aware that they have reservations about the method. Second, provide accurate information about the risks of OCs. Patients should be warned about the dangers of cigarette smoking if they smoke and be encouraged to quit. Third, provide clear instructions about how to take the pill.

Examples of Noncompliance

- Not filling or refilling OC prescriptions
- Forgetting to take pills
- Running out of pills
- Starting next pack late
- Taking pills incorrectly
- Using sporadically
- Not using backup method when needed

Clear Pill-Use Instructions

Success with pill taking will decrease if patients are not instructed about what to do if they miss pills, or if these instructions are unclear or misunderstood. "Missed pills," in this context, refer to any pills that are taken 24 or more hours late. Missing pills during any portion of the cycle may result in breakthrough bleeding; however, there is an increased risk of follicular development and possibly ovulation and pregnancy if pills are missed at the beginning of a new cycle. Most women do not understand that extending the pill-free interval beyond the usual 7 days is particularly critical. Many women believe—incorrectly—that pills missed at midcycle carry the greatest risk. In fact, missing even one at the beginning or end of a cycle may increase the risk of follicular development and possible escape ovulation.

During the pill-free interval, there is a fairly rapid return of pituitary function, with a rise in levels of follicle-stimulating hormone (FSH) and estradiol. By the seventh pill-free day, levels of FSH, luteinizing hormone (LH) and estradiol are similar to those in nonusers of oral contraceptives in the early

Effective Patient Counseling Includes Uncovering and Addressing Fears about the Pill

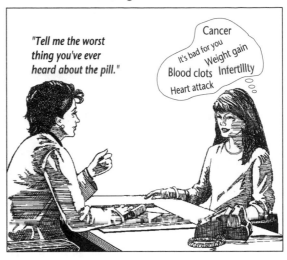

"Tell me the worst thing you've ever heard about the pill."

Cancer
It's bad for you
Weight gain
Blood clots Infertility
Heart attack

follicular phase of a normal ovulatory cycle. Thus, if pills are missed at the beginning or end of a packet, there is a risk that a subsequent LH surge could act on the primed ovary to produce ovulation.[16]

Careful instructions—both oral *and* written—regarding how to use the specific brand of pill prescribed may help to reduce confusion and improve compliance. Providing a patient with samples of the pill packet she will be using and showing her how to take the pills are important to ensure correct use from the outset.

Manufacturers provide some practical, compliance-related educational materials for new oral contraceptive users. These educational aids include pill-taking reminders, tips on side effects management, convenient instructions on how to deal with missed pills (such as those printed on a small, wallet-sized card) and information on the health benefits of the pill. Practitioners should review these materials with patients and encourage them to call the office or clinic if any questions arise.

When patients do call with questions or concerns about oral contraceptive use, listening to the problem and providing reassurance, when appropriate, are important. Listening to the patient is an essential first step. Phone calls may provide an ideal opportunity for further education and reinforcement; for example, if a woman calls "just to be sure" about an episode of breakthrough bleeding, the clinician may want to ask whether she's been taking her pills at the same time every day and suggest a strategy that will help her do so.

Compliance among Teens

Teenagers present a special challenge because adolescents often do not understand how important it is to take pills exactly as prescribed. Teens may have more trouble taking OCs correctly than do older women and many teenage pill users quit after a relatively brief period of time. Practitioners must dispel notions that lack foundation,

Clinical Recommendations for Improving Oral Contraceptive Compliance

1. All oral contraceptive users should know three things before they start taking their pills:

   a. How to take the oral contraceptive prescribed;

   b. What to do if they miss a pill or pills;

   c. Which side effects are common and usually transient (breakthrough bleeding and nausea), and which are potentially serious and should be brought immediately to their clinician's attention.

2. Simple instructions should be provided to all patients both verbally and in writing; a copy of written instructions should be discussed with the patient point by point during the visit. Another copy of written instructions should be offered at each follow-up visit.

3. Show each patient who is starting a new brand of pill (and especially first-time oral contraceptive users) how to use the specific package being prescribed. Use of the 28-day package enhances compliance.

4. Help women select a specific time of day to take their pills; a brief discussion of their daily schedules may help identify an optimal time of day. Taking the pill after dinner or with a bedtime snack lessens the possibility of nausea.

5. The refill prescription should include an additional cycle to accommodate missed pills or lost packets.

6. The use of a backup method and the availability of emergency contraception should be discussed.

7. Discuss prevention of sexually transmitted diseases. Provide the OC user with a condom and discuss its proper use.

8. On follow-up visits, ask patients if they have had any problems taking their pills; ask what they did when they missed pills.

9. Oral contraceptive users who have repeated difficulty remembering to take their pills or other serious compliance problems should be counseled about other available methods.

---

such as the belief that the pill causes weight gain or leads to lasting infertility or birth defects.

Teens benefit from verbal instruction about OC use because written instructions are often discarded from fear that parents may discover the teen is sexually active. On the other hand, when parental knowledge is not a concern, involving the teen's parents may enhance a teenager's compliance.[17]

Clinicians should encourage teens to ask questions *before* they leave the office or clinic. Teens should be urged to call immediately if any questions arise—rather than consulting friends or other pill users. The name and phone number of the health care provider to call should be given to the patient; she should also meet the staff member in person, if possible. In addition, practitioners also need to schedule more frequent visits with teenage patients than with adults.

Paula J.A. Hillard, MD, Associate Editor of *The Contraception Report*, raises another important issue for teens: "Other compliance problems concern logistical factors for teens who may be limited by their health plans or may only have enough money to get 1 month's supply at a time. Sunday-start pills may also be a problem for those who run out of the pill over the weekend and may or may not be able to contact their prescribers to get a refill.

"One other reason given for discontinuation is inconvenience. We tend to think of the pill as a fairly convenient method of contraception, but adolescents may not have the ordered lives that some older women do. This is particularly true if her parents are divorced and she is spending weekends at a different home or, in the case of an older teen, if she is spending the night at her boyfriend's," states Dr. Hillard.

Stressing Health Benefits

Counseling regarding health benefits may help to improve continuation with the pill. For example, a patient who breaks up with her boyfriend may stop taking the pill because she does not anticipate having sexual intercourse in the next few weeks or months. Women who understand that the pill has substantial health benefits, however, may continue to take the pill even if they perceive themselves as not needing it for contraception. Continuing to take the pill is important because many women do not switch to another effective method when they stop taking the pill and resumption of coitus may be unpredictable.

Menstrual Cycle Benefits

Counseling about menstrual cycle benefits may also help to improve compliance. Many women find cycle regularity, lighter periods and relief of dysmenorrhea welcome effects of the pill. Relief of dysmenorrhea, in particular, is one health benefit that may help adolescents (and adult women) continue to take their pills successfully.[18]

Taking the time to discuss these benefits with patients will reinforce the positive aspects of oral contraceptive use. An integrated counseling approach—one that includes discussions of health benefits, proper OC use and appropriate side effects management—will play a critical role in reducing the number of unintended pregnancies associated with OC discontinuation and noncompliance.

References

1. Trussell J, Hatcher RA, Cates W Jr., et al. Contraceptive failure in the United States: an update. *Stud Fam Plann* 1990;21:51-54.

2. Hillard PJA. Oral contraception noncompliance: the extent of the problem. *Adv Contracept* 1992;8(suppl 1):13-20.

3. Finlay IG, Scott MGB. Patterns of contraceptive pill taking in an inner city practice. *BMJ* 1986;293:601-602.

4. Oakley D, Parent J. A scale to measure microbehaviors of oral contraceptive pill use. *Social Biology* 1990;37:215-222.

5. Goldstuck ND, Hammar E, Butchart A. Use and misuse of oral contraceptives by adolescents attending a free-standing clinic. *Adv Contracept* 1987;3:335-339.

6. Brook SJ. Do combined oral contraceptive users know how to take their pill correctly? *Br J Fam Plann* 1991;17:18-20.

7. Potter L, Williams-Deane M. The importance of oral contraceptive compliance. *IPPF Bull* 1990;24:2-3.

8. The Gallup Organization. *Attitudes Toward Contraception.* A poll conducted for the American College of Obstetricians and Gynecologists. Princeton, NJ: March 1985.

9. American College of Obstetricians and Gynecologists. Poll shows women still skeptical of contraceptive safety (news release). January 20, 1994.

10. Peipert JF, Gutmann J. Oral contraceptive risk assessment: a survey of 247 educated women. *Obstet Gynecol* 1993;82:112-117.

11. Emans SJ, Grace E, Woods ER, et al. Adolescents' compliance with the use of oral contraceptives. *JAMA* 1987;257:3377-3381.

12. Zabin LS, Stark HA, Emerson MR. Reasons for delay in contraceptive clinic utilization. *J Adolesc Health* 1991;12:225-232.

13. Balassone ML. Risk of contraceptive discontinuation among adolescents. *J Adolesc Health Care* 1989;10:527-533.

14. Woods ER, Grace E, Havens KK, et al. Contraceptive compliance with a levonorgestrel triphasic and a norethindrone monophasic oral contraceptive in adolescent patients. *Am J Obstet Gynecol* 1992;166:901-907.

15. Pratt WF, Bachrach CA. What do women use when they stop using the pill? *Fam Plann Perspect* 1987;19:257-266.

16. Sapire KE, Belfield T, Guillebaud J, eds. *Contraception and Sexuality in Health and Disease.* UK Edition, London: McGraw-Hill Book Co. 1990:120-124.

17. Cromer BA. Behavioral strategies to increase compliance in adolescents. In: Cramer JA, Spilker B, eds. *Patient Compliance in Medical Practice and Clinical Trials.* New York: Raven Press, Ltd. 1991: 99-105.

18. Robinson JC, Plichta S, Weisman CS, et al. Dysmenorrhea and use of oral contraceptives in adolescent women attending a family planning clinic. *Am J Obstet Gynecol* 1992;166:578-583.

ii. Management of Breakthrough Bleeding

The evaluation and management of patients who have abnormal bleeding while taking oral contraceptives require thought and attention to the individual patient, rather than a standardized approach. One incorrect approach is simply to suggest a different formulation of pills. This frequently results in the patient who states that she's tried "all" the different types of pills, yet has had breakthrough bleeding with all of them. When questioned further, she may report that she took each type for only a few days or weeks before being switched to a different type. Three cycles of a given oral contraceptive are recommended to evaluate its effect.

Each patient who starts a new prescription for oral contraceptive pills should be told that a minority of women will experience breakthrough bleeding during the first few months of use. During the first month of use, up to 30% of women may have breakthrough bleeding; the proportion drops to less than 10% during the third month. If the patient does experience breakthrough bleeding, it is likely to resolve with time. Thus, the management of this side effect within the first 3 months of pill use consists simply of reassurance.

Try not to change the pill formulation by switching to a higher-dose pill or even to a different low-dose pill prior to 3 months of use. Regardless of formulation prescribed, one cannot predict for an individual woman whether or not she will experience breakthrough bleeding.

The issue of pill compliance should be explored when a patient experiences breakthrough bleeding. Missed pills are so common that the clinician should always inquire about missed pills first in relationship to breakthrough bleeding. The problem can be circular: missed pills result in breakthrough bleeding, which leads to more dissatisfaction with the pill, which may lead to more missed pills. The patient may be confused about whether or not the bleeding is a "real period" and when to take the pill. In addition, in adolescents experiencing breakthrough bleeding, clinicians should consider chlamydial infection and/or pregnancy.

If breakthrough bleeding persists after 3 months of oral contraceptive use, several management options are available. If the bleeding is slight, infrequent and not bothersome, no treatment may be necessary. If the bleeding is bothersome, additional estrogen to stabilize the endometrium may be appropriate. One approach includes the addition of oral estrogens to the patient's current pill formulation (1.25 mg conjugated equine estrogen or its equivalent daily for 1 week at the time the breakthrough bleeding occurs; repeated, if necessary).

Cycle of Breakthrough Bleeding, Missed Pills and OC Dissatisfaction

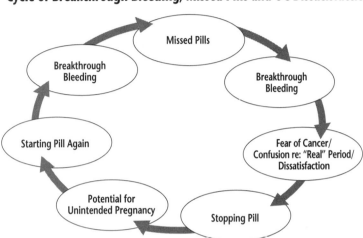

1.11: Drug Interactions

The possible interaction of oral contraceptives (OCs) with other drugs has been the subject of numerous case reports and clinical studies since the early 1970s. Some of these interactions are well documented and therapeutically relevant; others remain unproven or are the subject of continuing controversy. This section examines possible drug interactions among OCs and commonly (and not so commonly) prescribed medications (Figures 1-3).

Reports of drug interactions with OCs fall into two general categories: (1) the efficacy of oral contraceptive steroids may be affected by concomitant administration of other drugs, and (2) oral contraceptives may interfere with the metabolism of other agents. Interference from oral contraceptives can either increase or decrease the effectiveness of other drugs. Likewise, oral contraceptive efficacy may either be impaired or enhanced by concurrent drug therapy; impairment may result in breakthrough bleeding (and occasionally pregnancy), while enhancement of oral contraceptive efficacy may increase side effects.

Figure 1

Drugs That May Reduce Oral Contraceptive Efficacy

Interacting Drug	Documentation	Management
Antituberculosis (rifampin)	Established	Increase OC dose or change method
Antifungals (griseofulvin)	Strongly suspected	Increase OC dose
Anticonvulsants and Sedatives (phenytoin, ethotoin, mephenytoin, phenobarbital, primidone, carbamazepine, ethosuximide)	Strongly suspected; clinical trial data lacking	With spotting, increase OC dose; consult with neurologist to consider switch to sodium valproate
Antibiotics Tetracycline, doxycycline	Minimal, doubtful; two small studies find no association	None; with spotting, may increase OC dose
Penicillin (ampicillin)	Contradictory; information lacking	None; with spotting, may increase OC dose

Source: Adapted from Goldzieher JW, 1994 (see reference 3).

Figure 2

Drugs That May Enhance Oral Contraceptive Efficacy or Increase Related Side Effects

Interacting Drug	Effect
Co-trimoxazole	Increases ethinyl estradiol blood levels; norgestrel unaffected (data sparse)

Source: Adapted from Goldzieher JW, 1994 (see reference 3).

Drug Interactions Affecting Oral Contraceptive Efficacy

Anticonvulsant Drugs

The enzyme-inducing nature of a number of anticonvulsant drugs may increase the metabolism of OC steroids, resulting in insufficient levels of estrogen and/or progestin to prevent ovulation.[1] The most commonly implicated anticonvulsant agents are phenobarbital and phenytoin, although carbamazepine, primidone and ethosuximide have also been suspected of interfering with the efficacy of oral contraceptives.[2,3] On the other hand, the anticonvulsant drug sodium valproate has no enzyme-inducing properties and has not been shown to interfere with oral contraceptive efficacy.[2]

For OC users, the decrease in synthetic hormone levels as a result of enzyme-inducing anticonvulsant therapy can be countered by increasing the oral contraceptive dosage. The appropriate dosage is impossible to predict, however, because the extent of the enzyme-inducing effect varies greatly among individual patients. Several researchers have suggested starting with an intermediate dosage of 50 mcg ethinyl estradiol.[1] In the event of breakthrough bleeding, the amount can be increased incrementally up to 80 mcg, if necessary, by combining a 50 mcg preparation with a 30 mcg preparation.[1,4] Switching the anticonvulsant medication to sodium valproate and using a typical low-dose oral contraceptive may also be an option with some patients.[1-3] Some researchers have suggested decreasing the pill-free interval to 4 to 5 days.

Antibiotics

A widely accepted, but largely unproven, drug interaction involves the effect of antibiotics on OC efficacy. Researchers have suggested several mechanisms that may be responsible for this interference, including decreased enterohepatic recirculation, increased urinary or fecal excretion of the steroids, and increased liver degradation.[5]

Figure 3

Drugs Whose Activity May Be Modified by Oral Contraceptive Use

Interacting Drug	Documentation	Management
Analgesics Acetaminophen Aspirin Meperidine Morphine	Adequate Probable Suspected Probable	Larger doses of analgesic may be required Larger doses of analgesic may be required Decrease dose of analgesic Larger doses of analgesic may be required
Anticoagulants (dicumarol, warfarin)	Controversial	
Antidepressants Imipramine Other tricyclics	Suspected No data	Decrease dosage by about one-third

Tranquilizers
Diazepam,
  Alprazolam,
  Nitrazepam
Temazepam
Other
  benzodiazepines
	Suspected
	
	Possible
	
	Suspected
		Decrease dose
		
		May need to increase dose
		
		Observe for increased effect

Anti-inflammatories (corticosteroids)	Adequate	Watch for potentiation of effects, decrease dose accordingly

Bronchodilators
(aminophylline,
  theophylline,
  caffeine)
	Adequate	Reduce starting dose by one-third

Antihypertensives Cyclopenthiazide, guanethidine Metoprolol	Adequate Suspected	Increase dose May need to lower dose
Antibiotics Troleandomycin Cyclosporine	Suspected liver damage Possible	Avoid May use smaller dose

Source: Adapted from Goldzieher JW, 1994 (see reference 3).

Enterohepatic recirculation occurs when, following conjugation of contraceptive steroids in the liver and upper small intestine, conjugates pass through the bile into the colon. Bacterial enzymes in the colon then deconjugate the agents, which are then reabsorbed, presumably causing an increase in circulating ethinyl estradiol. Data from animal studies indicate that antibiotics can interrupt this process by killing the bacteria responsible for deconjugation in the colon, resulting in decreased hormone levels and reduced contraceptive efficacy.[2,4] Several studies involving human subjects have failed to support such an interaction.[5]

Likewise, other proposed mechanisms of interaction lack support from large, controlled studies. Thus, despite a number of case reports implicating penicillins, tetracyclines and other antibiotics in causing oral contraceptive failure, no firm pharmacokinetic evidence exists linking antibiotic administration with altered steroid blood concentrations.[2] In fact, two studies have shown no important interactions between oral contraceptives and tetracycline or doxycycline.[6,7] Given the huge number of subjects that would be needed for clinical trials addressing this issue, it is unlikely that a definitive answer will emerge.

Some researchers have recommended that patients taking antibiotics use an additional contraceptive method, such as a condom. This added precaution is probably unnecessary, however. Thirty years of experience with OCs have yielded a handful of case reports, but no clear controlled clinical data to suggest that antibiotics substantially interfere with pill efficacy.

Some have suggested that patients on long-term antibiotic therapy, such as oral antibiotics for the treatment of acne, be monitored for breakthrough bleeding, and pill dose be increased or a condom used if spotting occurs.[3] On the other hand, one might expect OC efficacy to stabilize over the course of long-term therapy as bacteria responsible for steroid deconjugation develop a resistance to the antibiotic. Thus, a gradual rise in contraceptive efficacy could follow the postulated initial drop in such patients.

Other Drugs

The effect of the antituberculosis drug rifampin on oral contraceptive efficacy was widely documented during the early and mid-1970s, when numerous pill failures were reported among tuberculosis patients.[2,4] Rifampin has potent enzyme-inducing properties and has caused a reduction in both progestogen and estrogen levels in clinical studies of oral contraceptive users.[2] As a result, patients simultaneously using rifampin and oral contraceptives will require an increased pill dosage. Since early reports of rifampin interference with oral contraceptives involved patients using intermediate-dose pills (50 mcg ethinyl estradiol), some women may require higher doses to maintain sufficient steroid levels.[4] Practitioners may wish to consider an alternative contraceptive method for rifampin patients.[3,4]

The antifungal drug griseofulvin has been associated with breakthrough bleeding and a small number of pregnancies among users of oral contraceptives.[2,8] Although the drug is known to modify hepatic enzyme activity in mice, evidence of a major enzyme-inducing effect in humans is lacking.[2] Patients using both OCs and griseofulvin may require a higher-dose pill to maintain optimum contraceptive efficacy.[3]

Oral Contraceptive Use Affecting Other Drugs

Benzodiazepines

Although documentation is not extensive, OC use may affect the activity of some benzodiazepine tranquilizers—either increasing or decreasing their efficacy. Oral contraceptives are suspected of reducing the clearance of certain benzodiazepines through the inhibition of enzyme activity. Studies have suggested that diazepam, chlordiazepoxide, alprazolam and nitrazepam are affected in this way[2]; lower dosages of these agents may be effective in oral contraceptive users.[3] On the other hand, the clearance of temazepam, a benzodiazepine that is metabolized by conjugation, may be increased and thus require increased dosage in oral contraceptive users.[2]

Corticosteroids

Simultaneous use of oral contraceptives and anti-inflammatory corticosteroids may result in an increased effect of the latter. A number of studies have reported decreased clearance and prolonged elimination half-life of prednisolone in pill users.[2] Patients undergoing corticosteroid therapy while using OCs should be closely monitored for increased effects; lower dosages may prove clinically effective in these patients.[2,3]

Theophylline

Bronchodilating agents, such as theophylline, aminophylline and the closely related compound caffeine, appear to be affected by oral contraceptive use.[2,3] Clearance of these drugs may be reduced between 30% and 40% in pill users, thus increasing their effect.[2] As a result, initial doses of theophylline and aminophylline should be reduced by one-third in patients using oral contraceptives.[3]

Analgesics

A number of studies have suggested an interaction between OCs and analgesic agents. Pill users may have less pain relief with acetaminophen. Although the evidence is contradictory, the effect of aspirin may also be reduced by oral contraceptive use. The pain-relieving response should be monitored in oral contraceptive users taking analgesic medications and the dosage increased, if necessary.[3]

Other Drugs

Antihypertensive agents, such as cyclopenthiazide and guanethidine, may require increased doses in oral contraceptive users.[3] On the other hand, the effect of the antihypertensive metoprolol may be enhanced and require a decreased dosage.[2,3] Plasma concentrations of cyclosporin are reported to be elevated in OC users, as well.[2]

Conclusion

Strong evidence suggests griseofulvin, rifampin and anticonvulsants that induce hepatic enzymes decrease the effect of OCs. Patients on these medications should be monitored for breakthrough bleeding and have their OC dosage adjusted, if necessary. No sound evidence suggests that other antibiotics decrease the efficacy of OCs; extra precautions are probably not warranted, but have been suggested by some. Other drugs that interact with OCs include some bronchodilators, antihypertensives and analgesics. Clinicians should be aware of possible interactions, monitor patients for signs of drug interaction and take appropriate steps to avoid potential adverse effects.

References

1. Mattson RH, Cramer JA, Darney PD, et al. Use of oral contraceptives by women with epilepsy. *JAMA* 1986;256:238-240.

2. Back DJ, Orme MLE. Pharmacokinetic drug interactions with oral contraceptives. *Clin Pharmacokinet* 1990;18:472-484.

3. Goldzieher JW. *Hormonal Contraception: Pills, Injections & Implants*. Third edition. London, Ontario: EMIS-Canada. 1994:52-57.

4. Fraser IS, Jansen RPS. Why do inadvertent pregnancies occur in oral contraceptive users? Effectiveness of oral contraceptive regimens and interfering factors. *Contraception* 1983;27: 531-551.

5. Fleischer AB Jr., Resnick SD. The effect of antibiotics on the efficacy of oral contraceptives. *Arch Dermatol* 1989;125:1582-1584.

6. Murphy AA, Zacur HA, Charache P, et al. The effect of tetracycline on levels of oral contraceptives. *Am J Obstet Gynecol* 1991;164:28-33.

7. Neely JL, Abate M, Swinker M, et al. The effect of doxycycline on serum levels of ethinyl estradiol, norethindrone, and endogenous progesterone. *Obstet Gynecol* 1991;77:416-20.

8. Van Dijke CPH, Weber JCP. Interaction between oral contraceptives and griseofulvin. *BMJ* 1984;288:1125-1126.

1.12: Delay of Pelvic Exam

On May 20, 1993, the Food and Drug Administration's (FDA) Fertility and Maternal Health Drugs Advisory Committee voted in favor of giving patients seeking oral contraceptives (OCs) the option of deferring physical examination without being denied a prescription. The change in prescribing protocol had been proposed by the Planned Parenthood® Federation of America, which asserted that the pelvic exam requirement was outdated and might be a barrier to OC access for many women. Based on the committee's recommendation, the FDA approved changes in OC labeling—both physician prescribing information and patient package insert— to allow patient deferral of the exam if deemed appropriate by the prescriber.

Examining the Issues

Prior to making its recommendation, the FDA advisory committee weighed the potential implications of allowing deferral of the exam. Testimony delivered at the committee meeting addressed these issues and provided valuable advice for practitioners with regard to counseling and follow-up in the wake of the new OC guidelines.

Michael Policar, MD, Vice President of Medical Affairs at Planned Parenthood Federation of America, outlined Planned Parenthood's rationale for changing OC labeling. "Primarily, we believe that the current guidelines, as stated in the package insert, are outdated at this point," Dr. Policar explained. "We have more than 30 years of experience with oral contraceptives now, and we feel that the caution of the 1960s and 1970s, while still important, may be relaxed to some degree, now that we're much more familiar with pill pharmacology and clinical effects."

Changes to OC Labeling

Physician Prescribing Information

Previous text:

"A complete medical history and physical examination should be taken prior to the initiation or reinstitution of oral contraceptives, and at least annually during the use of oral contraceptives."[1]

Revised text:

"Physical examination may be deferred until after initiation of oral contraceptives if requested by the woman and judged appropriate by the clinician."[2]

Patient Package Insert

Added text:

"The physical examination may be delayed to another time if you request it and the health care provider believes that it is good medical practice to postpone it."[2]

In explaining the Planned Parenthood proposal, Dr. Policar stressed that "we are not suggesting a waiver of the physical examination. We are certainly not suggesting that the physical examination is unnecessary or simply should be done away with." He emphasized that the proposed guidelines would give patients the option to defer the physical exam, but only if deemed appropriate by the provider. While the exam may be deferred, it should certainly be performed at the earliest opportunity.

Reasons for Deferral

Dr. Policar cited three situations in which women seeking oral contraceptives might want to defer the pelvic exam. He explained that the first of these instances involves teenagers—especially young teenagers—who wish to use oral contraceptives, but have avoided going to a clinic or physician's office out of fear of a pelvic examination.

"Second," Dr. Policar continued, "some women are seen for medical care during their menstrual period, and often the advice of the clinician is to avoid a full physical exam, including a pelvic exam, because of the interference of menstrual blood with cervical cytological sampling. Oftentimes, a woman has to reschedule her visit for a full physical exam and is not able to use oral contraceptives during that period.

"Third, there are some women who wish to initiate oral contraceptive use, but who are subject to long delays in the scheduling of an appointment for a full physical examination. If those women were able to have a shorter visit where a medical history was taken, informed consent was given and pill use was initiated, followed by deferral of the pelvic examination, those women would have access to oral contraceptives earlier than they might have had otherwise."

Dr. Policar pointed out that Planned Parenthood revised its own medical standards in August of 1992 to allow a 3-month deferral of the pelvic examination. "Since this change in standards was instituted," he said, "the response from Planned Parenthood affiliates has been enthusiastic. No important medical problems arising from this policy have been reported."

The Smart Start Project

Dr. Policar explained that Planned Parenthood's change in OC prescribing standards was based on data from a program called Smart Start,[3] initiated in Philadelphia in 1986 by the Family Planning Council of Southeastern Pennsylvania. The Smart Start project assessed the impact of allowing a deferral of the pelvic exam for teenagers wishing to use OCs.

Kay Armstrong, MS, Director of Research at the Family Planning Council, described the Smart Start project to the FDA committee and presented the results of the study. She began by explaining that many Philadelphia teenagers have expressed fears about the pelvic exam. The Smart Start model was designed to overcome these fears.

Ms. Armstrong explained, "A nationwide survey done in 1986 found that 69% of teens said they perceived the pelvic exam to be a barrier for accessing family planning services.[4] We very much wanted to reduce such barriers. We wanted teens who were sexually active to come in earlier. We also wanted to help educate teens and other women about the pelvic exam."

Results of the Study

According to Armstrong, the Smart Start program was offered to nonpregnant teens under age 18. The teens were given the option to delay the pelvic exam, but also received interactive counseling that helped them understand exactly what the exam entailed. Complete data, including a medical chart record, were obtained for 151 of the 390 teens who participated.

Of the 151 teens, 40 opted to delay having the pelvic exam performed at the time of the initial visit. "Of the teens who delayed," Armstrong noted, "69% came back and had their pelvic exams at the 3-month visit. ...[And] 78% of the teens in the delay group returned to the family planning clinic within the 6-month time frame."

With regard to improving access to OCs, Armstrong explained that "there were more teens coming in to delay after word of mouth had occurred," implying that teens who might have been avoiding OC use were coming to the clinic after learning that the pelvic exam was not required. Armstrong concluded, "Both the teens and the clinic staff are very supportive of Smart Start. They feel it really empowered the teens by offering them an option. As one teen said when she was asked to comment on Smart Start, 'What I liked most about my clinic visit was that I had a choice about the exam.' "

Support from ACOG and AFS

Planned Parenthood's labeling change proposal received support from both the American College of Obstetricians and Gynecologists (ACOG) and the American Fertility Society (AFS) [now known as the American Society for Reproductive Medicine]. Speaking on behalf of ACOG, then President-Elect William Andrews, MD, Professor of Obstetrics and Gynecology at Eastern Virginia Medical School, told the committee that deferring the pelvic exam "can be done safely, particularly in the case of teenage women, and may help reduce one of the barriers to oral contraceptives in this age group."

Dr. Andrews explained that "the absolute and relative contraindications to prescribing [OCs] can be obtained by taking a history, measuring the patient's blood pressure and, if indicated, performing a sensitive pregnancy test. There is virtually no information gained from the pelvic examination that would prevent a decision to prescribe oral contraceptives in young women.

"Clearly, the most compelling reason to perform a pelvic exam on a sexually active adolescent is to diagnose and treat sexually transmitted disease. This need, however, does not require a pelvic examination prior to prescribing OCs. The presence of a sexually transmitted disease is not a contraindication for OCs. It is a separate reason for doing the examination."

Representing AFS, Ann Davis, MD, Assistant Professor of Obstetrics and Gynecology and Assistant Professor of Pediatrics at Tufts University School of Medicine, expressed the society's support for the proposed changes in OC prescribing guidelines. Noting that the pelvic exam should not be a prerequisite to the prescription of OCs, she also asserted that "delaying the pelvic exam may help eliminate barriers to access. This, in turn, may reduce adolescent pregnancy. But, for this favorable cascade to occur, we must publicize that deferring pelvic examinations is an option."

Concerns

Although much support for the proposed OC labeling changes was expressed at the advisory committee meeting, concerns were also raised. Luz Alvarez Martinez, Director of the National Latino Health Organization, questioned whether women would try to defer the pelvic exam indefinitely under the new guidelines. "If the labeling is changed," noted Martinez, "the message is being given that medical exams and Pap smears are not necessary when young women begin using birth control. If women truly are anxious about having Pap smears, they may not come back after they complete their cycle of birth control pills. Women may go to a different clinic for subsequent oral contraceptive prescriptions and again pass up the opportunity for a medical exam."

Another concern was raised regarding whether the ability to defer the physical exam would include deferral of breast examination. Deferral of the breast exam, it was noted, could delay the diagnosis of preexisting malignancy. A third major concern was that by deferring the pelvic examination, the likelihood of detecting sexually transmitted disease would be decreased. In the absence of the pelvic exam, the patient history becomes the sole means by which to identify the presence of disease, a poor indicator. In addition, an adolescent who delays her examination may have more anxiety in the intervening 1 week to 3 months than if she had felt supported and comfortable enough at the initial visit to have the exam. It is particularly important to exclude pregnancy at the initial visit.

Advice for Providers

By voting in favor of allowing a deferral of the physical exam for women seeking OC prescriptions, the FDA advisory committee judged that the benefits of improving access to this contraceptive method outweighed any potential drawbacks. Nevertheless, it acknowledged that providers need to be aware of the concerns raised and should take steps to ensure that appropriate counseling and care are given to women opting to defer physical examination.

With regard to breast examination, Dr. Policar explained that Planned Parenthood's policy requires women over 30 to have a breast examination prior to receiving an OC prescription, even if the pelvic exam is postponed. Dr. Andrews agreed that practitioners should perform a breast exam and counsel patients on self-examination, especially older women. "In the vast majority of cases," he noted, "the [breast] examination should be performed…particularly as women pass the teen years."

The need for providers to take a detailed history and be alert for signs of sexually transmitted disease is especially important in the wake of the new OC guidelines. In addition, women need to be thoroughly counseled about the risk of disease and means of prevention, and patients must be familiar with disease symptoms to ensure accurate self-reporting in the absence of a pelvic exam.

Importance of Follow-Up

To help ensure that women opting to defer ultimately receive an examination, Dr. Andrews stressed the importance of thorough counseling and dedicated follow-up. "Deciding to provide oral contraceptives without a pelvic exam," he noted, "will require adequate follow-up procedures to ensure that women receive the necessary examination in a timely fashion and are not lost to care. It also requires adequate and age-appropriate counseling and health education so that they can both avoid sexually transmitted disease and correctly use the method of contraception that has been prescribed." However, as S. Jean Emans, MD, Associate Editor of *The Contraception Report* points out, appropriate follow-up may be difficult due to confidentiality concerns when contacting teens at home.

With regard to counseling patients—especially adolescents—on the pelvic exam, Dr. Davis offered practical advice to providers: "During a visit with an adolescent patient, I discuss the pelvic exam and I ask her what her concerns are about the exam. I try to always ask open-ended questions because if given an option, adolescents would much rather nod their heads 'yes' or 'no' than to interact, and only by interaction do we know what their concerns really are.

"Also, by asking what concerns they have about the pelvic exam, it implies that concerns are normal and we're able to engage in a conversation to address their exact fears. Those fears are both embarrassment about the exam and fear of pain. …[An effective] way to alleviate fear is to discuss the sensory perception that the patient will have during the procedure. After trying to alleviate her fears regarding the examination, she is given a choice."

References

1.   Food and Drug Administration. Fertility and Maternal Health Drugs Advisory Committee (meeting transcript). Washington, DC: U.S. Department of Health and Human Services; May 20, 1993.

2.   *F-D-C Reports*. Oral contraceptive labeling change modifying physical exam requirement. August 23, 1993:T&G1-2.

3.   Donovan P. Delaying pelvic exams to encourage contraceptive use. *Fam Plann Perspect* 1992;24:136-144.

4.   Lou Harris & Associates. *American Teens Speak: Sex, Myths, T.V. and Birth Control, 1986.* Survey conducted on behalf of Planned Parenthood® Federation of America.

1.13: Headache and Migraine

If a patient presents with a history of migraines, may oral contraceptives (OCs) be prescribed? Do OCs make migraines worse? In a patient with migraines, will the use of OCs increase her risk of having a cerebrovascular accident (CVA)? These are some of the questions that are often raised regarding OCs and headaches.

The origin of the concern regarding OCs and headaches dates back to the early studies of the pill in the 1960s and 1970s. During this time, a relationship was described between pill use and such cardiovascular events as thromboembolism, stroke and myocardial infarction.[1-4] Because stroke may be preceded by headache, a concern developed about whether prescribing OCs for women with headaches could precipitate a CVA. Smoking in combination with use of higher-dose pills increased the risk of cardiovascular complications for women participating in these early studies.[5] Screening for risk factors, such as smoking, family history of premature death from myocardial infarction, diabetes and hypertension, as well as using low-dose pills, has greatly reduced the risk of cardiovascular complications in OC users.[6,7]

Epidemiology of Headaches

Headache is the seventh leading presenting complaint for ambulatory care encounters in the United States. A telephone survey of over 10,000 residents in Maryland ages 12 through 29 years found that 77% of women reported that their most recent headache had occurred within the previous 4 weeks and 95% had experienced headache during their lifetime.[8] Fourteen percent had experienced four or more headaches in the preceding month. In addition, 7% of females were considered to have suffered a migraine headache in the month before the interview. In a survey of middle school students, 30% of girls reported at least weekly headaches.[9] A longitudinal study of Finnish pupils reported that by age 14, 15% of girls had experienced a migraine headache.[10] Thus, many candidates for oral contraceptives will need evaluation of this common complaint.

At the initial visit, clinicians should try to determine which type of headache the patient has experienced in the past, and the frequency and severity of the problem. Certain symptoms are indicative of a particular headache, although patients may experience a mixture of types of headaches (Figures 1A-1D). Patients may also not be clear about the type of headache they have. The word "migraine" is often used

---

Figure 1A

Symptoms of Migraine with Aura (Classic Migraine)

- Visual aura (prodrome)

- Throbbing, unilateral pain

- Photophobia/phonophobia

- Nausea/vomiting/anorexia

- Neurological symptoms during, but not after, headache

- Triggered by food, alcohol

- May be related to onset of menses

- Often a family history of vascular headache

Figure 1B

Symptoms of Migraine without Aura (Common Migraine)

- Throbbing, bilateral pain
- Photophobia/phonophobia
- Nausea/vomiting/anorexia
- Triggered by food, alcohol

Figure 1C

Symptoms of Tension Headache

- Steady, dull ache
- Bilateral pain
- Relief with aspirin or acetaminophen
- Pain waxes and wanes
- Long, protracted episodes
- Tense shoulder/neck muscles

Figure 1D

Symptoms Suggesting Intracranial Pathology

- Neurological symptoms during and after headache
- "Worst headache of my life"
- New onset of headache in patient over age 40
- Increased blood pressure
- Loss of consciousness

---

by patients simply to designate a severe headache. This can create confusion. A headache history is an important diagnostic tool that will help with the differential diagnosis.

Types of Headaches

Several types of headaches are common: migraine with aura (also known as classic migraine), migraine without aura (common migraine) and tension headaches. Less common are cluster headaches, posttraumatic headaches, headaches associated with vascular disorders (such as stroke, hematoma and hypertension) and headaches from intracranial pathology. A new classification was published in 1988.[11]

Migraine Headache

Migraine headaches are a type of vascular headache. Typically, they are recurrent episodes of throbbing pain accompanied by nausea, vomiting and/or anorexia.[12] There is frequently a family history of migraine; the majority of sufferers are women. In fact, migraine headaches are more common in females than males by an approximate 2:1 ratio.[12]

Migraine with aura is most often unilateral, throbbing pain accompanied by prodromal symptoms that occur just prior to or during the attack, usually developing over 5 to 20 minutes and lasting less than 60 minutes. These symptoms are distinct focal neurological deficits, such as visual disturbances: scotomata (isolated areas within the visual field in which vision is absent or depressed); specifically, scintillating scotomata or fortification spectra (zig-zag lines). Unilateral weakness or numbness, dizziness, photophobia and phonophobia can also occur. Importantly, however, the neurological symptoms resolve when the headache subsides.

In contrast, migraine without aura is *not* accompanied by focal neurological symptoms and is more commonly characterized by bilateral pain than is classic migraine. This variety of migraine is seen more frequently in the general population than is classic migraine.[12] Many patients report that fatigue, bright light, certain foods or beverages (aged cheese or alcohol, for example) and weather changes trigger both types of migraine episodes.

The etiology of migraine is not fully understood. A hormonal mechanism may be involved; many women report that migraine episodes are linked to their menstrual cycle. "Menstrual" migraine has been defined as a migraine that occurs prior to or during menstruation, but not at other times. Falling levels of female sex hormones may trigger the migraine with onset of menses or during the hormone-free interval of OCs.

Tension Headache

The most common type of headache is "muscle-contraction" or tension headache. A tension headache is often associated with depression, anxiety, emotional upset or stress and is characterized by bilateral pain and a tight band-like sensation.[12] Often, the neck and shoulder muscles are tight. The pain is usually described as a dull, steady ache. Importantly, there are no neurological deficits and the pain may be alleviated by the administration of aspirin, acetaminophen, nonsteroidal anti-inflammatories or muscle relaxants.

Data on Oral Contraceptives and Headaches

In the 1988 classification system, the International Headache Society listed a category entitled *"Birth control pill or estrogens"* with the comment, "The literature on this subject is conflicting. Further study is needed."[11] The package insert on oral contraceptives states, "The onset or exacerbation of migraine or development of headache with a new pattern which is recurrent, persistent, or severe requires discontinuation of oral contraceptives and evaluation of the cause."[13]

A comprehensive review of the literature found virtually no evidence to support a relationship between OCs and migraine. Benson and Rebar found that the available evidence "does not support the belief that those women who use oral contraceptives have a higher incidence of migraine headache...[and the data] do not indicate that migraine headache is necessarily a contraindication to prescribing oral contraceptives."[14]

Few studies have looked at whether or not OCs increase the risk of migraine occurrence. Furthermore, most studies of OCs fail to look at symptoms before the study is initiated. A Hungarian study of women with menstrual migraine headaches found that some worsened, but many improved or ceased to have headaches.[15] Other studies have had methodological problems, such as ascertainment bias and a nonblind protocol, so that a definite conclusion regarding the relationship of OCs to migraine could not be drawn.[14] A large, prospective cohort trial, the Walnut Creek Contraceptive Drug Study, did not find any evidence of a higher risk of either tension or migraine headaches among OC users.[16] "Thus," Benson and Rebar conclude, "the evidence that suggests that the pill exacerbates migraine headache in terms of either frequency or severity is weak at best."[14] However, experiencing an increased number or severity of headaches can be a cause for noncompliance with OCs in teens, whatever the cause of the headaches.[17]

Migraine, OCs and Risk of CVA

No conclusive evidence exists that women with migraine headaches who use OCs are more likely to develop a CVA than are nonusers. In 1975, the Collaborative Group for the Study of Stroke in Young Women published a case-control study of 568 young women hospitalized for stroke.[18] Only 30 patients had both migraine headaches and were OC users. Because of the differences between risks for hospital controls and neighborhood controls, the presence of migraine as a risk factor was viewed by the authors as inconclusive. "Our data do not confirm previous reports suggesting that migraine may increase the risk of stroke in women using oral contraceptives."

The International Headache Society has noted that "no causal relationship" has been established between migraine without aura and cerebral infarction. Increased risk for stroke in migraine patients has not been found in population-based studies, indicating that stroke is a rare complication of migraine."[11]

Clinical Guidelines

Given the common presentation of headache in clinical practice and the conflicting literature on OCs and migraine, which guidelines are useful for clinicians? Making the distinction between migraine with aura, migraine without aura and tension headache is relevant because each type of headache suggests different contraceptive management (Figure 2).

The potential for increased risks to patients who experience migraine headaches with aura should be carefully explained and alternative methods of contraception explored. Some physicians feel that migraine with aura, especially with pronounced visual or hemiplegic symptoms, is a strong contraindication to OC use; others balance risks for the individual patient (smoking, age, etc) with the risk of pregnancy. This decision must be weighed with care if the patient has factors that might predispose her to a high-risk pregnancy should she use a less-effective contraceptive method and conceive. How often the patient experiences a migraine should also be taken into consideration when evaluating the risk-to-benefit ratio.

In the case of migraine without aura, there is no evidence to suggest that OCs should not be used. Tension headaches also present no contraindication to initiating oral contraceptives, nor do they

---

Figure 2

Clinical Recommendations

Classic migraine (with aura)
- Avoid use of OC if patient can use alternative method of contraception
- Consider frequency of headache

Common migraine (without aura)
- No contraindication to OC use
- Further evaluate if headaches change to include neurological symptoms, especially double vision or loss of vision

Tension headache
- No contraindication to OC use
- May want to lower estrogen/ progestin dose
- Encourage patient to manage stress/tension

---

warrant discontinuation of OCs in a current user. The patient would probably benefit from knowing that her OC is not responsible for her headaches and should be directed to look for ways to manage stress.

For women who are taking OCs and develop headaches, one way to assess the potential role of the oral contraceptive is to use a nonhormonal contraceptive for a month or two and monitor the effect on the headaches. The physician may wish to change to a pill formulation with the lowest estrogen dose possible. A progestin-only pill, subdermal implants or injectable contraception could also be used.

When to Evaluate Headaches in OC Users

A worsening of migraine headaches, either in severity or frequency, or the new onset of headaches requires an evaluation (including blood pressure measurement). Headaches that are severe, persistent or of sudden onset, abnormal neurological signs that persist after a headache has resolved and headaches that are qualitatively different than the type normally experienced by the patient should be evaluated and would warrant discontinuing OCs, at least temporarily, until the situation is resolved (Figure 3) or an alternative diagnosis is made. If OCs are discontinued, practitioners should counsel patients about alternative methods of contraception.

Figure 3

Headaches Requiring Further Evaluation

- Previously existing migraines suddenly worsen or change
- Headaches of unusual severity and sudden onset
- Headaches followed by persistent abnormal neurological findings
- Headaches much worse when recumbent or with coughing, sneezing or valsalva maneuver
- Headache wakes patient from sleep
- Headaches begin at an older age without a previous history or positive family history

---

Source: Adapted from Digre K, 1987, et al (see reference 12).

References

1.	Mann JI, Vessey MP, Thorogood M, et al. Myocardial infarction in young women with special reference to oral contraceptive practice. *BMJ* 1975;2:241-244.

2.	Mann JI, Inman WHW. Oral contraceptives and death from myocardial infarction. *BMJ* 1975;2:245.

3.	Beral V. Mortality among oral contraceptive users: Royal College of General Practitioners' Oral Contraception Study. *Lancet* 1977;2:727.

4.	Vessey MP. Female hormones and vascular disease: an epidemiological overview. *Br J Fam Plann* 1980;6(suppl):1-12.

5.	Croft P, Hannaford PC. Risk factors for acute myocardial infarction in women: evidence from the Royal College of General Practitioners' oral contraception study. *BMJ* 1989;298:165-168.

6.	Stampfer MJ, Willett WC, Colditz GA, et al. Past use of oral contraceptives and cardiovascular disease: a meta-analysis in the context of the Nurses' Health Study. *Am J Obstet Gynecol* 1990;163:285-291.

7.	Porter JB, Hunter JR, Jick H, et al. Oral contraceptives and nonfatal vascular disease. *Obstet Gynecol* 1985;66:1-4.

8.	Linet MS, Stewart WF, Celentano DD, et al. An epidemiologic study of headache among adolescents and young adults. *JAMA* 1989;261:2211-2216.

9. Beiter M, Ingersoll G, Ganser J, et al. Relationships of somatic symptoms to behavioral and emotional risk in young adolescents. *J Pediatr* 1991;118:473-478.

10. Sillanpaa M. Changes in the prevalence of migraine and other headaches during the first seven school years. *Headache* 1983;23:15-19.

11. International Headache Society. Classification and diagnostic criteria for headache disorders, cranial neuralgias and facial pain. *Cephalalgia* 1988;8(suppl 7):1-96.

12. Digre K, Damasio H. Menstrual migraine: differential diagnosis, evaluation and treatment. *Clin Obstet Gynecol* 1987;30:417-430.

13. *Physicians' Desk Reference*. Oradell, NJ: Medical Economics Company, Inc., 1991.

14. Benson MD, Rebar RW. Relationship of migraine headache and stroke to oral contraceptive use. *J Reprod Med* 1986;31:1082-1088.

15. Karsay K. The relationship between vascular headaches and low-dose oral contraceptives. *Therapia Hungarica* 1990;38:181-185.

16. Ramcharan S, Pellegrin FA, Ray RM, et al. The Walnut Creek Contraceptive Drug Study. *J Reprod Med* 1980;25:346.

17. Emans SJ, Grace E, Woods ER, et al. Adolescents' compliance with the use of oral contraceptives. *JAMA* 1987;257:3377-3381.

18. Vessey MP, McPherson K, Yeates D. Oral contraceptives and stroke in young women: associated risk factors. *JAMA* 1975;75:718.

■2 Injectable Contraception

In late 1992, the Food and Drug Administration (FDA) approved depot medroxyproges-terone acetate (DMPA)—the first injectable contraceptive available in the United States. This highly effective, safe and long-term method of contraception requires user compliance only once every 13 weeks and can be used by many women in whom estrogen is contraindicated. Although the major concern regarding DMPA's effect on breast cancer has been researched for over 20 years, concern has been raised most recently over the potential impact of DMPA on bone mineral density, particularly among adolescents. As a result, more research is currently being conducted into this possible adverse effect. The first section of this chapter consists of an overview of the method and its long and arduous path to regulatory approval.

In the several years following, as U.S. clinicians gained more experience with the method, counseling issues came to the forefront. How could clinicians help women cope with menstrual changes and their potential impact on sexual relations? What about amenorrhea, the delay in return to fertility and weight gain? These and other issues are covered in the second section of this chapter, which provides an in-depth look at various counseling issues and gives suggestions as to how to address them.

2.1: Overview of FDA Approval

On October 29, 1992, the FDA approved DMPA as a long-acting injectable progestational contraceptive. The drug, previously approved in the U.S. for the treatment of endometrial and renal cancers, had been recommended for approval as a contraceptive by Fertility and Maternal Health Drugs Advisory Committees twice in the past (1973 and 1975); however, the FDA overruled these previous recommendations citing several safety concerns, most notably a possible increased breast cancer risk. The final approval recommendation, issued June 19, 1992, followed the publication of World Health Organization (WHO) data suggesting that women using DMPA have no overall increased risk of cancers.[1]

Use, Method of Action and Efficacy

Over the past 20 years, 30 million women in over 90 countries have used DMPA.[2,3] Women using the drug as a contraceptive usually receive a 150 mg dose every 13 weeks via intramuscular injection. DMPA is delivered in the form of microcrystals suspended in an aqueous solution, which slowly dissolve and release the drug into the body. Contraceptive levels of progestogen are maintained for up to 4 months following injection; however, clinicians should perform a pregnancy test if the patient returns for the next injection after the recommended 13 weeks.

In women using DMPA, circulating levels of progestogen are adequate to block the luteinizing hormone surge; thus, the method works primarily by suppressing ovulation. Secondary mechanisms of action include thickening of the cervical mucus and alteration of the endometrium, serving as barriers to sperm penetration and ovum implantation, respectively. The combined effect of these mechanisms makes DMPA a highly effective form of contraception—the expected failure rate is less than 1%. Moreover, because the method requires no daily compliance, the typical failure rate with DMPA is below 1% as well.[4]

DMPA in the U.S.

Safety concerns surrounding DMPA were first raised in the early 1970s, when toxicology studies in beagle dogs and rhesus monkeys found an increase in mammary gland tumors and endometrial cancer, respectively. Questioning the relevance of these findings to humans, in 1973 the FDA's Obstetrics and Gynecology Advisory Committee recommended approval of DMPA as a contraceptive for a subgroup of women unable to use reliable alternative methods. The committee again recommended DMPA for this limited patient population in 1975, following congressional hearings that had placed the drug's expected approval on hold. In 1978, however, the FDA denied approval, citing safety concerns that again included breast cancer as reported in the controversial beagle study. Three years later, the FDA appointed a public board of inquiry to conduct a scientific review of safety issues surrounding DMPA. The board's conclusion, submitted in 1984, stated

Figure 1

DMPA in the United States: Historical Perspective

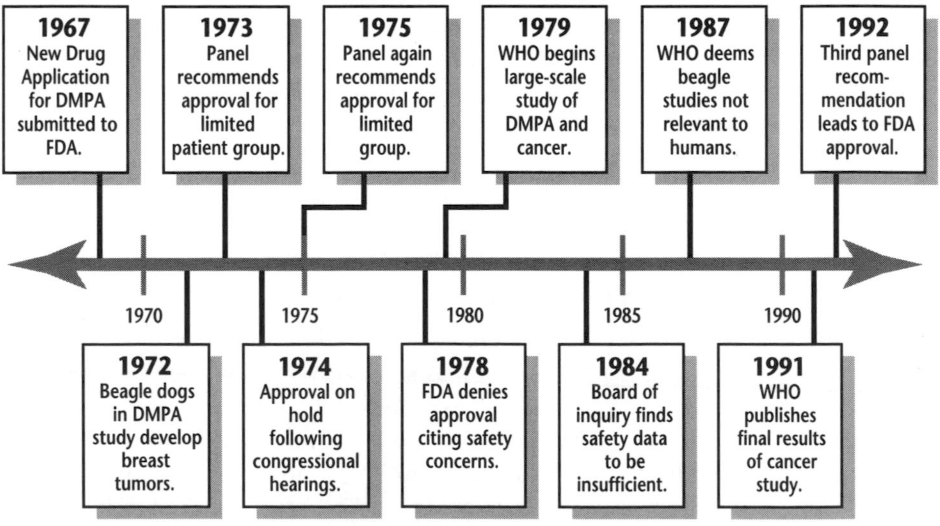

1967	1973	1975	1979	1987	1992
New Drug Application for DMPA submitted to FDA.	Panel recommends approval for limited patient group.	Panel again recommends approval for limited group.	WHO begins large-scale study of DMPA and cancer.	WHO deems beagle studies not relevant to humans.	Third panel recommendation leads to FDA approval.

	1970	1975	1980	1985	1990

1972	1974	1978	1984	1991
Beagle dogs in DMPA study develop breast tumors.	Approval on hold following congressional hearings.	FDA denies approval citing safety concerns.	Board of inquiry finds safety data to be insufficient.	WHO publishes final results of cancer study.

Source: Based on information presented at FDA advisory panel meeting, 1992 (see reference 6).

that existing data were insufficient to support FDA approval for broad-population use of DMPA as a contraceptive.[2]

In 1979, the year after the FDA denied approval, WHO began a large, hospital-based, case-control study of DMPA and cancer risk that spanned the following decade.[1] Subsequent to the reporting of the WHO study's final results on DMPA and breast cancer late in 1991, a third FDA advisory panel met to reexamine the 20-year-old question.[5] The committee reviewed evidence and listened to testimony regarding the safety concerns, side effects and benefits associated with DMPA. Figure 1 provides an overview of the drug's path to approval.

Breast Cancer

In terms of safety concerns with DMPA, the most attention over the past 2 decades has been devoted to the issue of breast cancer risk. Although originally cited as a reason for the 1978 FDA denial of approval for DMPA, the beagle dog toxicological study that first raised the breast cancer issue was eventually acknowledged by the FDA as not relevant to humans. Consequently, beagle and monkey studies are no longer required by the FDA for approval of steroid contraceptives. Addressing the advisory committee at the June 1992 meeting, FDA supervisory pharmacologist Alexander Jordan, PhD, admitted that "there are fundamentally different mechanisms operating in dogs and humans. ... It is now well known that the progesterone receptor in beagle dogs is not identical to the progesterone receptor in humans, such that certain steroids have a higher affinity for the progesterone receptor in dogs than in humans."[6] Dr. Jordan also noted that the extreme dose in the 1972 beagle study—25 times the human contraceptive dose—was largely responsible for the outcome.

The WHO Study

Dismissing the relevance of past animal studies, the FDA instructed the committee to take into consideration only the more recent human trials—specifically, the recently concluded WHO study. FDA Division of Metabolism and Endocrine Drugs Director Solomon Sobel, MD, explained that "the crucial studies are the epidemiologic studies of the World Health Organization, and these are the studies that I think are the most important ones for the committee to consider."[6]

David Thomas, MD, MPH, Professor and Head of the Program in Epidemiology at the Fred Hutchinson Cancer Research Center in Seattle and coordinator of the WHO Collaborative Study of Neoplasia and Steroid Contraceptives, presented the results of the study. With regard to epithelial ovarian cancer, liver cancer and invasive squamous cell cervical cancer, the researchers found no statistically significant alteration of risk associated with use of DMPA. As for endometrial cancer, Dr. Thomas noted that DMPA use was associated with a reduction in risk similar to that observed with oral contraceptives.[1]

Presenting and analyzing the findings for breast cancer, Dr. Thomas noted that the overall relative risk (RR) in ever-users of DMPA was 1.2 (95% confidence interval [CI], 1.0-1.5). He also noted that the risk estimates were elevated in short-term users as well as in women under age 35 (Table 1).[1,6]

Table 1

Relative Risk of Breast Cancer in DMPA Users

Feature of use	Age at Diagnosis ≤34 years	All ages
Any use	1.4 (0.9–2.2)	1.2 (1.0–1.5)
Months of use		
≤3	1.4 (0.6–3.2)	1.7 (1.1–2.6)
4–12	1.3 (0.6–2.7)	1.2 (0.8–1.7)
13–36	1.5 (0.7–3.1)	1.3 (0.8–1.9)
≥37	1.5 (0.7–3.3)	0.9 (0.6–1.4)

( )=95% confidence interval

Source: Adapted from WHO, 1991 (see reference 1).

"The breast cancer risk was highest," explained Dr. Thomas, "in women who used DMPA for less than or equal to 3 months—that is to say, with a single injection. And, the risk actually decreased—at least, these estimates decreased—with additional months of use. So, it appears to be a phenomenon in short-term users." Dr. Thomas went on to explain that, in his view, the increase in relative risk in women under age 35 was probably caused by the increased likelihood of finding recent users in this younger age group: "My interpretation of the age effect is that it has to do with there being more recent users in the younger age group—and it is really a recency of use effect." He noted that this phenomenon also was seen in a recent New Zealand study, the results of which were comparable to the WHO study.[7] (In 1995, researchers pooled WHO and New Zealand data and found no overall increased risk of breast cancer in ever-users of DMPA.[8] See summary that follows.)

According to Dr. Thomas and the WHO researchers, since an increase in breast cancer risk is noted soon after initiation of DMPA use and the overall risk does not increase over time, DMPA appears, if anything, to stimulate the growth of existing tumors rather than promote the formation of new ones—the latter being a far greater cause for concern.[1,6] Dr. Thomas concluded that the "risks of cancer associated with use of DMPA are low and are no greater than cancer risks associated with use of oral contraceptives. As with all other contraceptives, the risks and benefits of DMPA should be made known to women so that they can make their own informed decisions."[6]

Other Safety Concerns

In addition to the breast cancer issue, the FDA asked the advisory panel to examine recent evidence involving DMPA's possible association with osteoporosis and low birth weight.

Breast Cancer Risk and DMPA

Pooled results from two case-control studies suggest no overall increased risk of breast cancer among women who have ever used DMPA.[8] The analysis pooled results from a trial conducted by the World Health Organization and a trial with similar design features conducted in New Zealand. The pooled data suggested no elevated breast cancer risk for women who had ever used DMPA (RR=1.1; 95% CI, 0.97-1.4). In addition, no increase in risk occurred with increasing durations of DMPA use. Similar reassuring findings have been reported from many large studies, including those conducted over a decade ago by the Centers for Disease Control and Prevention and Emory University School of Medicine.[9,10]

Relative risk estimates were higher in certain subgroups (Figure 2). For example, women who had started using DMPA within the previous 5 years were estimated to have a RR of 2.0 (95% CI, 1.5-2.8), while current users of DMPA younger than 35 years of age had a RR of 2.1 (95% CI, 1.1-3.8). These findings may well be due to enhanced detection of breast tumors in recent or current users. The study authors concluded, "The increased risk of breast cancer observed in recent (or current) users could be due to enhanced detection of breast tumors in women using DMPA or to acceleration of the growth of preexisting tumors. Women who had used DMPA more than 5 years previously had no increase in risk of breast cancer, regardless of duration of use."

Figure 2

Relative Risk of Breast Cancer with DMPA Use: Pooled Results from World Health Organization and New Zealand Studies

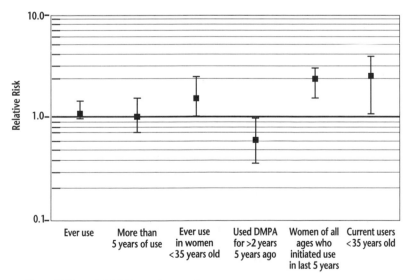

Source: Skegg DCG, et al, 1995 (see reference 8).

Addressing the issue of osteoporosis, Tim Cundy, MD, of the Department of Medicine at Auckland Hospital in New Zealand, discussed the findings of a study he and his colleagues published in 1991 on decreased bone density in DMPA users. The study compared women who had been using DMPA for at least 5 years with two control groups—premenopausal and postmenopausal women.[11] Bone density for each of the three groups was measured at the lumbar spine and the femoral neck. According to Dr. Cundy, in terms of bone density, "at the lumbar spine, the DMPA users were, on average, 7.5% lower than premenopausal controls, and at the femoral neck they were, on average, 6.5% lower than premenopausal controls." He noted that postmenopausal controls had a greater degree of bone density loss than the DMPA users.

Dr. Cundy pointed out that although lower density was associated with DMPA use, this effect did not increase with long-term use: "The deficit of bone density does not appear to get any larger with continued use of DMPA. There is no relationship here between years of DMPA use and apparent deficit in bone density." Furthermore, referring to preliminary findings from a prospective study still in progress [now published], Dr. Cundy noted that the loss in bone density associated with DMPA use appears to be reversible.[12] Dr. Cundy noted that following termination of DMPA use, "the average increase in bone density at the first year was 3%... at the end of 2 years, it was 6%." Based on this information, the panel recommended that research continue in the area of bone density and DMPA use, and that product labeling address this potential adverse effect; however, it concluded that the overall risk/benefit balance was not seriously affected by the issue. (Editor's note: Research is ongoing, particularly concerning the effect of DMPA on bone density during adolescence. For further discussion, see section 2.2 in this chapter.)

Ronald Gray, MD, of The Johns Hopkins School of Hygiene and Public Health, addressed the panel on the topic of low birth weight in infants exposed to DMPA during pregnancy. Dr. Gray explained the results of a cohort study he and his colleagues performed in Thailand.[13] The study found that "among those pregnancies estimated to have occurred within the first 4 weeks after a [DMPA] injection, there was a twofold increased risk of low birth weight and that risk diminished as we moved further away from time of injection to estimated time of conception."

Dr. Gray concluded that the attributable risks of low birth weight were "very, very small" and did not constitute an important problem with DMPA. He also pointed out the "if the first injection of DMPA is given within 5 days of the onset of the last regular menstrual period, then one can avoid giving the drug to already pregnant women. ...Similarly, if repeat injections are within 14 weeks, we can avoid accidental pregnancies." The panel's recommendations took this into account, as committee chairwoman Barbara Hulka, MD, MPH, Kenan Professor and Chair of the Department of Epidemiology at the University of North Carolina School of Public Health, stated, "the committee recommends, in terms of the infant birth weight issue, that the labeling be very clear about timing of the injection during the menstrual cycle so that no pregnant women get DMPA." (In 1995, the manufacturer of DMPA instituted labeling changes to clarify questions concerning the timing of injections. For further discussion, see section 2.2 in this chapter.)

DMPA Side Effects

The most widely noted short-term side effects of DMPA use are menstrual changes.[14,15] Although these changes are unpredictable, they are universal in users of injectable progestogen contraception. Irregular bleeding and spotting are common during the first few months of DMPA use; these episodes may last 7 days or more. With increased duration of use, bleeding and spotting episodes occur less frequently and are shorter in length. Amenorrhea is common following 9 to 12 months of DMPA use. Irregular bleeding patterns and amenorrhea are also the most frequent reasons for method discontinuation. A 1986 multicenter study by WHO found cumulative discontinuation rates at 12 months for women using DMPA (150 mg) to be slightly more than 13% for bleeding-related reasons and just under 13% for amenorrhea.[14]

Bleeding irregularities associated with DMPA are similar to those noted with other progestin-only contraceptive methods, although the incidence of amenorrhea is markedly different. Responding to a question about the differences between injectable and implantable progestational contraceptives in terms of menstrual changes and amenorrhea, Andrew Kaunitz, MD, Associate Professor of Obstetrics and Gynecology at the University of Florida Health Science Center at Jacksonville, explained that "with long-term use, women using DMPA tend to experience amenorrhea, with 50% incidence of amenorrhea with 1 year of use. Then, the incidence of amenorrhea with more prolonged use increases beyond that. ...The incidence of amenorrhea in women using subdermal progestin implants long term is less than 10%." Dr. Kaunitz noted, however, that not all women consider amenorrhea to be a negative consequence of DMPA therapy—some consider it a desirable effect. He stressed the need for appropriate patient selection and proper counseling with regard to menstrual changes to encourage compliance and continuation.

Other side effects noted with DMPA use include weight gain, headache, breast tenderness and psychological effects, such as loss of libido, depression, nervousness and fatigue.[14,15] Of these, weight gain is the most common. The package insert lists an approximate weight gain of 5 pounds at 1 year, 8 pounds at 2 years, 14 pounds at 4 years and 17 pounds at 6 years. The amount of weight gain may also depend on individual differences. Committee members expressed concern that the size of the weight gain might be a deterrent for some women.[6]

Some data published since the time of the FDA meeting, however, suggest DMPA may not cause significant weight gain, at least during the first year of use.[16,17] In a small randomized trial (71 women), Mainwaring et al found no significant weight gain at 1 year among users of levonorgestrel subdermal implants, DMPA or oral norethindrone.[16] Moore et al performed a retrospective chart review of 50 patients each using oral contraceptives, subdermal implants or DMPA. At 1 year, no significant weight change occurred in any of the treatment groups.[17] (For further discussion concerning counseling patients regarding weight gain, see section 2.2 in this chapter.)

An additional concern that has been raised regarding DMPA use is return of fertility. Following a 150 mg injection of the drug, the mean interval before return of ovulation is 4.5 months. The delay to conception is approximately 9 months following the last

DMPA injection and is unaffected by duration of use.[15,18] There is no evidence of any change in fertility 2 years after discontinuation of DMPA.

Benefits of DMPA Use

Weighed against the potential risks and side effects of DMPA are a number of substantial benefits—both contraceptive and noncontraceptive. The method is highly effective, with failure rates below 1%.[4] The panel had high regard for DMPA's effectiveness: "I am impressed first by the unchallenged efficacy of the drug," noted committee member Ezra Davidson, MD, Professor and Chair of the Department of Obstetrics and Gynecology at the Charles D. Drew Postgraduate Medical School in Los Angeles. Other contraceptive benefits of DMPA include its lack of interference with intercourse, long-acting nature, virtual freedom from compliance concerns and lack of estrogen-related side effects. This last benefit allows DMPA to be considered for patients with a history of thromboembolism, women over 35 who smoke, and certain congenital heart disease patients.

In patients with sickle-cell disease, a noncontraceptive benefit of DMPA is that it may inhibit intravascular sickling and increase hemoglobin and red blood cell survival.[19] Other noncontraceptive benefits of the drug include evidence that DMPA may increase the quantity and protein content of milk in breastfeeding mothers,[20] and prolong the length of time a woman is able to nurse her child.[21] While DMPA neither increases nor decreases a woman's risk of epithelial ovarian cancer,[22] the hormone does reduce the risk of endometrial cancer.[23] Furthermore, DMPA likely has the same benefits associated with the progestin element of oral contraceptives: less pelvic inflammatory disease (PID),[24] fewer ectopic pregnancies and less endometriosis.[13] In fact, DMPA has been used as a treatment for endometriosis.

An additional benefit of DMPA is potential long-term cost-effectiveness. Addressing the panel on behalf of Jacqueline Darroch Forrest, PhD, Vice President for Research at the Alan Guttmacher Institute (AGI) in New York, Lisa Kaeser (also from AGI) compared DMPA to other cost-effective, long-acting contraceptives. She noted that DMPA and other "long-acting reversible methods, like [subdermal implants] and the [copper] IUD, can be very cost-efficient over the long run."

Patient Selection

Patients who are seeking reliable, long-term reversible contraception—especially those for whom other reversible methods are problematic—are suitable candidates for DMPA use. Problems with other reversible methods may include a contraindication to the estrogen in oral contraceptives, medical factors that preclude the use of intrauterine contraception, and difficulty with compliance or side effects. It is important for practitioners to inform potential users adequately of possible short- and long-term side effects, with particular emphasis on those most closely associated with discontinuation (ie, menstrual disturbances). Appropriate patient selection practices should be complemented by easy access to follow-up counseling, ensuring the highest degree of patient comfort, reassurance and satisfaction with the method.

Conclusion

After considering many aspects of DMPA and weighing the risks and benefits of the drug's use as a contraceptive, the Fertility and Maternal Health Drugs Advisory Committee voted 7-0 in favor of recommending FDA approval of DMPA for this purpose. Regarding the issue of osteoporosis, the panel recommended additional studies be performed to determine DMPA's effect on bone density. The committee also stressed the need for inclusion of the potential osteoporosis risk in product labeling and on informed consent documents. Additional research and clear product labeling were also recommended with regard to the infant birth weight issue. The advisory committee's third unanimous recommendation for approval of DMPA as a contraceptive—and the FDA's subsequent decision to approve the drug for this purpose—demonstrated a conviction that any potential safety concerns with DMPA were outweighed by the drug's benefits as an additional contraceptive choice for women in the U.S.

References

1. WHO Collaborative Study of Neoplasia and Steroid Contraceptives. Breast cancer and depot-medroxyprogesterone acetate: a multinational study. *Lancet* 1991;338:833-838.

2. Kaunitz AM. Injectable contraception. *Clin Obstet Gynecol* 1989;32:356-367.

3. Upjohn's *Depo-Provera C-150* long-acting injectable contraceptive recommended for approval by advisory committee after almost 20 years of FDA consideration. *F-D-C Reports, "The Pink Sheet"* 1992;54(25):3-4.

4. Trussell J, Hatcher RA, Cates W Jr., et al. Contraceptive failure in the United States: an update. *Stud Fam Plann* 1990;21:51-54.

5. Upjohn *Depo-Provera* benefits outweigh risks of osteoporosis and low birthweight, FDA cmte. concludes; Women's Health Network opposes approval. *F-D-C Reports, "The Pink Sheet"* 1992;54(26):8-9.

6. Food and Drug Administration. Fertility and Maternal Health Drugs Advisory Committee (meeting transcript). Washington, DC: U.S. Department of Health and Human Services; 1992.

7. Paul C, Skegg DCG, Spears GFS. Depot medroxyprogesterone (Depo-Provera) and risk of breast cancer. *BMJ* 1989;299:759-762.

8. Skegg DCG, Noonan EA, Paul C, et al. Depot medroxyprogesterone acetate and breast cancer. A pooled analysis of the World Health Organization and New Zealand studies. *JAMA* 1995;273: 799-804.

9. Greenspan AR, Hatcher RA, Moore M, et al. The association of depo-medroxyprogesterone acetate and breast cancer. *Contraception* 1980;21:563-569.

10. Liang AP, Greenspan Levenson A, Layde PM, et al. Risk of breast, uterine corpus, and ovarian cancer in women receiving medroxyprogesterone injections. *JAMA* 1983;249:2909-2912.

11. Cundy T, Evans M, Roberts H, et al. Bone density in women receiving depot medroxyprogesterone acetate for contraception. *BMJ* 1991;303:13-16.

12. Cundy T, Cornish J, Evans MC, et al. Recovery of bone density in women who stop using medroxy- progesterone acetate. *BMJ* 1994;308:247-248.

13. Gray R, Pardthaisong T. In utero exposure to steroid contraceptives and survival during infancy. *Am J Epidemiol* 1991;134:804-811.

14. World Health Organization. A multi-centered phase III comparative clinical trial of depot-medroxyprogesterone acetate given three-monthly at doses of 100 mg or 150 mg: I. Contraceptive efficacy and side effects. *Contraception* 1986;34:223-235.

15. Lande RE. New era for injectables. *Population Reports* August 1995;Volume 23, Number 2.

16. Pardthaisong T. Return of fertility after use of the injectable contraceptive Depo Provera: up-dated analysis. *J Biosoc Sci* 1984;16:23-34.

17. Mainwaring R, Hales HA, Stevenson K, et al. Metabolic parameter, bleeding, and weight changes in U.S. women using progestin only contraceptives. *Contraception* 1995;51:149-153.

18. Moore LL, Valuck R, McDougall C, et al. A comparative study of one-year weight gain among users of medroxyprogesterone acetate, levonorgestrel implants, and oral contraceptives. *Contraception* 1995;52:215-220.

19. De Ceulaer K, Gruber C, Hayes R, et al. Medroxyprogesterone acetate and homozygous sickle-cell disease. *Lancet* 1982;2:229-231.

20. Costa TH, Dorea JG. Concentration of fat, protein, lactose and energy in milk of mothers using hormonal contraceptives. *Ann Trop Paediatr* 1992;12:203-209.

21. Briend A, Fauveau V, Chakraborty J. Contraceptive use and breast-feeding duration in rural Bangladesh. *Eur J Clin Nutr* 1991;45:341-346.

22. Stanford JL, Thomas DB. Depot-medroxyprogesterone acetate (DMPA) and risk of epithelial ovarian cancer. *Int J Cancer* 1991;49:191-195.

23. Thomas DB, Ray RM. Depot-medroxyprogesterone acetate (DMPA) and risk of endometrial cancer. *Int J Cancer* 1991;49:186-190.

24. Gray RH. Reduced risk of pelvic inflammatory disease with injectable contraceptives. *Lancet* 1985;1:1046.

2.2: Patient Counseling

Depot medroxyprogesterone acetate (DMPA) was approved by the Food and Drug Administration (FDA) for use as a contraceptive in the United States in October 1992 after almost 25 years of investigation and debate. The U.S. was the 92nd country to approve DMPA for contraception. Since then, many American clinicians have acquired experience in counseling patients about the method.

Introduction

The availability of long-acting methods has given family planning providers an impetus to refine their counseling skills. This is the message of Linda Dominguez, CNP, Senior Nurse Practitioner at Planned Parenthood of New Mexico in Albuquerque: "One of my main messages to providers is that DMPA has offered us an opportunity to refresh our family planning message. We've had to assess both the kind of information we provide and the manner in which it is given in order to determine whether we're enhancing the patient's success with the method. For example, if a woman was unhappy with a short-acting method, such as the pill, she could easily stop using it— she had control over when to stop and start. With a long-acting method, such as DMPA, however, because it can't be taken out once it's been given, the quality of our counseling and the quality of the patient's understanding have become that much more important."

Offering All Options

Women should be aware of all the methods available to them. Paula J. A. Hillard, MD, Associate Editor of *The Contraception Report*, explained that "Even if a woman comes to me asking specifically for DMPA, I make sure to backtrack and cover other options. For example, if she's an appropriate candidate for the intrauterine device (IUD) I'll ask her, 'Do you know the IUD is available? Have you ever considered the

IUD as a contraceptive method?' It's important to make sure the woman knows about all her options and their specific advantages and disadvantages.

"We're getting a lot of referrals from adolescents who are telling their friends about DMPA. Particularly for adolescents who have had problems taking the pill or who have been dissatisfied with barrier methods, the convenience of 'the shot' (DMPA) is attractive," Dr. Hillard said. In fact, one study of 536 women attending 17 family planning clinics in Texas found that the main source of information about DMPA was friends (42%), followed by health care providers (37%) and family members (16%).[1]

Interestingly, media-fostered misperceptions do not seem widespread concerning DMPA. The study of Texan women found that only 10% received their information on DMPA from media sources.[1] Dr. Hillard commented, "Even though DMPA has been on the market for a long time for other indications and has been available in other countries, recently it hasn't gotten the kind of press that the pill has gotten. So, today's women do not seem to have the concerns about its safety or the misunderstandings about the method they tend to have with the pill.

"One misperception I've encountered among some clinicians," Dr. Hillard continued, "has been that DMPA can be relied upon to induce amenorrhea. Although DMPA has been used to suppress menses, it's not a guarantee. Of course, longer durations of use result in a greater likelihood of amenorrhea; however, the percentage of patients who become amenorrheic is only about 50% during the first year."

Menstrual Changes

The major side effects of DMPA are menstrual disturbances, weight gain and a delay in the return of fertility. These side effects, particularly changes in menstruation, can have a substantial impact on a woman's decision initially to select and to continue with the method.

Almost all women using DMPA will experience spotting, irregular or prolonged bleeding, particularly during the first few months of use.[2,3] Amenorrhea occurs in about half of women by the end of 1 year and increasingly thereafter.[4] Changes in menstrual patterns and their implications need to be thoroughly explained to women prior to the first injection because they constitute the primary cause of discontinuation.

Why are menstrual changes disturbing for women? From the time young women begin to menstruate, they learn that periods are generally supposed to come on a regular basis and that a lack of menses may mean they are pregnant. Variations in regularity may not be considered "normal." Although changes in menstrual patterns are not medically serious, they have psychological and sociological implications.

Cultural factors influence the meaning of menses to women and their perceptions of themselves while they are bleeding. For example, menstruating women may be prohibited from participating in food preparation if they are Hindu or from prayer if they are Muslim.[5] Some religions (Orthodox Judaism, Hinduism and the Muslim religions) prohibit intercourse during vaginal bleeding, thus affecting the couple's sex life.[6] Furthermore, many consider intercourse during menses or any vaginal bleeding unhygienic. Men's beliefs about menstruation also may influence how women perceive changes in their menstrual patterns.

A Chilean study of about 500 men and women found that the majority avoid sexual intercourse during menses or spotting.[6] The most common reason cited was that sexual relations during menstruation are "not hygienic" (46% of women and 37% of men), followed by "uncomfortable" (41% of women and 38% of men) and "it's dirty" (16% of women and 16% of men).

Menstrual changes also can be inconvenient or embarrassing. The woman may need more sanitary supplies, become more self-conscious or change the way she dresses. Visiting the bathroom frequently may not be convenient or feasible.

Knowledge of the Menstrual Cycle

Basic knowledge about the menstrual cycle may help women accept bleeding changes induced by DMPA. According to Linda Dominguez, one way to enhance acceptance of the method is by briefly reviewing some basic reproductive anatomy and physiology with the patient. She explained, "If the woman does not have a core understanding of her normal menstrual cycle, then she is less likely to accept your reassurances that changes in her menses are okay.

"Remember that women may believe certain myths about menses and menstrual blood. For example, here in the Southwest it's a commonly held perception that women of color—Hispanic, Native American and African-American women—believe that if they don't bleed for a certain number of days that it's harmful. The myth is that 'unclean vapors' or 'bad blood' builds up inside the body. But, I have found that all women have concrete, fundamental beliefs about the way they're supposed to bleed. What I've found is that a disturbance in a woman's menstrual pattern often creates a disturbance in her identity, her psyche, her feeling of well-being.

"What I like to do," Ms. Dominguez continued, "is to spend a few minutes explaining the normal menstrual cycle to women. I use concrete terms they can understand. During my explanation, I link ovulation and the endometrial lining together and make a simple drawing of the uterus and ovaries."

Menstrual Irregularities and Sexual Activity

Bleeding irregularities may affect a woman's sex life. Ms. Dominguez emphasized, "One reason for discontinuing DMPA is that menstrual irregularities interfere with the couple's lovemaking. This is often an *unspoken* reason for discontinuation. After talking to women about bleeding patterns, I naturally move into this subject. I ask: 'If you have this kind of bleeding, is that going to be a problem for you and your sexual partner?' Often, clinicians don't ask this question and the woman may not make the connection herself. If the woman realizes that her partner is not going to touch her while she's bleeding, she may decide to choose another method. You need to reassure her that breakthrough bleeding does not mean she's bleeding to death, is hemorrhaging, has cancer or is going to get cancer. But, while you're trying to reassure her about irregular bleeding, if it's going to be a problem with her sexual partner, all your reassurances won't matter. The client may return later, unhappy with the method, but not telling you the real reason why."

While menstrual irregularities are to be expected, persistent or heavy bleeding should be investigated. Dr. Hillard advised, "Although heavy bleeding may be due to DMPA, we must not forget that our patients are sexually active and at risk for sexually transmitted diseases (STDs). STDs and other pathology need to be ruled out if a patient complains of unusually heavy or persistent bleeding."

Amenorrhea

About half of women will experience amenorrhea within the first year. Some women find the side effect problematic; others welcome it. Becky Schroder, ARNP, MSN, and Supervisor of Women's Health Research in the Department of Obstetrics and Gynecology at the University of Florida Health Science Center in Jacksonville, shared her experience regarding DMPA and its side effects. Ms. Schroder, who is helping to conduct a study on DMPA and has used the method herself, said, "We need to be realistic with patients and let them know that not everyone will experience amenorrhea. Patients need to understand that bleeding patterns vary greatly and they may not be among the group that stops bleeding."

Ms. Schroder also cautioned that women need to fully understand that amenorrhea does not mean they are pregnant. She shared, "Even though I have a medical background and was very familiar with DMPA, the first month I didn't get my period I was concerned that I might be pregnant. Most women will need a lot of reassurance about this particular side effect."

Management of Bleeding Irregularities

The primary management of menstrual irregularities consists of reassurance from the clinician. According to Dr. Hillard, "Tell patients if they experience side effects that they should call, they don't have to suffer. It's important for patients to know the name of the person they can call if they have questions or concerns. This contact person may be the physician, nurse or resident who's been following the patient. A large part of management is reassurance; however, the effectiveness of the reassurance depends, in part, on the development of a trusting relationship with the patient.

"Time is also on the patient's side. Patients should be told that irregular bleeding is likely to decrease the longer they use DMPA. For some women, reassurance that there is nothing medically wrong is enough, while others may need more concrete intervention."

Management strategies vary (Figure 1). The clinician may want to prescribe a short course of estrogen, one or two cycles of oral contraceptives (OCs), or a non-steroidal anti-inflammatory other than aspirin. Dr. Hillard explained, "A short course of estrogen can be given for up to 3 weeks to help stabilize the endometrium; this will often help stop the bleeding. Patients need to be aware, however, that the bleeding may return when the medication is discontinued. Or, clinicians can prescribe one or two cycles of OCs.

"One study evaluated the effect of levonorgestrel, estrogen or ibuprofen on breakthrough bleeding in women using subdermal implants.[7] That study found that all three treatments reduced breakthrough bleeding compared to placebo. The use of

Figure 1

Strategies for Management of Irregular Bleeding with DMPA

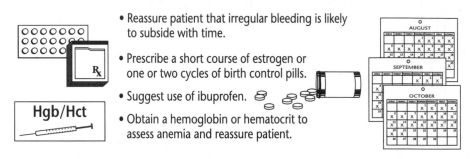

- Reassure patient that irregular bleeding is likely to subside with time.

- Prescribe a short course of estrogen or one or two cycles of birth control pills.

- Suggest use of ibuprofen.

- Obtain a hemoglobin or hematocrit to assess anemia and reassure patient.

ibuprofen 800 mg three times per day for 5 days reduced breakthrough bleeding by 27%; it has been suggested that nonsteroidal anti-inflammatory drugs also may help DMPA users. In addition to medical management, sometimes I will do a hemoglobin or hematocrit to provide reassurance for the patient. Having an objective measurement that she is not anemic will often help alleviate her anxiety."

Another strategy that has been suggested is giving the next injection before 3 months are up. Although no randomized trials confirm the efficacy of this approach, some clinicians suggest giving the next injection early may help to bring about amenorrhea sooner.[8] One study, however, found that giving the next injection early did not alter bleeding episodes.[9]

Ms. Lybia Burgos, CRNP, emphasized the importance of the clinician's commitment to providing ongoing counseling. Ms. Burgos is the Director of Special Medical Services at Planned Parenthood of New York City. In August 1995, she spoke about counseling strategies for long-acting methods of contraception at a workshop sponsored by the Center for Population Research of the National Institute for Child Health and Human Development. She told the conference participants, "When you provide long-acting contraception, you have to be ready to commit yourself to counseling women before, during and after method use. With the two long-acting methods, we [Planned Parenthood of NYC] provide [injectables and implants], we talk to patients on the telephone and see them quite frequently. Counseling before DMPA must be thorough and help patients anticipate how menstrual irregularities may affect them. During use, women usually need reassurance about menstrual changes.

"Why do you need to counsel women *after* they stop using DMPA? If the patient's been amenorrheic and she doesn't get her period right away, often she'll call the clinic and ask, 'When am I going to get my period? Aren't you going to give me something to bring it on?' What I'd like to emphasize is that counseling requires a commitment throughout use; just because the woman stops using DMPA doesn't mean that she stops having concerns or questions."

DMPA Discontinuation Rates

About one-third of patients stop using DMPA by the end of 1 year; about one-half do so by the end of 2 years. Adolescent discontinuation rates appear similar. One study of 50 teens using DMPA found that a little over two-thirds used the drug for 1 year.[10] At 2 years, about half were using the drug; by the end of 3 years only 18% continued to use DMPA (Figure 2). Although amenorrhea has been cited as a common reason for discontinuation among adult women, this side effect was well tolerated by the adolescents; 72% of those experiencing amenorrhea were happy about it.

Finding another contraceptive option for women who discontinue DMPA is important to prevent unintended pregnancy. Women who express dissatisfaction with bleeding irregularities probably should be encouraged to use another method that will not interfere with regular menstrual cycles. For example, subdermal implants are probably not the ideal choice for a woman who disliked irregular bleeding with injectable contraception. "On the other hand," Dr. Hillard suggested, "a logical choice for women discontinuing DMPA is the pill. Because cycle regularity is likely to be very important to these women, clinicians should find a pill formulation that gives the patient good cycle control with minimal breakthrough bleeding."

Women who discontinue DMPA and switch to the pill probably will need help to take it correctly and consistently. Often, women who have chosen DMPA have done so because of problems with compliance. In fact, in a prospective study of teens using either DMPA, subdermal implants or OCs, almost 90% of young women using DMPA

Figure 2

Continuation Rates among Adolescents Using DMPA

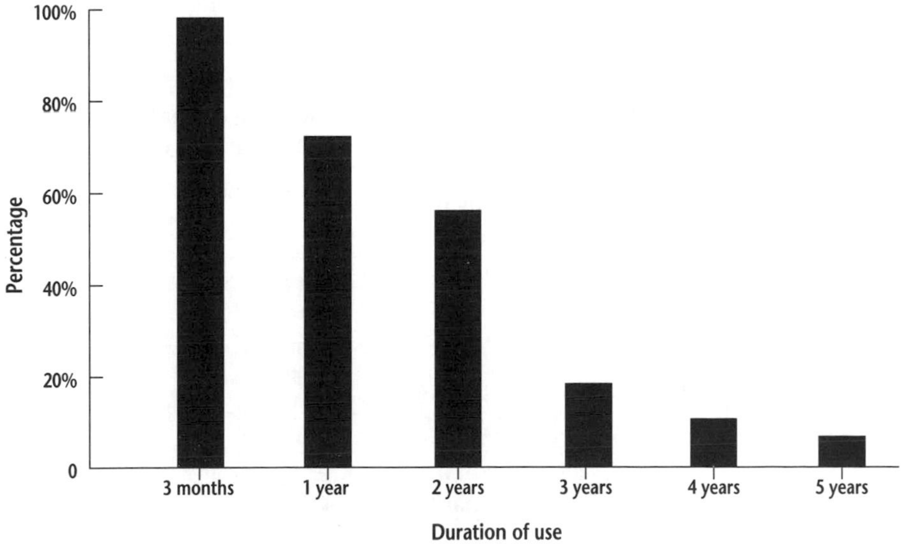

Source: Smith RD, et al, 1995 (see reference 10).

liked the fact that they didn't have to remember to use it.[11] It's a good idea to help women associate pill-taking with a routine activity, such as eating breakfast, brushing the teeth or going to bed. Other compliance aids include providing clear, written instructions and making sure to tell the patient to take one pill every day.

Knowledge about the normal menstrual cycle may help to prevent women from discontinuing DMPA and switching to less effective methods or no method. Ms. Dominguez commented, "Frequently patients tell me after they've been on a hormonal method, 'I'm going to use condoms because I need to get everything out of my system.' I think if we've done our job well of explaining the normal menstrual cycle and how it's altered with long-acting hormonal methods, the patient's not as likely to have the idea that somehow her system needs to be 'cleaned' or 'purged.' Hopefully she'll not be as likely to make a big leap from hormonal contraception to using nothing, or to less-effective methods like condoms alone or to condoms only occasionally."

Weight Gain

Women need to be told about the likelihood of weight gain. The average weight gain with DMPA is as much as four to five pounds per year over 3 years, which then stabilizes. "The possibility of weight gain must be addressed with patients," Dr. Hillard stated. "Weight gain frequently occurs and patients must be made aware of it. There are women who may not be bothered by it; some cultures are more accepting of heavier women. For women who decide to use DMPA who are overweight to begin with, I'd refer them to a dietitian at the start to try to improve their chances of maintaining appropriate weight through proper diet and exercise."

Delay in Return of Fertility

A delay in the return of fertility, but not permanent impairment of fertility, occurs with DMPA.[12] Compared to users of other methods or no method, DMPA users have been found to have about a 9-month delay to restore full fertility after the last DMPA injection.

The importance of a delay in the return of fertility will vary among patients. According to Dr. Hillard, "With adolescents, I mention the delay in return to fertility, but it probably doesn't need to be emphasized. On the other hand, women who may want to become pregnant in the next year or two need to understand clearly what that delay means. I often explain it by telling patients, 'If 85% of women not using birth control get pregnant in 1 year, 85% of DMPA users will get pregnant within 2 years after they stop using it.'"

Helping Patients Manage Weight Gain with DMPA

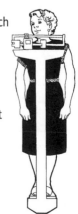

- Advise patient that weight gain of as much as 4 to 5 pounds per year is common with DMPA

- Inform patient that a healthy, balanced diet may help prevent weight gain

- Refer to dietitian if appropriate

- Encourage patient to exercise

Other Side Effects

Depression, headaches and premenstrual-like symptoms have been reported with DMPA. These side effects occur relatively infrequently, but need to be addressed. According to Dr. Hillard, "I don't see these symptoms very often. I see it less with the injectable formulation than I do with even short courses of oral medroxyprogesterone acetate."

Another side effect that patients may be worried about is decreased libido. Clinicians can address this concern by providing reassurance. According to Lybia Burgos, "It's important to remember that you need to respond to how the woman is *feeling*, not just her words. If she's worried that she might be losing her sex drive, it's important to listen. When we offer patients this kind of support, it's not unusual to have them come back for their next injections and say that 'their sexual feelings are better.'"

Ideally, a baseline assessment should be made of the patient's level of sexual activity before use of DMPA. "Patients can become concerned when they read that they might experience a loss of libido," Linda Dominguez explained. "They might come in and say, 'I need something else because I have less sex drive.' It's important to assess the patient's prior sexual history. During my initial counseling I'll ask the patient, 'Tell me how you feel about sex. Are you comfortable with sex? Is it enjoyable for you?' If she says yes, good. If she says no, then I say, 'Well, this [DMPA] may not make it any better!' Then, I need to assess the reasons why she may be having difficulty with sex. If the patient complains of a loss of libido, how can you determine whether the effect is real or not if you haven't gotten some baseline information about her sex drive? It's important to obtain at least a brief sexual history during initial patient counseling."

Bone Density

One potential side effect of DMPA under investigation is loss of bone density. A small cross-sectional study published in 1991 first drew attention to the issue.[13] In a small follow-up study, the investigators found that the loss of bone density appears to be reversible.[14]

Methodological problems warrant cautious interpretation of these data. First, only cross-sectional data were obtained; no data were available on bone mineral densities before the use of DMPA. Ideally, because women vary so much in their bone densities, a baseline assessment of each individual's bone density should be made and then the women should be followed over time. Second, smoking may be confounding the results.[15] More women using DMPA were smokers, a known risk factor for osteoporosis. In addition, factors such as diet, exercise, prior pregnancy and history of amenorrhea all influence bone density and represent potential confounding variables in studies of this type.

Some clinicians feel that the potential for bone loss warrants cautious use in younger adolescents. S. Jean Emans, MD, Associate Editor of *The Contraception Report*, avoids the use of DMPA in adolescents 12 to 14 years of age. "Because young adolescents are gaining most of their bone mineralization for their lifetimes during this period, until we know more, I would not use DMPA as a first choice in this age group. Studies of adolescents are urgently needed."

Others argue that the benefits among young adolescents probably outweigh the risk of future osteoporosis. Joseph Goldzieher, MD, Associate Editor of *The Contraception Report*, explained that "Estrogen levels in DMPA users tend to be in the follicular-phase level, which is much more than in young amenorrheic athletes who do tend to osteopenia. In addition, pregnancy (as in the event of contraceptive failure) causes a tremendous drain on bone mineral. Bone gain and loss are much more active in adolescence, and rapid repair can be expected. For example, rapid repair occurs after immobilization in young people and after weightlessness. Furthermore, diet is crucial. A recent study showed that giving adolescents 500 mg/day of calcium supplements (as citrate) produced an astounding further increase in bone mineral deposition of 1.3% per year.[16] So, I think we really need to balance the risks and benefits for young women who are considering using this contraceptive."

Barbara Cromer, MD, just completed a small prospective study of bone density among adolescents using three different forms of hormonal contraceptives.[17] Dr. Cromer, Associate Professor of Pediatrics at The Ohio State University College of Medicine, and her colleagues found that bone density significantly decreased in young women using DMPA compared with adolescents using either the pill, levonorgestrel subdermal implants or no hormones. DMPA users had a 1.5% decrease in bone density over 1 year, while young women in the other groups experienced bone density increases of up to 2.9%. At 2 years, DMPA users experienced a 3% bone density loss, compared to a bone gain of 9% and 10% in implant and control subjects, respectively. Measurement of bone density at 2 years was not possible in the OC group because no users continued with the method for this long. The young women in the study were between the ages of 12 and 21; the mean age was between 14 and 15 years.

Dr. Cromer explained that this magnitude of bone loss is substantial. "After women reach their peak bone mass," she said, "which is reached in some parts of the body during late adolescence and in other parts by the end of the third decade, they naturally lose bone at about 1% per year. So, the girls on DMPA lost bone as if they were women who had reached their peak bone mass.

"The concern is that adolescents who are supposed to be increasing bone density may actually be losing it, and we're not sure whether they'll get it back when they discontinue DMPA. The younger the adolescent, the greater the concern. It's theorized that higher progestin levels seen with DMPA use keep a woman's natural estrogen level from having peaks throughout the menstrual cycle; estrogen levels consistently remain at a low level.

"Interestingly," she continued, "our study found *increased* bone density among levonorgestrel subdermal implant users. Several factors may explain the disparity between these two progestin-only methods: the progestins are different, with levonorgestrel a closer relative to testosterone; and the constant level of progestin with implants is lower than that seen with DMPA. Previous research has indicated that women using levonorgestrel implants experience wider variability, including higher levels, of circulating estrogen.

"It's essential to put the issue in proper context. At this time, we do not know enough about potential bone loss with DMPA to warrant any change in prescribing or to consider it a contraindication for use. We don't have long-term data, and we don't know what happens when women stop using the drug. Perhaps the bone density is regained as if they had never taken it; we don't know. My message to clinicians is that more study needs to be done and that we should adopt a wait-and-see attitude. Young women for whom I would hesitate to use DMPA would be those who naturally may already have low bone density—those with chronic renal disease, who are wheelchair-bound, or who have had chronic amenorrhea." Dr. Cromer emphasized that her findings include fewer than 50 young women, and that the issue must be further studied before conclusions can be drawn and recommendations made.

DMPA Labeling Clarification

In June 1995, the manufacturer of DMPA strengthened package insert labeling to clarify the timing of initial and subsequent injections. The clarifications focused on:

1) Providing a consistent definition of the 3-month dosing interval.

2) Emphasizing the need to rule out pregnancy prior to administration of the first dose.

Manufacturer Labeling Clarification for DMPA Dosing and Administration

1. The dosing interval between injections should be 3 months (13 weeks).

2. If the interval between injections is greater than 13 weeks (91 days), the clinician should determine that the patient is not pregnant before administering the drug.

The labeling clarification was prompted not by new scientific data but by reports of varying administration practices.

According to the manufacturer, "The updated labeling defines the 3-month dosing interval as 13 weeks, specifically 91 days. During clinical trials, researchers gathered data on pregnancy rates for women receiving the injection every 90 +/– 7 days, 90 +/– 5 days and 84 days +/– 5 days. The occurrence of pregnancy in relationship to the dosing interval was not studied. Data from studies investigating return to ovulation showed that the median number of months from the last injection to conception was 10 months, with a range of 4 to 31 months. Thus, data from the clinical trials regarding the dosing interval and studies addressing the time interval for return to fertility support a 3-month (13-week) interval, but at the same time do not exclude a 14-week interval. However, in order to encourage the use of a dosing schedule that reflects the experience in the clinical trials, is less cumbersome to calculate when the next injection is due and is consistently stated throughout the package insert, the recommended dosing interval is 13 weeks (91 days)."

The manufacturer also made changes in labeling regarding the need to exclude pregnancy before the first injection. The new labeling adds emphasis to the admonition to give the first injection during the first 5 days of the normal menstrual period. It states, "...to ensure that the patient is not pregnant at the time of the first injection, the first injection MUST be given ONLY during the first 5 days of a normal menstrual period; ONLY within the first 5 days postpartum if not breastfeeding; and if exclusively breastfeeding, ONLY at the sixth postpartum week."

Dr. Barbara Cromer explained the first DMPA injection protocol used at her institution. "We developed a protocol that we have found very successful. If the adolescent is not in the first 5 days of her menstrual cycle, we do a pregnancy test that day. If it's negative, then we give her monophasic pills for 2 weeks. Then, she comes back and we repeat the pregnancy test. If it's still negative, then we go ahead and give the injection. This helps rule out a false-negative first pregnancy test," she explained.

Variability of Absorption

Clinicians should ensure that DMPA is given intramuscularly to avoid variability of absorption. Dr. Hillard explained, "We need to ensure that the drug is given in the muscle for consistent absorption. For example, an injection in the buttocks of a heavy woman might only reach the subcutaneous tissue. In that case, it may be better to give the injection in the deltoid muscle." In addition, clinicians and patients should avoid massaging the injection site, as this can cause accelerated absorption.[18]

Compliance Considerations

One advantage of DMPA is the need to comply only once every 13 weeks. Nonetheless, clinicians need to make sure patients return on time for the next injection. Several strategies may be helpful. First, make sure the patient has her next appointment before she leaves the office. Second, help the patient associate the date of her next injection with a familiar date she'll remember—an anniversary or birthday.

Becky Schroder explained the anniversary strategy. "I got my first injection on Valentine's Day and made an anniversary of it. I use this approach with patients. I'll say, 'Do you know anyone whose birthday is this month? Is there an important event that happens this month? If so, you can use that as a reminder that you need to return within 3 months for your next injection.'"

Reminder cards can be sent, but confidentiality issues warrant clearing this with the patient first. "Especially with adolescents," Dr. Hillard cautioned, "confidentiality is important. We don't routinely send reminder cards; we make sure the woman leaves with her next appointment. Reminder cards may break the confidentiality of women who are using DMPA, but don't want their parents or others to know."

Teens who desire confidentiality may face another source of discovery—supplies of tampons and sanitary napkins. Linda Dominguez asks teen patients whether their mothers know they are using contraception. If the teen says no and she doesn't want her to find out, Linda explains that her mother may wonder why she is using so many or so few tampons or pads.

Protection Against STDs

DMPA is not known to provide protection against STDs, although it may help prevent pelvic inflammatory disease (PID). One WHO study found that the risk of acute PID among DMPA users was half that among nonusers (RR=0.5; 95% CI, 0.25-1.0); however, the difference in risk was not significant due to a small sample size.[19] DMPA may protect users from PID by thickening cervical mucus and preventing the ascension of STD organisms into the upper reproductive tract.

How DMPA may affect the likelihood of HIV (human immunodeficiency virus) acquisition is not known. All women at risk of STDs, however, need to know how to protect themselves. Clinicians should try to help women understand their risk of acquiring STDs, including HIV, and counsel them about using male latex condoms. If a male partner refuses to use a latex condom, the woman may wish to use a female condom to help protect herself against infection.

Questions about condom use need to be part of a routine sexual history-taking. According to Linda Dominguez, asking patients about their sexual behavior is no longer optional. "If I see that a woman has indicated on the sexual history form that she only occasionally or never uses condoms, I'll question her further. 'Tell me why you only use condoms sometimes or never. What has been your experience with condoms?' And then, depending on her answer, I'll try and help her understand her risk and link her positive choice of using birth control with another positive choice—protecting herself against infection.

"Good counseling really must include a sexual history. With HIV and the other sexually transmitted infections that are out there, we cannot avoid talking about patients' sexual behaviors. With teenagers, in particular, more frequent visits and reinforcing the message about condom use are essential. As clinicians, we must address our own sensitivities about sex and talking with patients about the specifics of their sexual lives—often, clinicians don't have an easy time in this area."

The Art of Counseling

Counseling patients has two components: the art and the science. According to Linda Dominguez, "Providing patients with the science is the easy part. The DMPA patient booklet and package information contain all the scientific facts the patient will need. I think clinicians can help patients even more by practicing the 'art' of counseling. What I mean by the 'art' is counseling patients in such a way that they see how their contraceptive choices work in their lives. I like to help women understand how successful use of contraception can impact other aspects of their lives—work, future goals, health etc.

"Family planning differs from many other types of health care delivery. Women come for contraception because they've decided that family planning will have a positive impact on their lives. Family planning providers aren't doing something to the patient because she's sick. We're supporting the patient and bridging the gap between the woman's choice to use contraception and the knowledge and skills she needs to make her eventual contraceptive choice.

"First, I like to support the patient with praise that she's made the choice. I praise her for making the decision to use contraception and then I attempt to link her choice with the other goals in her life. When I take a patient history, for example, I ask what the woman does for a living, whether she's in school, and try to get an idea of what goals she may have. Then, during the counseling process, I try to reinforce that family planning is a decision that will help her in other areas of her life. I see it as helping the patient take a success with family planning and build it into other successes. Choosing contraception is not just about preventing a pregnancy, it's about creating the life she wants for herself.

121

"I support the patient with praise, information and options. The information part comes from written materials, as well as our discussions. Good written materials are very important for reinforcement of the discussions. The option aspect pertains to her contraceptive choices, but also to her diet, smoking etc. For example, if I've seen the patient for a while and she's telling me she'd like to stop smoking cigarettes, I can use her positive experience with contraception to bridge into another lifestyle success, like quitting smoking.

"That's what family planners can do: We can help telescope contraceptive successes into other successes. The success may be one family planning success leading into another family planning success, or a family planning success leading into success in another area of the patient's life.

"We also need to let the patient know that we are working on this issue together as partners. If for any reason she feels the method is not working for her, she must feel free to come back and discuss it. Presentation is very important. If I 'sell' the method and say, 'I've got such a great method. It's nearly 100% effective and all my patients do really well with it,' then, if she has problems, she may feel that she's disappointed me or that somehow she's failed. So, we need to let the patient know that if the method doesn't work out for her that other methods are available and that she hasn't failed. It's particularly important to help patients be successful with the method they've chosen because often their experience with one method influences how they feel about all other methods. If they have a bad experience with one method, they may have a tainted view of all contraceptives.

"Family planning can help a woman choose a method that's appropriate for a particular slice in time. No one method probably will suit her for her lifetime. Let's say the patient has used DMPA for 1 year and decides it's not for her anymore. I like to emphasize her success with DMPA as I introduce her to other methods. For example, I'll say, 'DMPA did exactly for you what you wanted it to do—it kept you from getting pregnant for the time you were on it. And, at some time in the future, you may want to use this method again. Now, let's talk about other options, because the choice is yours to make.'"

References

1. Sangi-Haghpeykar H, Poindexter AN 3rd, Moseley DC, et al. Characteristics of injectable contraceptive users in a low-income population in Texas. *Fam Plann Perspect* 1995;27:208-211, 225.

2. World Health Organization. A multi-centered phase III comparative clinical trial of depot-medroxyprogesterone acetate given three-monthly at doses of 100 mg or 150 mg: I. Contraceptive efficacy and side effects. *Contraception* 1986;34:223-235.

3. Kaunitz AM. Long-acting injectable contraception with depot medroxyprogesterone acetate. *Am J Obstet Gynecol* 1994;170:1543-1549.

4. Belsey EM. Vaginal bleeding patterns among women using one natural and eight hormonal methods of contraception. *Contraception* 1988;38:181-206.

5. Finger WR. Method choice involves many factors. *Network* December 1994;15:14-17. *Network* is published by Family Health International, PO Box 13950, Research Triangle Park, NC, 27709.

6. Barnhart K, Furman I, Devoto L. Attitudes and practice of couples regarding sexual relations during the menses and spotting. *Contraception* 1995;51:93-98.

7. Diaz S, Croxatto NB, Pavez M, et al. Clinical assessment of treatments for prolonged bleeding in users of Norplant implants. *Contraception* 1990;42:97-109.

8. Stubblefield PG. Menstrual impact of contraception. *Am J Obstet Gynecol* 1994;170:1513-1522.

9. Harel Z, Biro FM, Kollar LM. Depo-Provera in adolescents: effects of early second injection or prior oral contraception. *J Adolesc Health* 1995;16:379-384.

10. Smith RD, Cromer BA, Hayes JR, et al. Medroxyprogesterone acetate (Depo-Provera) use in adolescents: uterine bleeding and blood pressure patterns, patient satisfaction, and continuation rates. *Adolesc Pediatr Gynecol* 1995;8:24-28.

11. Cromer BA, Smith RD, McArdle Blair J, et al. A prospective study of adolescents who choose among levonorgestrel implant (Norplant), medroxyprogesterone acetate (Depo-Provera), or the combined oral contraceptive pill as contraception. *Pediatrics* 1994;94:687-694.

12. Pardthaisong T. Return of fertility after use of the injectable contraceptive Depo Provera: up-dated data analysis. *J Biosoc Sci* 1984;16:23-34.

13. Cundy T, Evans M, Roberts H, et al. Bone density in women receiving depot medroxyprogesterone acetate for contraception. *BMJ* 1991;303:13-16.

14. Cundy T, Cornish J, Evans MC, et al. Recovery of bone density in women who stop using medroxyprogesterone acetate. *BMJ* 1994;308:247-248.

15. Sharma JB, Newman MRB, Smith RJ. Depot medroxyprogesterone acetate and osteoporosis. Smoking may explain findings. *BMJ* 1994;308:1567. Letter.

16. Lloyd T, Andon MB, Rollings N, et al. Calcium supplementation and bone mineral density in adolescent girls. *JAMA* 1993;270:841-844.

17. Cromer BA, Blair JM, Mahan JD, et al. A prospective comparison of bone density in adolescent girls receiving depot medroxyprogesterone acetate (Depo-Provera), levonorgestrel (Norplant), or oral contraceptives. *J Pediatr* 1996;129:671-676.

18. Lande RE. New era for injectables. *Population Reports* August 1995:K-5:1-32. *Population Reports* is published by The Johns Hopkins School of Hygiene and Public Health, 111 Market Place, Suite 310, Baltimore, MD, 21202-4012.

19. Gray RH. Reduced risk of pelvic inflammatory disease with injectable contraceptives. *Lancet* 1985;1:1046. Letter.

■3 Subdermal Implants

Levonorgestrel subdermal implants came to the United States market in early 1991. The implants offer a highly effective, long-term, reversible option with few adverse effects. The first section of this chapter provides an overview of the method and includes information about how the silicone rod delivery system was developed. In the second and third sections of the chapter, U.S. nurse practitioners who participated in clinical trials share their insights into patient counseling and the basic insertion and removal process.

Since their introduction, however, implants have been besieged by highly publicized reports of difficult removals and claims of serious side effects. Although difficult removals occur, they do so only in a small minority of patients. This prompted an updated look at insertion and removal, which includes interviews with clinicians around the world who are exploring variations in technique in order to make removals simpler. Section four highlights the Pop-Out method, the Emory method and the "U" technique.

3.1: Overview

In December 1990, the first subdermal contraceptive implant was approved for use in the United States. The method uses the synthetic progestin levonorgestrel, which is a component of many combination oral contraceptives (OCs). Unlike OCs, however, levonorgestrel implants require no daily compliance after insertion. The implants were studied in clinical trials including 55,000 women in 44 countries before introduction in the U.S.

Historical Background

The idea of using subdermal capsules for contraceptive steroid delivery evolved from observing the fact that Silastic® tubing could be used as a reservoir for the prolonged release of a variety of lipophilic drugs. The Population Council, a nonprofit organization located in New York, began researching subdermal implants in 1966.[1] The Council's International Committee for Contraception Research led the biochemical and clinical investigations into the safety and efficacy of the method.

Several progestational agents were used in the early attempts to develop subdermal implants. These included megestrol acetate, norethindrone, norgestrienone and levonorgestrel.[1] Although norethindrone was promising, sufficient levels of the progestin could not be delivered through the tubing to provide contraceptive efficacy. Both norgestrienone and levonorgestrel were efficacious; however, only 1 year of contraceptive protection could be expected with norgestrienone. The decision was made to use levonorgestrel for two reasons: sustained release could be maintained for 5 years, and extensive safety data were available on levonorgestrel because it had been used widely in OCs for many years.[1,2]

The hormone is contained in six flexible closed capsules made of Silastic tubing. These capsules are implanted in a fan-like pattern beneath the skin of the woman's upper arm. There they slowly release levonorgestrel, which provides protection that begins within 24 hours of insertion and lasts up to 5 years.

The six capsules that comprise the system each contain 36 mg of crystalline levonorgestrel and are 34 mm long and 2.4 mm in diameter.[3] An average of 30 mcg of progestin is released into the bloodstream each day. Initial mean plasma levels of levonorgestrel are about 1,600 pg/ml. After 3 months, levels fall to approximately 400 pg/ml and level off at about 300 pg/ml after the first year and continue for at least 5 years.

Efficacy

There are at least two known mechanisms of action of levonorgestrel implants: ovulation inhibition and thickening of the cervical mucus. There is evidence to indicate that the implants also interfere with the luteal phase hormonal milieu and suppress development and growth of the endometrium. During the first year, the typical failure rate is 0.2%. Overall annual pregnancy rates, derived from studies conducted during the 1980s in 11 countries, are 0.2%, 0.9%, 0.5% and 1.1% in the second through fifth years, respectively. Some studies documented failure rates of 0% in the first year.[4]

Phenytoin decreases the efficacy of subdermal implants.[5] This may be true of other hepatic enzyme-inducing anticonvulsants, as well.

Return to Fertility

Fertility promptly returns to preinsertion levels once implants are removed.[4,6-8] In addition, the return to fertility is unrelated to duration of use. In one Chilean study, by the end of 12 months, 86% of implant users and 89% of Copper T IUD users were pregnant.[6] An Indonesian study found no difference in conception rates after discontinuing implants, the IUD or injectable contraception.[7]

Side Effects

The primary adverse effects consist of menstrual irregularities, although headache and acne also occur. Menstrual irregularities include prolonged bleeding, spotting, amenorrhea, irregular onsets of bleeding and an increase in spotting/bleeding days. These pattern changes predominate in the first year of use. Although the total number of days of bleeding increases, overall blood loss may be less and hemoglobin levels are more likely to increase rather than decrease.[9] Weight gain or loss, nausea and depression have also been reported; however, it is not known if these occur more often than in women not using subdermal implants. Infection at the implant site is uncommon (0.7%), as is expulsion of the capsules.[3]

There are few contraindications to the use of levonorgestrel implants (Figure 1). Careful follow-up and management are advised for women who smoke heavily, have high blood pressure, or history of thrombophlebitis, cardiovascular disease and diabetes. These warnings are similar to the cautions given for OC use, but their relevance to levonorgestrel implants, a progestin-only method, is questionable. In

Figure 1

Contraindications for Levonorgestrel Subdermal Implants

- Active thrombophlebitis
- Undiagnosed abnormal genital bleeding
- Acute liver disease
- Known or suspected carcinoma of the breast
- Known or suspected pregnancy

Source: Levonorgestrel subdermal implants package insert.

fact, levonorgestrel implants have the advantage of containing only progestin and therefore being an alternative for women in whom estrogen is contraindicated. In addition, the total progestin dose is lower than that with OCs, and peak and trough levels of the progestin are avoided.

Continuation Rates

First-year continuation is high when compared to continuation rates with methods such as OCs and barrier methods (Figure 2). According to early data from preintroduction international trials, in the first year of use, 90% of women continue with the method.[10] Data gathered from American women after U.S. market introduction suggest that at least 85% continue with the method at 1 year.[11-15] Discontinuation rates increase during the second through fifth years of use, making it particularly important to provide thorough counseling before insertion. The age of the user does not appear to affect requests for removal; at least one study has found that both adolescents and adults continue at about equal rates (see Chapter 7 on adolescents).[11] It should be noted that continuation rates with

Figure 2

Percentage of Couples Who Are Continuing to Use a Birth Control Method at 1 Year

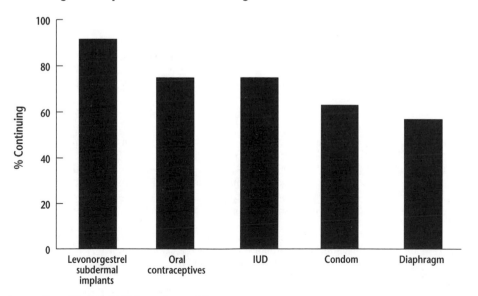

Source: Trussell J, et al, 1990 (see reference 10).

127

methods requiring ongoing compliance may be much lower than shown in Figure 2, especially in selected populations such as adolescents.

The most common reason for discontinuation during the first 2 years is menstrual irregularities. To address this issue, some clinicians provide potential implant users with an injection of depot medroxyprogesterone acetate (DMPA). DMPA induces menstrual irregularities similar to those of implants, but its action is short term (3 months) and reversible. This short-term trial allows the woman to evaluate whether she (and her sexual partner) will be able to tolerate menstrual disturbances induced by implants prior to having them inserted. Others prescribe a trial of a progestin-only pill for the same purpose.

User Perceptions

A San Francisco study of 205 women found that over 75% reported the ease of use of subdermal implants to be the contraceptive's most attractive feature.[16] Second, women cited the high effectiveness, and third, its long-term contraceptive protection. Of the 140 women still using the implants at the end of the study, 88% rated themselves as very satisfied with the method, and 74% said they would use it again.

The study also looked at women's concerns about the method. Of those who reported anxiety about using implants, the most frequent concern was fear of pain with insertion; however, 87% of women interviewed said they had either no or only slight discomfort during the procedure. Furthermore, 91% reported that they were able to go back to their daily activities immediately after the insertion. Most of the remainder were able to return to their routine 1 day after insertion.

Importantly, user perceptions may be influenced by the media, friends and family, whose information may not be accurate. Thorough patient counseling is essential to provide a balanced perspective on the risks and benefits of this contraceptive method.

References

1. Segal SJ. The development of NORPLANT® implants. *Stud Fam Plann* 1983;14:159-163.

2. Segal S. A new delivery system for contraceptive steroids. *Am J Obstet Gynceol* 1987;157: 1090-1092.

3. Population Council. Summary of clinical findings on NORPLANT® subdermal contraceptive implants. New York: January 1989.

4. Sivin I. International experience with NORPLANT® and NORPLANT®-2 contraceptives. *Stud Fam Plann* 1988;19:81-94.

5. Haukkamaa M. Contraception by NORPLANT® capsules is not reliable in epileptic patients on anticonvulsant treatment. *Contraception* 1986;33:559-565.

6. Diaz S, Pavez M, Cardenas H, et al. Recovery of fertility and outcome of planned pregnancies after the removal of NORPLANT® subdermal implants or Copper-T IUDs. *Contraception* 1987;35:569-579.

7. Affandi B, Santoso SS, Djajadilaga, et al. Pregnancy after removal of NORPLANT® implants contraceptive. *Contraception* 1987;36:203-209.

8. Kurunmaki H, Toivonen J, Lahteenmaki PL, et al. Immediate postabortal contraception with NORPLANT®: levonorgestrel, gonadotropin, estradiol, and progesterone levels over two postabortal months and return of fertility after removal of NORPLANT® capsules. *Contraception* 1984;30:431-442

9. Shoupe D, Mishell DR. NORPLANT®: subdermal implant system for long-term contraception. *Am J Obstet Gynecol* 1989;160:1286-1292.

10. Trussell J, Hatcher RA, Cates W Jr., et al. Contraceptive failure in the United States: an update. *Stud Fam Plann* 1990;21:51-54.

11. Cullins VE, Remsburg RE, Blumenthal PD, et al. Comparison of adolescent and adult experiences with NORPLANT® levonorgestrel contraceptive implants. *Obstet Gynecol* 1994;83:1026-1032.

12. Dugoff L, Jones OW 3rd, Allen-Davis J, et al. Assessing the acceptability of NORPLANT® contraceptive in four patient populations. *Contraception* 1995;52:45-49.

13. Frank ML, Poindexter AN 3rd, Cornin LM, et al. One-year experience with subdermal contraceptive implants in the United States. *Contraception* 1993;48:229-243.

14. Gerber S, Westhoff C, Lopez M, et al. Use of NORPLANT® implants in a New York City clinic population. *Contraception* 1994;49:557-564.

15. Blumenthal PD, Wilson LE, Remsburg RE, et al. Contraceptive outcomes among postpartum and postabortal adolescents. *Contraception* 1994;50:451-460.

16. Darney PD, Atkinson E, Tanner S, et al. Acceptance and perceptions of NORPLANT® among users in San Francisco, USA. *Stud Fam Plann* 1990;21:152-160.

3.2: Patient Counseling

All patients need careful counseling prior to insertion and ongoing counseling when side effects occur. An ideal candidate is a woman with no contraindications, who does not desire children for at least 3 to 5 years, desires a highly effective, convenient birth control method and who agrees to undergo a simple insertion procedure.

Counseling should be an ongoing process throughout implant use. It is important to provide patients with the name and telephone number of a contact person if they have questions or concerns about their implants. Women who experience side effects may require reassurance. It is important to offer removal as an option at any time.

For women who experience a predictable bleeding pattern, a change from this pattern and/or amenorrhea after regular bleeding may indicate pregnancy. A change in bleeding pattern coupled with abdominal pain may indicate an ectopic pregnancy. Women should be advised to contact their practitioner if they experience these symptoms.

At the time of removal, it is important to stress that as soon as the implants are taken out the woman is no longer protected against pregnancy. An alternative method of contraception should be initiated immediately if the patient does not want to become pregnant.

What general information should be included in a counseling session for women considering the use of subdermal implants?

1. *Provide a general description of the implants:* Implants consist of six soft, flexible Silastic capsules containing levonorgestrel (a synthetic progestin commonly used in birth control pills) placed just under the skin in the upper inner arm. The implants contain no "new" drugs and do not contain estrogen.

2. *Describe the mechanisms of action:* Implants prevent ovulation in about 50% of cycles, alter the luteal phase hormonal environment, thicken cervical mucus, and may suppress development and growth of the endometrium.

3. *Compare and contrast advantages and disadvantages of subdermal implants with other methods of contraception:*

Advantages

- Highly effective, continuous progestin-only birth control method lasting up to 5 years.
- Convenient, noncoital method requiring no compliance.
- Prompt return of fertility after discontinuation.
- Cost-effective when used for several years.

Disadvantages

- Progestin-related side effects, including bleeding changes (particularly irregular bleeding), weight gain, acne, headache and mood changes.
- Requires a minor procedure for initiation and discontinuation.
- High initial start-up costs in relation to other temporary methods.
- No documentation of protection against sexually transmitted diseases.
- Contour of implants may be visible beneath the skin.

4. *Describe the procedures used for insertion and removal. Include information on:*

- Techniques for placement and removal.
- Sensations associated with procedures.
- Duration of the procedures. This averages 10 to 15 minutes for insertion and 15 to 30 minutes for removal.
- Potential complications. With insertion these include infection, expulsion, hematoma/bleeding and scarring. For removal, potential complications include infection, hematoma/bleeding, scarring, breakage of implants and the need for a second incision.

What kinds of questions should I ask a woman who is considering subdermal implants?

1. *What are your reproductive plans for the next 5 years?* It is important to stress that the implant system is intended to provide long-term contraceptive protection and is most cost-effective when used for at least 3 to 5 years. Patients interested in birth control for only 1 or 2 years should be encouraged to consider other appropriate methods.
2. *What methods of birth control have you used in the past, and did you have any problems with them (eg, a contraceptive failure or unintended pregnancy)?* This will give you an idea as to why she is interested in using implants and may also bring up a history of past OC use, which may help predict tolerance of some of the progestin-related side effects associated with the use of subdermal implants.

3. *How would you and your partner tolerate irregular or prolonged episodes of spotting or bleeding?* The most common side effect associated with implant use is change in menstrual bleeding patterns. The changes range from irregular or prolonged spotting or bleeding to no change, to amenorrhea. Bleeding is usually light, does not signify a health problem, but may require the use of a sanitary napkin or tampon. There is no way to predict whether a woman will experience side effects or if her bleeding pattern will alter. Bleeding alterations are experienced by a majority of women; however, you can reassure the patient that bleeding changes and other nuisance side effects tend to resolve after the first year of use.

A frank discussion of side effects will help women develop realistic expectations about the method and help to encourage appropriate contraceptive selection. For those women who would find menstrual changes or one of the other side effects unacceptable, another contraceptive method should be strongly encouraged. For the woman who cannot tolerate irregular bleeding, for example, an OC with good cycle control may be a better option. Proper counseling can enhance user satisfaction and acceptance and help improve continuation rates.

What kinds of questions do women ask about implants?

1. *Are the implants visible?* In the majority of women, the contours of the implants are not visible under the skin, although they are more likely to be visible in thin women. A hyperpigmentation of the skin may develop directly over the implants in women with darker skin tones, but most women are not bothered by this. It resolves after removal.

2. *Can you feel the implants?* Yes.

3. *Will there be a large scar?* No, the scars for both insertion and removal should be no larger than 3 to 5 mm, and keloid formation has not been reported as a problem.

4. *Will the implants break or be damaged if I bump into something, carry my child or someone grabs my arm where the implants are placed?* No, the arm would have to be subjected to trauma, such as a laceration, severe enough to damage the underlying tissues.

5. *Will the implants move under my skin?* No, once in place under the skin, the implants generally do not move. It is possible that during the period initially following insertion, the implants could shift position slightly. This may be because the fibrous sheath that holds each implant in place does not form immediately; however, most reports indicate that any displacement of the capsules from their original position is minor (less than one inch).

What should I tell women after the insertion procedure?

For the next 24 hours, patients should leave the dressing in place, keep the area clean and dry, and avoid heavy lifting or vigorous activity. An ice pack may be applied to the area and a mild analgesic may be taken, if needed.

After the first 24 hours, women should apply warm, moist heat to the area to enhance reabsorption of bruising, which usually resolves in 7 to 10 days. The area may be tender to touch or with motion of the arm for 7 to 10 days. Patients should leave the adhesive strips in place for 3 to 4 days, unless blistering or itching occurs around them. Blistering or itching may indicate an allergic reaction to the adhesive. Patients should notify their practitioner should this occur.

Women should watch for signs and symptoms of infection, expulsion and failure to heal, and call the office/clinic if these symptoms occur. The practitioner may want to provide written instructions with the name and phone number of the appropriate person to contact if the patient has a question.

These counseling strategies are based on the experience of several nurses involved with implant research done in the United States:

Sandy Kelly Gonzalez, RNC
Robert Wood Johnson Hospital
New Brunswick, NJ

Cindy Klaisle, MSN, NP
University of California -
San Francisco
San Francisco, CA

Maria Lacarra, RN
Los Angeles County – University of
Southern California Medical Center
Los Angeles, CA

If the implants have been inserted in the first 7 days of the menstrual cycle, no back-up method of contraception is needed.

What should I tell women after the removal procedure?

Patients should be advised to follow the same post-procedure instructions as for insertion and be reminded of the prompt return to fertility.

Patients should be shown the six capsules to assure them that all implants have been removed. Women should be reminded that the fibrous sheaths in the arm may be felt, but that all implants have been removed and this sensation will resolve during the next few months.

3.3: Basic Insertion and Removal

Adequate training and knowledge about what to expect during insertion and removal of implants facilitates both processes. This section provides an overview of the basic insertion and removal procedures and tips on how to make both easier.

Insertion

If there is any possibility that the woman may be pregnant, a pregnancy test should be performed prior to insertion. Insertion can take place immediately after abortion and in postpartum women after lactation is established.

Providers should be trained by an experienced clinician before attempting insertion and removal independently. Proper insertion facilitates easier removal. The procedure requires a specially marked trocar and obturator (Figure 1). The insertion site is the inner aspect of the nondominant arm, approximately 8 to 10 cm above the elbow crease. The six capsules are inserted in a fan-like pattern of approximately 75° angle,

Figure 1

**Trocar and Obturator
Used for Implant Insertion**

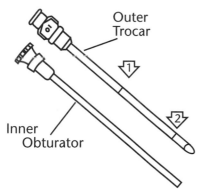

Outer
Trocar

Inner
Obturator

The trocar has two marks on it. Mark #1 is closer to the hub and indicates how far the trocar should be introduced under the skin before the loading of each capsule. Mark #2 is close to the tip and indicates how much of the trocar should remain under the skin following the insertion of each capsule.

leaving approximately 15° between each capsule (Figure 2). The capsules should be placed close to the surface of the skin and on the same plane. Inserting the capsules too deeply encourages development of excessive scar tissue and can contribute to a difficult removal. Depending on the experience and skill of the practitioner, insertion usually takes 10 to 15 minutes. Removal can take longer, depending on the practitioner's skill and the degree of tissue scarring around the end of the capsules.

Figure 3A shows the proper positioning of the patient. The patient lies supine with the arm flexed at the elbow and externally rotated such that her hand is by her head. The area is prepared with antiseptic and draped. The insertion area should be anesthetized with approximately 5 ml of anesthetic (Figure 3B). The anesthetic should be injected into the six tracks in the fan-like pattern that the capsules will

Figure 2

**Position of Properly Inserted Subdermal Implants
(top view and side view)**

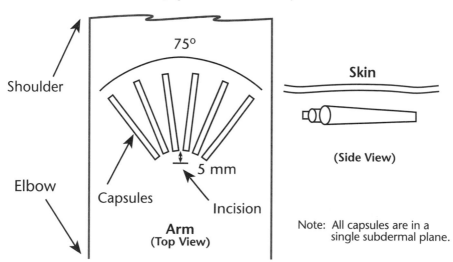

75°

Skin

Shoulder

Elbow

Capsules

5 mm

Incision

Arm
(Top View)

(Side View)

Note: All capsules are in a
single subdermal plane.

Source: Wehrle KE. The Norplant System: easy to insert, easy to remove. Nurse Practitioner 1994;19(4):47-54. Reproduced with permission of the publisher, Elsevier Science Inc.

Figure 3

Insertion

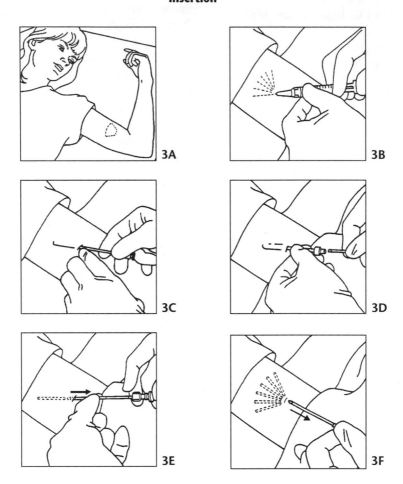

3A

3B

3C

3D

3E

3F

follow. The trocar, with the obturator in place, is inserted through a 2 to 4 mm incision; the trocar should be inserted up to mark #1 near the hub of the trocar (Figure 3C). The obturator is removed. Then, the capsule is loaded into the trocar (Figure 3D). The obturator should be used to advance the capsule to the end of the trocar. While holding the obturator steady, gently *pull back on the trocar* until the distal mark on the trocar appears (mark #2), depositing the capsule in the appropriate position (Figure 3E). Without removing the trocar from the incision, redirect the trocar about 15° away and repeat the steps above until all six capsules have been inserted.

The trocar should not be completely removed from the incision site until all capsules have been placed. After insertion of all the capsules, all six are palpated and the trocar is removed (Figure 3F). Apply firm pressure to the site of implant placement. The incision should be closed with adhesive strips and a dry sterile dressing. A simple

Figure 4

Removal

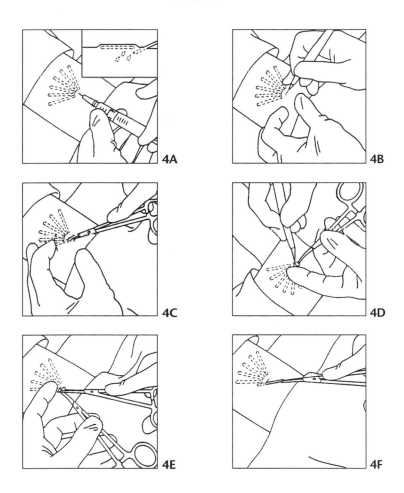

drawing of the placement of the capsules should be included in the patient's chart in order to document their location.

Removal

In general, removal will take more time than insertion. The patient should be placed in the same position as for insertion. After palpating the area to locate the capsules, apply a small amount of anesthetic (usually 3 ml) *under* the capsules (Figure 4A). A 3 to 5 mm incision should be adequate to remove the capsules (Figure 4B). With the fingers, gently push a capsule toward the incision site and grasp the tip with the forceps (Figure 4C). Open the fibrous sheath that will have formed around the capsule with either the scalpel or another mosquito forceps (Figure 4D). Remove the capsule with the second pair of forceps (Figures 4E & 4F). After removal, if a new set of implants is desired, they can be inserted through the same incision, in the same or opposite direction as the previous set. Adhesive strips should be used to close the incision and a dry sterile dressing applied. The patient should be advised to keep the area clean and dry for a few days. If it is difficult to remove some of the capsules, have the patient return for another visit in 4 to 6 weeks to have the remaining capsule(s) taken out.

Tips on Insertion and Removal

Insertion

1. Educate the patient as to what to expect in order to relieve any anxiety she may have. This will help facilitate insertion.

2. Proper insertion is the key to a smooth and uncomplicated removal.

3. Place the capsules at the appropriate level in the subcutaneous tissue just under the surface of the skin. Placing the capsules too deeply is the most common error.

4. Do not force the trocar. Direct it firmly, but gently.

5. Keep the trocar bevel up at all times, making sure to tent the skin upward.

6. Make sure the previous implant is stabilized by gently palpating the capsule with your index finger. Keep this finger on the previously placed implant while redirecting the trocar and starting the next track. This reduces the risk of implant fracture or poor placement.

7. Always keep the trocar in the incision until all capsules are inserted (this will help to keep all the capsules in the same plane). Removal and reinsertion of the trocar will result in unevenly placed capsules at different depths and will make removal more difficult.

8. Adhesive strips are sufficient to close the incision. A sterile dressing is recommended to keep the area clean and dry, and to act as a reminder to the patient to follow postinsertion instructions.

Removal

1. Removal differs from insertion because a fibrous sheath has formed around each capsule.

2. Make sure to inject the anesthetic *underneath* the capsules, not above them. Placing the anesthetic *under* the capsules pushes them up toward the surface of the skin.

3. A large incision will not necessarily make removal easier because each capsule must still be located and the sheath removed.

4. Each capsule can be pushed toward the incision slightly by applying gentle pressure on the distal end.

5. A scalpel or straight mosquito forceps can be used to strip the fibrous sheath off the tips of the capsules.

6. If you cannot remove all the capsules in one sitting, close the incision and have the patient return in about 4 to 6 weeks. The remaining capsules are usually easier to remove at the second visit because swelling present at the previous removal has dissipated. Be sure to remind the patient to use another method of contraception if she does not desire pregnancy.

3.4: Update on Insertion and Removal

Removal of subdermal implants is a simple, office-based procedure, but one that needs to be learned. Training is an essential element, both for proper insertion and removal. Modified approaches to removals have been proposed by various researchers to help clinicians find a method that works for them. These include the Pop-Out method, the Emory method and the "U" technique.

Introduction

In December 1990, the Food and Drug Administration approved the use of contraceptive levonorgestrel subdermal implants in the United States. During the next few years, over 750,000 women decided to use implants. Although the contraceptive effect lasts for up to 5 years, a woman may request removal at any time. Thus, as more than 5 years have passed since introduction, requests for removal are increasing. This is true particularly in areas where large numbers of insertions have been performed.

For example, in Indonesia, levonorgestrel subdermal implants have been available for 10 years. Over 1.5 million Indonesian women have used subdermal implants. Now, a steady state has been reached whereby requests for insertion about equal or exceed requests for removal.[1]

Removal is usually a simple, office-based procedure. However, challenging removals do occur. Proper preparation for removing implants, particularly those that may be deeply embedded in the subcutaneous tissue, bent or broken, is essential.

If clinicians are overly concerned about removing implants, several things may happen: clinicians may not offer removal services to patients; uncertainty about removing implants may result in a reluctance to insert them; and removals that take a long time may cause delays in busy family planning clinics.

Removal Difficulty

Removal of subdermal implants varies in difficulty. One evaluation of 1,253 removal procedures at 15 clinical settings in Texas found about half of the removals were completed in less than 30 minutes.[2] However, about 19% of removals lasted for over 1 hour. Nine women had to return for a second removal procedure. One removal took 215 minutes. About one-quarter of the women reported substantial pain.

As experience with removals increases, researchers have begun to propose modified removal techniques. One goal is to shorten the time needed for removal. Another is to reduce the occurrence of broken capsules. Other goals include decreasing the need for second incisions or additional patient visits, and decreasing pain and bleeding.

Factors Associated with Difficult Removals

Researchers at Family Health International performed a retrospective analysis of 3,416 subdermal implant removals.[3] They included women from 11 countries who participated in clinical trials. Just under 5% of these women experienced difficult or complicated removals. The majority of complicated removals were due to the implants being broken during the removal procedure, followed by embedding or displacement of the implants. A multivariate logistic regression model analyzed potential risk factors leading to complicated removal. The clinical factors of having had a complication at insertion or having an infection at the implant site at the time of removal significantly increased one's chances of having a complicated removal. Women with one of these factors had a fourfold increased risk of complicated removal. The mean removal time for complicated procedures was almost 30 minutes, as compared to 12 minutes for uncomplicated removals.

Randy Dunson, MS, Senior Research Associate, Clinical Trials Division at Family Health International, spoke to *The Contraception Report* about the results. "We chose to perform this analysis because there was no comprehensive report in the literature about implant removal complications. We wanted to present a clinical summary of complicated implant removals as well as to suggest potential risk factors that might be associated with difficult removals," he said. "Our results emphasize the role of proper insertion. The greatest influence on the ease of removal was whether capsules were deeply embedded, displaced or broken. Our model suggests that acquiring an infection at the time of insertion or experiencing a complication at insertion is associated with four times the risk of having a complicated removal. The association between infection and complicated removal may be due to induration of the tissue surrounding the implants. It is important to note, however, that among women experiencing complicated removals, the overall incidence of infection at the implant site at removal was very small, less than 4%," he added.

Proper Insertion Facilitates Removal

Robert Hatcher, MD, Director, Family Planning Program at Emory University, emphasized several points concerning insertions. He commented, "One, insertions should generally be done by clinicians who are also performing removals. This is important because when you have experience with removals, you understand how improper insertion can lead to removal difficulties. That knowledge, in turn, makes the clinician more careful during insertions. Two, implants should be inserted with a template. A template, or plastic stencil, outlines the fan pattern of implants. Clinicians can use the stencil and a marker to draw the correct pattern on the patient's skin, which will help guide the insertion process. Three, implants must not be too deeply embedded, but they also should not be too superficially placed. Insertion into the dermis can make removal difficult as well. Fourth, during insertion the outer trocar should be withdrawn in order to place the capsule, rather than plunging in the inner obturator. If the obturator is used to push the capsule in, the implant will be pushed too far away from the incision site."

Francisco Alvarez-Sanchez, MD, Director of the Biomedical Research Department at Profamilia in the Dominican Republic, has been working with subdermal implants since 1975. He helped to conduct the multinational Phase III clinical trial of subdermal implants. Dr. Alvarez-Sanchez echoed the sentiments of many clinicians, "The most important aspect of a smooth and easy removal is proper insertion. I insist that any discussion of removal include insertions, because that is where many of the problems begin."

Modified Insertion Technique

Some clinicians have proposed a modified, no-scalpel insertion technique that eliminates the need for an initial incision. A group of Brazilian investigators performed subdermal implant insertions with and without a scalpel to see if either presented a benefit to the patient.[4] Insertions without the scalpel use the sharpened trocar to make a puncture in the skin. The original Population Council method, recommended by the manufacturer, calls for using a scalpel to make a 4 mm incision prior to insertion.

The Brazilian study randomly assigned implant acceptors to receive implants using a technique with or without a scalpel. The scalpel method was used for 420 women, the no-scalpel method for 423. Local signs and symptoms were evaluated at 7 and 30 days after insertion to determine whether one method was preferable.

Investigators found no important differences between the two groups in pain, tenderness, edema, bruising or scarring. Based on these findings, they recommended using only the trocar to insert the capsules through the trocar puncture. They cautioned that sharpened trocars must be available to facilitate this type of insertion. Participating investigators reported a preference for the puncture method because less bleeding occurred.

Training

Training of clinicians is important for ensuring uncomplicated implant removals. A retrospective study of 338 Indonesian women found that trained providers removed implants in significantly less time than untrained providers ($p<0.001$).[5] Although different clinicians may prefer slightly modified procedures to remove the capsules, all agree that adequate training makes removal much easier.

Having a well-defined plan before attempting removal facilitates the process. Seshu P. Sarma, MD, Medical Director of the Family Planning/Women's Health Care Clinic at Emory University School of Medicine in Atlanta, Georgia, comments, "It is essential that the clinician have a plan, know what instruments are needed and know each next logical step. A step-by-step procedure will help clinicians who are faced with an unusual or difficult removal. If you spend more than 20 to 30 minutes attempting removal, too much frustration builds on the part of the clinician. The tissues become swollen and make the procedure more difficult. You should stop after about 30 minutes and try again at another time."

Dr. Hatcher believes that training for both insertion and removal procedures should take place at the same time. "In the ideal situation," he explained, "clinicians would receive training in both insertions and removals so that they could see the impact of the insertion technique on removal. This is only possible, however, in centers where enough insertions have been done to generate a steady stream of patients requesting removal. In our area, we've done over 3,000 insertions, so we have quite a few patients coming in to request removal. We also receive many requests for removal from clinicians in the surrounding area."

The Population Council or "Standard" Method

During clinical trials, the Population Council developed the insertion and removal techniques recommended by the manufacturer (see *Basic Insertion and Removal*, section 3.3, in this chapter). Insertions are done through a 4 mm incision, using a specially marked trocar and obturator. Removals are performed by making a 3 to 5 mm incision with a scalpel, approximately 0.5 cm away from the ends of the capsules. The incision should be made close to all six implant tips.

Recommended instruments include a #11 scalpel, and one straight and one curved mosquito forceps. The mosquito clamp is used to find and hold the implant, while gauze or the scalpel is used to scrape away or incise the fibrous sheath surrounding the implant. The straight mosquito clamp can dissect the fibrous tissue before grasping and removing the implant.

Modified Removal Techniques

As clinicians gain more experience with removals, suggestions are appearing for modified versions of the standard technique. Three modified methods (from that originally developed by the Population Council) include the Pop-Out method, the Emory method and the "U" technique. The methods vary by the size and location of the incision, the instruments used and the approach to removing the capsules.

The Pop-Out Method

The Pop-Out method of implant removal is appropriate for situations in which the implants are palpable and superficially located. The method differs from the standard Population Council approach in several ways. Primarily, the method uses less anesthetic, a smaller incision and eliminates the use of hemostats.[6] Fingers and a scalpel are all that are needed. Eliminating the need for instruments decreases pain and trauma at the site, and avoids the risk of fracture. The removal incision is less than 4 mm long, providing better cosmetic results. Instead of using the mosquito clamp to grasp the implant, one uses fingers to direct the implant into the incision, while the scalpel is used to incise the fibrous sheath surrounding the implant. After the fibrous sheath is incised, the implant pops out through the small incision, where it can be grasped easily and removed.

Clinicians at San Francisco General Hospital performed either an 'instrument' or Pop-Out removal for 102 women.[7] They found that women who had the Pop-Out method reported less immediate and subsequent discomfort (Table 1). Mean time for removal using the Pop-Out method was 23 minutes, slightly faster than for instrument removals. One consideration with the Pop-Out method is that deeply placed,

Table 1

Time Required, Incision Length and Pain with Pop-Out vs Instrument Removal, San Francisco General Hospital

	Pop-Out (n=40)	Instrument (n=62)
Minutes required for removal	23.5	32.4
Incision length (mm)	3.3	3.9
Pain – none to slight	97%	62%
Pain – moderate to severe	3%	38%

Source: Darney PD, et al, 1992 (see reference 7) and personal communication.

immobile implants are not as likely to come out. (For information on how to obtain a videotape showing both the standard and Pop-Out methods, see the Note to Clinicians box at the end of this chapter.)

Researchers continue to investigate and evaluate the Pop-Out method. According to Cindy Klaisle, MSN, NP, a clinician who has been researching implants for many years and has removed over 500 sets of implants, "I think that clinicians should be familiar with the different removal techniques and use the method they are most proficient and comfortable with. The Pop-Out method has the advantage of potentially eliminating or at least reducing the need for forceps, causing fewer of the problems that can be associated with instruments. These problems include damaging implants, bleeding, bruising, pain and swelling.

"I like to remove as many capsules as possible using the Pop-Out technique and then use the standard method on any capsules that cannot be retrieved. The use of instruments is rare for properly inserted implants, that is, those placed in a fan shape just beneath the dermis. The Pop-Out method is inappropriate for implants that are inserted deeply or difficult to palpate. Of course, proper insertion of implants is the key to easy removal, no matter which technique is utilized."

Pop-Out Method: Key Points

1. Prep the removal site. Raise a wheal in the dermis using 1/2 cc of anesthetic (1% lidocaine with 1:100,000 epinephrine).

2. Make a small incision with the scalpel (<4 mm) at the ends of the implants.

3. Use the fingers of both hands to direct the implant into the incision.

4. Incise the fibrous sheath with the scalpel.

5. The implant will pop out easily when the fibrous sheath is incised.

6. Grasp and remove the implant with the fingers.

The Emory Method

The Emory method of implant removal is a modified approach that differs from the standard approach in three key ways: more anesthetic is recommended; a larger incision (0.8 cm to 1 cm, rather than 4 mm) is made; a curved, 5" Halstead mosquito forceps is used to dissect the subcutaneous tissues under the proximal ends of each implant.

Dr. Seshu Sarma developed the modified method in late 1992. She and Dr. Hatcher evaluated this method in 50 patients.[8] Using the Emory method, 88% of removals were successfully completed in less than 10 minutes. The mean time of removal was 8 minutes. (See the Note to Clinicians box for details on how to obtain an instructional video of the Emory method.)

According to Dr. Sarma, the Emory method has two main advantages: removal is faster; and the slightly larger incision and dissection of the tissue under the capsules facilitate removal of deeply or poorly placed capsules. The larger incision allows the mosquito forceps to be moved laterally or more deeply with greater ease. "We've taught this method to many clinicians, including residents, interns, physician assistants and nurse practitioners, and they can usually perform removals in 10 minutes or less," said Dr. Sarma. "It is important to have an incision long enough to insert the curved mosquito forceps well into the incision, dissect the tissue under the implants and grasp the implants. I recommend grasping the capsules about one-third of the way up, not just at the tip of the implant. They're too difficult to hold only at the tip."

Emory Method: Key Points
(Modified from reference 8)

1. Draw up 6 cc of 1% lidocaine. (The Population Council method calls for 3 cc lidocaine.)

2. Inject about 1 cc at the incision site and 3/4 cc underneath the lower (proximal) half of each implant.

3. Make a superficial, horizontal incision about 1 cm long at the original incision site or close to the distal ends of the implants (those closest to the elbow). (The Population Council method calls for an incision of 3 to 4 mm.)

4. The incision should cut through the skin and stop in the subcutaneous tissue.

5. Introduce the curved mosquito forceps into the incision and gently dissect the subcutaneous tissues under the proximal ends of each implant for about 20 seconds. (The Population Council method suggests pushing the implant gently toward the incision until the tip is visible and to clear the fibrous sheath over the tip of the implant using the gauze or the scalpel.)

6. The dissection should be vigorous enough to break the tissue encapsulation under the implants.

7. While pushing the distal end of the implant toward the incision with the index finger, grasp the implant from underneath with the curved mosquito forceps.

8. With the help of the straight mosquito forceps, grasp the implant alone, without holding any of the surrounding tissues.

9. Remove the curved mosquito forceps and pull the implant with the straight mosquito forceps.

Dr. Hatcher added, "Dr. Sarma's modification to the removal method has taken advantage of the first rule of surgery, 'adequate exposure.' Increasing the incision length to 0.8 cm to 1 cm provides greater visualization. There are clinicians who may be having difficulty with a smaller incision and they should be aware that this method is another option. Although the incision is a bit larger, in our experience, the scar has been cosmetically acceptable. As with the standard method, the incision does not require sutures." Dr. Sarma added, "In my experience, a 1 cm incision, when healed, leaves a minimal scar, which has been very well accepted by all of the patients for whom I've used this technique."

The "U" Technique

The "U" technique differs from other methods in several ways. One, the incision site is uniquely positioned. All other methods described, to date, have relied upon an incision made perpendicular to the tips of the implants. This method calls for an incision made parallel to the implants, between the third and fourth implant (Figure 1). A 4 mm incision is made about 0.5 cm from the distal ends of the capsules (those closest to the elbow crease). One advantage of the location of the incision is that it improves the chances that all six capsules will be within 1 cm of the incision.

The second way that the method differs is by use of a modified instrument. The "U" technique relies upon a modified vas deferens holding forceps. The ring at the tip of the vas deferens forceps measures 2.2 mm, the diameter of subdermal implant capsules. This instrument is now available from the manufacturer (see box at the end of this section for details on how to order the instrument and updated video on insertion and removal). The "U" technique also includes the use of mosquito forceps and a scalpel.

The third major difference from other methods is the approach to grasping the capsules. Unlike any other method, the "U" technique advocates using the modified forceps to grasp the implants from the side rather than at the tip (Figure 2). Grasping the implants laterally is easier than grasping them at the tip, which may be more slippery and harder to hold. The modified forceps also allow the clinician to snugly grasp the capsule without applying too much pressure. The snugly fitting ring decreases breakage of implants.

Between June 1991 and May 1992, Praptohardjo and Wibowo compared the "U" technique to the standard method.[1] They enrolled 76 women requesting removals. Measured variables included the time required to

Figure 1

Size and Location of Removal Incision in Four Methods

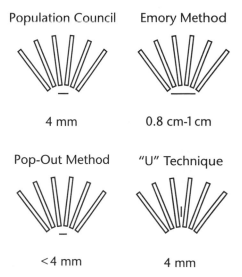

Population Council

4 mm

Emory Method

0.8 cm-1 cm

Pop-Out Method

<4 mm

"U" Technique

4 mm

Figure 2

**Approach to Grasping Implants
with the Modified Holding Forceps
in the "U" Technique**

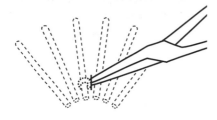

complete removal, number of unbroken capsules and number of incisions required. The assessment included only those women who had visible or palpable capsules. Approximately 14% of patients were ineligible because their implants were difficult to feel.

The results were promising. The "U" technique removals took significantly less time than those using the standard method (mean 7 minutes versus 20 minutes, p<0.0001). In addition, the "U" technique always recovered all six capsules during one sitting using a single incision, whereas removals performed with the standard technique sometimes did not recover all capsules during one sitting (p<0.01) and in five cases required a second incision.

The authors point out that the "U" technique presents advantages when removals are difficult. First, the "U" technique allows the long axis of the implant, rather than only the tip, to be grasped. The long axis often has less fibrous tissue. Second, the authors state that the position of the incision site increases the chances that distant capsules are within 1 cm of the incision site. When capsules are further than 1 cm away, they are grasped more easily with the modified forceps. Third, the forceps grasp the implants firmly, but gently, reducing the chance of breakage.

A second study of the "U" technique performed between June 1992 and July 1993 included women with hard-to-palpate capsules.[9] The study of 181 women found that the mean time to remove easily palpated capsules was about 7 minutes, compared to 9 minutes for hard-to-palpate capsules. In one case (0.5%), the "U" technique damaged a capsule.

The "U" Technique: Key Points

1. Make a 4 mm longitudinal incision between capsules three and four, starting approximately 0.5 cm above the distal ends of the capsules.

2. Insert the modified forceps through the incision to the nearest capsule.

3. Stabilize the capsule by placing the index finger just lateral and parallel to the long axis of the capsule.

4. Grasp the capsule with the modified ring at right angles to the long axis, and within 5 mm of the distal tip.

5. Gently grasp and pull the capsule toward the incision.

6. Rotate the handle of the forceps toward the client's shoulder, bringing the tip of the implant into view of the incision.

7. Clean and open the tissue surrounding the capsule with gauze or scalpel.

8. Use the mosquito forceps to grasp the exposed tip of the capsule and remove it.

Suggested Advantages and Disadvantages of Modified Approaches to Implant Removal

	Pop-Out Method	Emory Method	"U" Technique
Advantages	• Decreased pain • Small incision • No tissue trauma • No risk of fracture or implant damage	• Increased ability to move forceps laterally and more deeply to locate hard-to-find implants • Shorter removal time	• Snug grip of implant with modified instrument • Lateral grasp of implants • Few broken implants
Disadvantages	• Possibly longer removal time • Good only for palpable, superficially located implants	• Longer incision needed	• Need modified instrument
Differences from Standard Population Council Method	• No hemostats • Less local anesthetic • Smaller incision	• More anesthetic (6 cc vs 3 cc) • Longer incision • Disruption of subcutaneous tissue	• Modified instrument • Parallel incision between third and fourth capsule

Additional Techniques

Sometimes, clinicians may encounter capsules that are bent or misshapen, or encased in thick, fibrous tissue. Additional removal techniques may be helpful.[10]

Palpation of capsules may reveal a curved or U-shaped capsule. Palpation of the site will reveal five tips at the distal side and seven proximally. To remove a bent capsule, a second incision is generally needed at the proximal tip of the bent capsule. This approach may also be useful in the case of a misshapen, broken or corkscrew-shaped capsule.

If the clinician cannot locate an implant, he or she can use plain film x-ray to help find the capsule. Some clinicians have also suggested the use of ultrasound or fluoroscopy to help guide the capsule through thick fibrous tissue.[11] Convenience and cost may make use of plain film x-ray more feasible than fluoroscopy.

One other technique employs a curved hemostat without serrations, in place of the #11 scalpel, to enter the fibrous tissue capsule. Blanchard and Kellerman recommend first grasping the tip of the implant in the usual manner with the curved forceps, and then introducing a closed dissecting hemostat into the fibrous capsule.[12] Second, gently open the blades of the clamp, spreading all layers down to the bare implant. Third, remove the implant with a straight hemostat. The physicians report that the procedure results in relatively little bleeding.

Note to Clinicians

A free videotape on patient management and the standard and Pop-Out removal techniques is available by writing to: The Implant Video, UCSF Department of OB-GYN, 6D, San Francisco General Hospital, San Francisco, CA 94110.

For readers who wish to learn more about the Emory method, a videotape is available for $25. For information, call (404) 373-0530.

The modified instrument used in the "U" technique and a four-volume video library, which includes a video of the alternative methods highlighted in this section, are available from Wyeth-Ayerst Laboratories. For more information about these and other support materials for clinicians and patients, call (800) 922-0877.

References

1. Praptohardjo U, Wibowo S. The "U" technique: a new method for NORPLANT® implants removal. *Contraception* 1993;48:526-536.

2. Frank ML, Poindexter AN, Cornin LM, et al. One-year experience with subdermal contraceptive implants in the United States. *Contraception* 1993;48:229-243.

3. Dunson TR, Amatya RN, Krueger SL. Complications and risk factors associated with the removal of NORPLANT® implants. *Obstet Gynecol* 1995;85:543-548.

4. Diaz J, Rubin J, Faundes A, et al. Comparison of local signs and symptoms after the insertion of NORPLANT® implants with and without a scalpel. *Contraception* 1991;44:217-221.

5. Noerpramana NP. The NORPLANT® removal training and service at Dr Kariadi Hospital, Semarang, Indonesia. *Adv Contraception* 1991;7:389-401.

6. Darney PD, Klaisle CM, Tanner S, et al. Sustained-release contraceptives. *Curr Prob Obstet Gynecol Fertil* 1990;13(3):88-125.

7. Darney PD, Klaisle CM, Walker DM. The Pop-Out method of NORPLANT® removal. *Adv Contracept* 1992;8:188-189.

8. Sarma SP, Hatcher R. The Emory method: a modified approach to NORPLANT® implants removal. *Contraception* 1994;49:551-556.

9. Praptohardjo U. One year experience for NORPLANT® implants removal by "U" technique. Abstract FC059.1. Presented at the XIV World Congress of Gynecology and Obstetrics, Montreal, Canada, September 24-30, 1994.

10. Wehrle KE. The NORPLANT® System: easy to insert, easy to remove. *Nurse Practitioner* 1994;19(4):47-54.

11. Kirk EP, Field CS. Difficult NORPLANT® removal facilitated by fluoroscopy. *Am J Obstet Gynecol* 1993;169:748. Letter to the Editor.

12. Blanchard PA, Kellerman RD. Alternative procedure for removal of NORPLANT®. *Am Fam Physician* 1994;49:1733.

4 The Intrauterine Device

The intrauterine device (IUD) is having a renaissance in the United States. Recent epidemiological studies have resolved earlier questions about the safety of this form of contraception. In addition, the cumulative failure rate with the Copper T 380A is almost as low as that achieved with sterilization.[1] As shown by Trussell and others, the 5-year costs of contraception with IUDs are among the lowest of all fertility control methods.[2,3] As concluded by a World Health Organization (WHO) Scientific Group, "The currently available copper and hormone-releasing IUDs, when properly used, are probably the most effective and reliable reversible method of fertility regulation."[4] This chapter provides an overview of such topics as how IUDs work, the safety of currently available devices, the role of the IUD tail and the likelihood of pelvic inflammatory disease (PID).

4.1: Highlights from an International Conference

On March 27-28, 1992, experts from around the world met in New York City to discuss and reexamine biomedical and programmatic issues surrounding the use of intrauterine contraceptives. The international conference—cosponsored by the Population Council and the journal Contraception—provided a forum for balancing the risks and benefits of IUD use and discussing the factors limiting the device's acceptability and accessibility in the U.S.

IUD Use

Worldwide use of IUDs has been rising steadily in recent years. In 1982, IUD users totaled some 60 million[5]; by 1987, this figure had risen to about 84 million.[6] According to W. Parker Mauldin, MA, Senior Associate at the Population Council, current worldwide IUD use is approaching 100 million.[7] During his presentation at the New York conference, Mauldin noted that IUD use is most prevalent in East Asia, with China accounting for two-thirds of all IUD users worldwide.[7]

While the IUD is used by over 40% of all contraceptors in China and by about 20% of all contraceptive users worldwide, the picture is radically different in the U.S. During the period when overall IUD use was increasing, U.S. use dropped from 2.2 million in 1982 to 700,000 in 1988.[8] According to Jacqueline Darroch Forrest, PhD, Vice President for Research at the Alan Guttmacher Institute, this figure has remained relatively constant during the past several years.[9] The method accounts for less than 2% of all contraceptive use in this country.[10]

Table 1
IUDs in the United States

Device*	Type	Introduced	Status
Lippes Loop	Nonmedicated	1964	Discontinued 1985
Saf-T-Coil	Nonmedicated	1967	Discontinued 1983
Dalkon Shield	Nonmedicated	1970	Discontinued 1975
Copper 7	Copper	1973	Discontinued 1986
Tatum T	Copper	1978	Discontinued 1986
Progestasert	Hormone-releasing	1976	Available
ParaGard	Copper	1988	Available

*Brand names are for identification purposes only and do not imply endorsement.

Source: Contraceptive Technology, *1990 (see reference 16).*

Decline in U.S. Accessibility

The rapid decline in IUD use in the U.S. during the 1980s coincided with a peak in IUD-related product liability litigation. Much of this litigation involved the Dalkon Shield IUD, which researchers had linked to a substantial increase in risk of PID.[11] The highly publicized controversy over the Dalkon Shield led many users to doubt the safety of IUDs in general, and many discontinued use of the IUD.

The combination of soaring litigation defense costs and a shrinking market caused several IUD manufacturers to discontinue marketing their products in the U.S. (Table 1). Of the five IUDs available in the early 1980s, only one—the hormone-releasing Progesterone T device—remained on the U.S. market by 1986. The Copper T 380A was introduced 2 years later, and these products remain the only IUDs available in the U.S. today. Some patients may be unaware that the IUD is still a contraceptive option.

Another factor affecting IUD accessibility in the U.S. is the insufficient amount of IUD insertion training received by gynecology residents. Carolyn Westhoff, MD, MSc, Assistant Professor of Obstetrics and Gynecology and Public Health at Columbia University in New York, presented the results of a survey on this topic. Dr. Westhoff's survey of the 272 U.S. obstetrics and gynecology residency programs had a 79% response rate and revealed that one-third of chief residents had never inserted an IUD. Another one-third reported having performed five or fewer insertions.[12]

According to the insertion and removal instructions found in the package inserts of both IUDs sold in the U.S., "It is probably wise to have done 15 to 25 insertions under supervision prior to inserting an IUD unsupervised. A practitioner with only four to six insertions would probably not have had adequate experience with difficult insertions." When viewed in conjunction with these insertion guidelines, Dr. Westhoff's study suggests that two-thirds of the potential IUD providers emerging from U.S. residency programs are not adequately prepared to perform IUD insertions—a substantial obstacle to IUD accessibility in this country.

Hormone-Releasing IUDs

Early IUDs sold in the U.S. were nonmedicated. In the late 1960s, however, a means of enabling IUDs to release a controlled amount of synthetic hormone was discovered.[13] In 1976, the hormone-releasing Progesterone T IUD was introduced in the U.S. The Progesterone T IUD releases progesterone into the uterine cavity at a rate of 65 mcg/day. The hormone diffuses through a permeable polymer membrane surrounding a 38 mg reservoir in the IUD's vertical stem (Figure 1). The device's 36 mm x 32 mm T-shaped frame is constructed of ethylene vinyl acetate copolymer, with barium sulfate added to render the IUD radiopaque. A monofilament nylon thread attached to the base of the vertical stem aids in removal of the Progesterone T.

Figure 1

The Progesterone T IUD

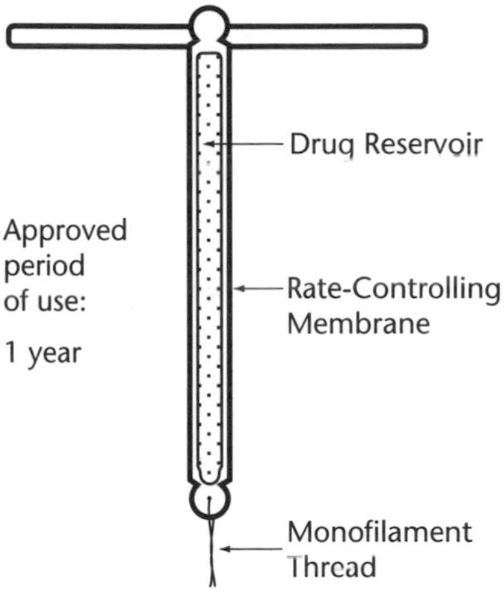

Drug Reservoir

Approved period of use:

1 year

Rate-Controlling Membrane

Monofilament Thread

Source: Alza Corporation, 1992.

The Progesterone T is an effective means of fertility control. The device has a first-year failure rate of 2.9%.[14] The Progesterone T must be replaced annually due to depletion of the hormone reservoir.

Copper-Containing IUDs

In the late 1960s, it was discovered that the use of copper in the construction of an IUD could improve the device's contraceptive efficacy.[15] The first copper IUD available in the U.S. was approved by the Food and Drug Administration (FDA) in 1973. Copper wire wrapped around the product's stem provided a medicated surface area of 200 mm².

The most recently developed and only copper IUD available in the U.S. is the Copper T 380A. Its flexible, 36 mm x 32 mm T-shaped frame is made of polyethylene and contains barium sulfate for radiopacity. Coiled around the Copper T 380A's vertical stem is 314 mm² of pure electrolytic copper wire, while an additional 66 mm² of copper surface area is provided by two sleeves

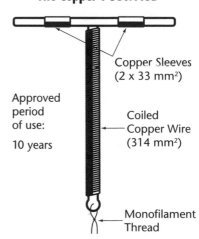

Figure 2

The Copper T 380A IUD

Copper Sleeves (2 x 33 mm²)

Approved period of use:

10 years

Coiled Copper Wire (314 mm²)

Monofilament Thread

Source: GynoPharma Inc., 1992.

attached to the horizontal arms of the device (Figure 2). The total copper surface area is 380 mm²—greater than any other IUD to date. A monofilament polyethylene thread is attached to a 3 mm ball at the tip of the vertical stem to facilitate removal of the IUD.

The Copper T 380A is a third-generation IUD and the most effective intrauterine contraceptive ever used in the U.S.[16] The device has a first-year failure rate of 0.5%.[14] Originally approved for 4 years of use, the Copper T 380A's duration of effectiveness was extended by the FDA to 6 years in 1989, 8 years in 1991 and 10 years in 1994.

New IUDs

Several new IUDs were discussed at the New York conference. While some are still in the clinical trial stage, others have already been approved for use in other countries. One unique copper device currently in clinical trials in the U.S. has no solid frame. Instead, six copper sleeves are strung on a monofilament thread for a total of 330 mm^2 of copper. The IUD is anchored to and suspended from the uterine fundus by pushing a knot into the myometrium using a specially designed inserter. The flexible design is expected to result in less pain and bleeding.

Another new IUD discussed at the conference is a levonorgestrel-releasing, T-shaped device that has been on the market in Finland since 1991. Much like the Progesterone T IUD, the levonorgestrel device has a reservoir in its vertical stem from which 20 mcg/day of the hormone is released. Levonorgestrel has been used safely and effectively for many years in oral contraceptives and, most recently, in subdermal contraceptive implants. The levonorgestrel IUD is reportedly also safe and very effective, with a first-year failure rate of 0.3%. Menstrual blood loss and dysmenorrhea are both reduced in users of the levonorgestrel device, while amenorrhea rates are higher than with other IUDs.[4]

Mechanism of Action

While the IUD's mechanism of action is not fully understood, it has long been hypothesized that the device inhibits fertility primarily by causing a pronounced foreign body reaction in the uterus, altering the endometrium and rendering it unsuitable for implantation.[17] Recent evidence, however, has provided new insight into the IUD's mechanism of action and strongly supports a true contraceptive effect in preventing fertilization.

First, hormonal surveillance for early pregnancy losses among IUD users has not supported the hypothesis that IUDs act as abortifacients. In fact, human chorionic gonadotropin (hCG) studies have suggested that women using no method of contraception experience embryonic loss at rates similar to or higher than IUD users.[18]

Second, the relative rarity of fertilized ova being found in the fallopian tubes of IUD users provides additional support for contraceptive effects of IUDs. Tubal flushings in a study by Alvarez et al not only failed to find any fertilized ova in the tubes of IUD users, but also recovered fewer unfertilized ova from IUD users (39%) compared to controls (56%) who used no contraceptive method.[17] In their study, Alvarez et al noted that uterine and tubal fluids are able to intermix, allowing cells and substances found in the uterus of the IUD user to migrate into the fallopian tubes. Leukocytes, or white blood cells, which are mobilized as part of the foreign body reaction elicited by an IUD *in situ*, are found in high concentrations in the uterine fluid of IUD users (as are copper ions in users of copper devices). Leukocytes, leukocyte degradation products and copper are all cytotoxic, and their presence in the fallopian tubes could lead to early destruction of the egg prior to fertilization.[18]

A third line of evidence pointing to the contraceptive effect of IUDs involves the scarcity of viable sperm in the fallopian tubes of women with an IUD *in situ*. The leukocytes elicited may have a cytotoxic effect on sperm. In addition, copper has a demonstrated spermicidal effect, and thickened cervical mucus inhibits sperm transport in users of hormone-releasing IUDs.[18] As a result, numerous studies have found a marked decrease in the number of oviductal sperm in IUD users, and in the case of Copper T IUDs, a large proportion of those sperm recovered from the tubes were damaged and incapable of fertilization.[18]

Speaking at the New York conference on the topic of IUD method of action, Horacio B. Croxatto, MD, of the Chilean Institute of Reproductive Medicine in Santiago, Chile, cited several studies relating to decreased proportions of viable sperm, reduced numbers of oviductal eggs and absence of fertilized ova in the uterus of IUD users. Dr. Croxatto concluded that loss of viability of the embryo in the uterus is not the IUD's primary mode of action; rather, the device interferes with the reproductive process prior to fertilization.[19]

IUDs and Ectopic Pregnancy

IUD use has an overall protective effect on the risk of ectopic pregnancy. Irving Sivin, MA, Senior Associate at the Population Council's Center for Biomedical Research in New York, addressed the conference on this often misunderstood benefit of IUD use.[20] When pregnancy occurs in an IUD user, the likelihood of that pregnancy being extrauterine is greater than among pregnant nonusers of contraception.[4] This fact has led many to mistakenly associate IUD use with increased risk of ectopic pregnancy. However, as with other methods of contraception, the overall risk of ectopic pregnancy among IUD users is *decreased* because the probability of pregnancy itself is greatly decreased. A 60% reduction in ectopic pregnancy risk has been reported among IUD users compared to women using no method of contraception.[21]

Sivin noted that copper IUDs have been shown to provide the greatest protection against ectopic pregnancy, in direct proportion to the device's total copper surface area. He also pointed out the prolonged use of IUDs does not affect the risk of ectopic pregnancy, and no increase in ectopic pregnancy risk has been found in women who become pregnant after discontinuing IUD use.[20] In fact, package labeling for the Copper T 380A IUD no longer lists a history of ectopic pregnancy as a contraindication to use.

Other Benefits of IUDs

Other benefits of IUD use discussed at the conference include ease of compliance, efficacy and safety. The IUD does not rely on regular user compliance. In addition, IUDs are highly effective at preventing pregnancy, with failure rates of U.S. devices between 0.5% and 2.9%.[14] The risk of death associated with IUD use is low, making it a safe method as well. Since 1977, there has not been an IUD-related spontaneous abortion death in the U.S., according to a conference presentation by Hani K. Atrash, MD, MPH, Chief of the Pregnancy and Infant Health Branch at the Centers for Disease Control and Prevention in Atlanta.[22]

IUDs and PID Risk

Although the IUD is a safe and effective method of contraception, it is not without certain risks. The most highly publicized and most widely misunderstood risk associated with IUD use is upper genital tract infection. Studies performed during the 1970s and early 1980s suggested an increased risk of PID in IUD users.[23] However, reanalysis of these early studies has brought to light several biases that exaggerated the risk of PID associated with IUDs.[21]

Reanalysis has shown that failure to separate Dalkon Shield users—known to be at higher risk of PID—from users of other IUDs in the study population biased the results of some early research.[23] Many studies also included users of other methods of contraception in control groups, which resulted in spuriously elevated PID risk among IUD users due to the protective effect associated with use of oral contraceptives and barrier methods. Ascertainment bias was also suspected in some studies, resulting from a lack of objective PID diagnosis criteria and the increased likelihood of physicians diagnosing PID in IUD users compared to nonusers with similar complaints and findings.[21] An elevated relative risk would result from this overdiagnosis of PID in IUD users.

Confounding factors, such as number of sexual partners and exposure to sexually transmitted diseases (STDs), have also been cited as contributing to inflated relative risk estimates in early studies.[21] Since bacteria such as *Neisseria gonorrhoeae* and *Chlamydia trachomatis* are reported to cause PID,[24] sexual behavior that increases the likelihood of contact with these bacteria would also increase the risk of PID. This was illustrated by an analysis from the Women's Health Study, in which the greater risk of PID in IUD users was found among never-married women, while no significant increase in PID risk was found among married or cohabiting IUD users with only one recent sexual partner.[25] A recent WHO review of IUD clinical trial data also suggested no increased risk of PID among IUD users who were at low risk for STDs.[23]

The risk of IUD-associated PID is related to the insertion process and not to the device or its string. Olav Meirik, MD, PhD, a medical officer with WHO and a coauthor of the 1992 WHO study on IUD use and PID, told the conference delegates that WHO data suggested a significant increase in PID risk during the first 20 days following IUD insertion. On the other hand, this risk was found to be low and uniform during all other times in the course of IUD use (Figure 3). According to Dr. Meirik, no increase in PID risk was associated with long-term use.[23]

The increased risk of PID found to occur during the first few weeks following insertion is likely the result of microbiological contamination of the uterine cavity during the insertion procedure. As a result, the WHO researchers recommended not only that insertion be performed under strict aseptic control, but also that IUDs be left *in situ* for their full lifespan rather than replaced at shorter intervals, thus reducing the number of insertion procedures required.[23]

Addressing the conference, David A. Grimes, MD, Executive Editor of *The Contraception Report*, also recommended the use of prophylactic antibiotics at the time of IUD insertion to diminish the risk of infection.[26] Dr. Grimes referred to a large randomized, controlled trial in Kenya, in which 200 mg of oral doxycycline was administered to

Figure 3
PID Incidence by Time Since Insertion

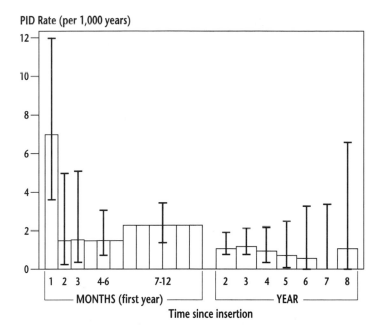

Source: Farley TMM, Rosenberg MJ, Rowe PJ, et al. *Intrauterine devices and pelvic inflammatory disease: an international perspective.* Lancet *1992;339:785-788. Reproduced with permission of the publisher, ©The Lancet Ltd.*

patients prior to IUD insertion, resulting in a one-third decrease in PID incidence.[27] This finding, however, was not corroborated in a smaller trial conducted in Nigeria.[28]

The identification of insertion as the major factor in PID risk among IUD users provides additional evidence against the role of the IUD tail in PID incidence. If the tail served as a bridge for bacteria, rates of infection would remain elevated throughout the use of the device. As evidenced by the WHO study, this does not occur.[23] Roberto Rivera, MD, Director of the Clinical Trials Division of Family Health International in Research Triangle Park, North Carolina, also pointed out that studies comparing tailed and tailless versions of the same IUD have failed to find an increased risk of PID with the tailed devices. Dr. Rivera concluded that, unlike the multifilament tail of the Dalkon Shield IUD, the monofilament tail of modern devices does not increase the risk of PID in IUD users.[29]

Other IUD Risks and Complications

In addition to PID, IUD use has several other potential complications. Uterine perforation at the time of insertion is a potentially serious complication, although the incidence is relatively low (one to three per 1,000 insertions) and is closely related to the ability of the individual inserting the IUD.[21] There is some evidence that insertion during lactation may increase the risk of perforation. In the event of perforation, the copper devices should be removed—usually by laparoscopy—to avoid further complications.[4] Evidence is lacking concerning the medical advisability of removing intraperitoneal IUDs that do not contain copper, although such devices are customarily removed in the U.S.

Complications surrounding pregnancy that occurs with an IUD *in situ* have also been documented. A 10-fold increase in the risk of second trimester spontaneous abortion is reported among women continuing a pregnancy with an IUD *in situ*.[4] Although no association between the IUD and congenital abnormalities has been found, the risks of premature delivery, low birth weight and stillbirth are all increased when the IUD is not removed in the first trimester.[21]

Pain and bleeding associated with IUD use are responsible for discontinuation of the method in 5% to 15% of women.[21] This complication was addressed at the conference by Goran Rybo, MD, Assistant Professor in the Department of Obstetrics and Gynecology at the University of Goteborg, Sweden, who reported that the amount of menstrual blood loss varies greatly with the type of IUD. According to Dr. Rybo, copper IUDs may cause a 50% to 75% increase in menstrual blood loss, while progestogen-releasing devices actually decrease the amount of bleeding due to endometrial suppression.[30] However, the duration of bleeding and incidence of spotting may be increased with progestogen IUDs.[21]

Dr. Rybo noted that iron supplementation can be used to prevent iron deficiency in the case of increased bleeding and stressed the importance of patient counseling both prior to insertion and when bleeding occurs.[30] Physicians should explain to patients that the amount of blood loss often decreases over time as the uterus adapts to the presence of the IUD.[21]

Another problem associated with IUD use is expulsion of the device. Reported expulsion rates vary by IUD type: the Copper T 380A ranges from 3.3 to 7.1 per 100 women at 1 year of use, while the Progesterone T ranges from 1.2 to 4.2 per 100 women at 1 year.[4] Other factors affecting the likelihood of expulsion include age and parity. Older, multiparous women experience fewer expulsions than younger, nulliparous IUD users.[4] Most expulsions occur within 3 months of insertion and are likely to take place during menstruation. Practitioners should instruct their patients to check for the IUD tail regularly—at least after each menstrual period—and may want to schedule a follow-up visit within the first 3 months to detect possible unnoticed expulsions.

Patient Selection

Many of the risks and complications associated with IUD use can be minimized or even avoided through appropriate patient selection. Absolute contraindications for IUD insertion include malignant disease of the corpus uteri or cervix, vaginal bleeding of unknown etiology, suspected pregnancy and active PID.[24] Conference Chairperson Daniel R. Mishell, Jr., MD, Lyle G. McNeile Professor and Chairman of the Department of Obstetrics and Gynecology at the USC School of Medicine in Los Angeles, agreed that these absolute contraindications are based on logic and good medical practice. Dr. Mishell noted, however, that there is some debate over the validity of certain relative contraindications, such as diabetes and history of PID, stating that they may be based more on supposition and concern over litigation than on clinical data.[31] On the other hand, relative contraindications, such as multiple sexual partners and risk of STD exposure, are clinically based and should be factors in determining IUD candidacy.

Conclusion

Use of an IUD for contraception has both benefits and risks. While the method is not suitable for every woman, careful screening can identify appropriate candidates. Parous women in mutually monogamous relationships are good candidates for IUD use—especially those for whom compliance with other methods of contraception has been a problem. Patient counseling prior to and following insertion is important and necessary to ease patient concerns and reduce discontinuation rates. To reduce the risk of infection, insertion should only be performed by individuals with adequate training and with sterile technique. In addition, once inserted, the device should not be replaced sooner than its recommended lifespan. The consensus among the delegates at the international IUD conference was that when used within these guidelines, the IUD is a safe, highly effective and cost-effective method of contraception.

The proceedings from the IUD conference are now available as a book for $85 (U.S.) from Butterworth-Heinemann. Call (800) 366-2665 to order.

Bardin CW, Mishell DR Jr., eds. *Proceedings from the Fourth International Conference on IUDs.* Boston: Butterworth-Heinemann, 1994.

References

1. Peterson HB, Xia Z, Hughes JM, et al. The risk of pregnancy after tubal sterilization: findings from the U.S. Collaborative Review of Sterilization. *Am J Obstet Gynecol* 1996;174:1161-1170.

2. Trussell J, Leveque JA, Koenig JD, et al. The economic value of contraception: a comparison of 15 methods. *Am J Public Health* 1995;85:494-503.

3. Ashraf T, Arnold SB, Maxfield M Jr. Cost-effectiveness of levonorgestrel subdermal implants. *J Reprod Med* 1994;39:791-798.

4. World Health Organization. Mechanism of action, safety and efficacy of intrauterine devices. *Technical Report Series* 1987;753:1-91. Geneva, Switzerland: World Health Organization.

5. Liskin L, Fox G. IUDs: an appropriate contraceptive for many women. *Population Reports* 1982;4:101-135. *Population Reports* is published by The Johns Hopkins School of Hygiene and Public Health, 111 Market Place, Suite 310, Baltimore, MD, 21202-4012.

6. Treiman K, Liskin L. IUDs: a new look. *Population Reports* 1988;16:1-31.

7. Mauldin WP, Segal SJ. IUD use throughout the world: past, present and future. Presented at *A New Look at IUDs—Advancing Contraceptive Choices*; March 27-28, 1992; New York, NY.

8. Mosher WD, Pratt WF. Use of contraception and family planning services in the United States, 1988. *Am J Public Health* 1990;9:1132-1133.

9. Forrest JD. Acceptability of IUDs in the United States. Presented at *A New Look at IUDs—Advancing Contraceptive Choices*; March 27-28, 1992; New York, NY.

10. Harlap S, Kost K, Forrest JD. *Preventing Pregnancy, Protecting Health: A New Look at Birth Control Choices in the United States.* New York: The Alan Guttmacher Institute;1991.

11. Burkman RT. Association between intrauterine device and pelvic inflammatory disease. *Obstet Gynecol* 1981;57:269-276.

12. Westhoff CL, Marks F, Rosenfield A. Physician factors limiting IUD use in the U.S. Presented at *A New Look at IUDs—Advancing Contraceptive Choices*; March 27-28, 1992;New York, NY.

13. Scommegna A, Pandya GN, Christ M, et al. Intrauterine administration of progesterone by a slow release device. *Fertil Steril* 1970;21:201-210.

14. Sivin I, Schmidt F. Effectiveness of IUDs: a review. *Contraception* 1987;36:55-84.

15. Zipper J, Medel M, Prager R. Suppression of fertility by intrauterine copper and zinc in rabbits: a new approach to intrauterine contraception. *Am J Obstet Gynecol* 1969;105:529-534.

16. Hatcher RA, Stewart FH, Trussell J, et al. *Contraceptive Technology 1990-1992*. 15th revised ed. New York: Irvington Publishers, Inc.;1990.

17. Alvarez F, Brache V, Fernandez E. New insights on the mode of action of intrauterine contraceptive devices in women. *Fertil Steril* 1988;49:768-773.

18. Sivin I. IUDs are contraceptives, not abortifacients: a comment on research and belief. *Stud Fam Plann* 1989;20:355-359.

19. Croxatto HB. IUD mechanisms of action. Presented at *A New Look at IUDs— Advancing Contraceptive Choices*; March 27-28, 1992; New York, NY.

20. Sivin I. Intrauterine devices reduce risks of ectopic pregnancy. Presented at *A New Look at IUDs—Advancing Contraceptive Choices*; March 27-28, 1992; New York, NY.

21. Grimes DA. Whither the intrauterine device? *Clin Obstet Gynecol* 1989;32:369-376.

22. Atrash HK, Frye AA. Incidence of morbidity/mortality with IUD *in situ*. Presented at *A New Look at IUDs—Advancing Contraceptive Choices*; March 27-28, 1992; New York, NY.

23. Farley TMM, Rosenberg MJ, Rowe PJ, et al. Intrauterine devices and pelvic inflammatory disease: an international perspective. *Lancet* 1992;339:785-788.

24. Diagnostic and therapeutic technology assessment (DATTA): intrauterine devices. *JAMA* 1989;261:2127-2130.

25. Lee NC, Rubin GL, Borucki R. The intrauterine device and pelvic inflammatory disease revisited: new results from the Women's Health Study. *Obstet Gynecol* 1988;72:1-6.

26. Grimes DA. Prophylactic antibiotics at IUD insertion. Presented at *A New Look at IUDs—Advancing Contraceptive Choices*; March 27-28, 1992; New York, NY.

27. Sinei SKA, Schulz KF, Lamptey PR, et al. Preventing IUCD-related pelvic infection: the efficacy of prophylactic doxycycline at insertion. *Br J Obstet Gynaecol* 1990;97:412-419.

28. Ladipo OA, Farr G, Otolorin E, et al. Prevention of IUD-related pelvic infection: the efficacy of prophylactic doxycycline at IUD insertion. *Adv Contraception* 1991;7:43-54.

29. Rivera R. Is there an effect of the IUD string in the development of pelvic inflammatory disease in IUD users? Presented at *A New Look at IUDs—Advancing Contraceptive Choices*; March 27-28, 1992; New York, NY.

30. Rybo G. IUD use and endometrial bleeding. Presented at *A New Look at IUDs—Advancing Contraceptive Choices*; March 27-28, 1992; New York, NY.

31. Mishell DR, Ballagh S, Kjos SL. Determining contraindications to IUDs. Presented at *A New Look at IUDs—Advancing Contraceptive Choices*; March 27-28, 1992; New York, NY.

5 The Female Condom

The year 1992 saw yet another approval for a birth control device—this time a new barrier method. The female condom, the first condom completely under the control of the woman, received a quick approval from the Food and Drug Administration (FDA) under new guidelines designed to hasten the introduction of products with the potential to stop the spread of sexually transmitted diseases (STDs). Made of polyurethane, a plastic with good heat transmitting properties, the condom was studied preclinically in the United States and Latin America. The first section of this chapter provides an overview of the product and its FDA review.

Early on, clinicians raised concerns about user acceptability. These concerns included the product's visibility outside the vagina, partner acceptance and ease of use. In August 1994, when the female condom became widely available across the U.S., the manufacturer launched an educational awareness campaign designed to familiarize women with the product. Women and clinicians needed answers to such questions as: When should it be inserted and removed? How much protection against pregnancy and STDs can be expected? What if the product becomes dislodged? What will it feel like during sex? The second section of this chapter covers these counseling issues, and the third provides a question and answer guide to help prepare clinicians for patient discussions.

5.1: Overview of FDA Approval

On January 31, 1992, the Obstetrics and Gynecology Devices Panel of the FDA, chaired by The Contraception Report editorial board member Elizabeth B. Connell, MD, and consisting of 14 experts in the field, recommended approval of a new female barrier contraceptive device—a disposable female condom. The female condom is designed to provide the same benefits as its male counterpart: pregnancy prevention and protection from STDs and acquired immunodeficiency syndrome (AIDS).

The Female Condom

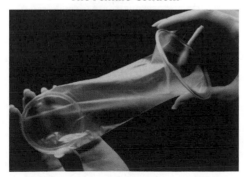

Expedited Review

Because of the device's potential role in preventing the spread of AIDS and STDs, the female condom set a precedent as the first product to receive an expedited review under new guidelines developed by the panel and approved by the FDA. During her introductory remarks on the purpose of the FDA panel meeting, Christine L. Brauer, a Reviewer with the Obstetrics and Gynecology

Devices Branch of the FDA's Office of Device Evaluation, noted that the female condom was "the first potential candidate to qualify and be evaluated according to the preclinical and clinical guidelines outlined in our guidelines, which are utilizing a surrogate study endpoint combined with elimination of a concurrent control."[1]

Description and Insertion Procedure

The female condom is a soft, thin polyurethane sheath with a flexible ring at each end. The ring that lies at the closed end of the sheath serves as the insertion mechanism (Figure 1A). This ring is pinched and inserted into the vagina much like a diaphragm (Figure 1B), where it expands to cover the cervix and holds the device in place (Figure 1C). The other ring, located at the sheath's external edge, lies outside the vagina after insertion and covers the labia (Figure 1D). The polyurethane sheath itself covers the cervix, lines the vaginal wall and extends out over the labia, forming a physical barrier between the two partners. Should the inner ring become dislodged during intercourse, the sheath continues to provide protection, moving with the penis much like a male condom.

The female condom can be inserted anywhere from several minutes to several hours prior to intercourse, although most women report inserting the female condom within 20 minutes before initiating intercourse.[2] The over-the-counter device is available in one size only and does not require fitting by a health care professional. The female condom comes prelubricated with silicone in packages of three, and each package contains extra water-soluble lubricant.

Insertion of the Female Condom

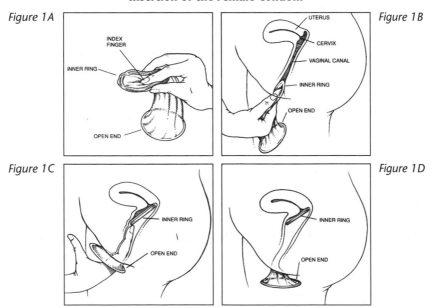

Figure 1A
Figure 1B
Figure 1C
Figure 1D

Source: The Female Health Company.

Contraceptive Efficacy

Results of a contraceptive effectiveness study performed by Family Health International (FHI) and the Contraceptive Research and Development (CONRAD) Program place the device on a par with other barrier methods.[1,3] During the FDA hearing, Gaston Farr, Associate Director of Clinical Trials at FHI, presented a summary of the preliminary results from a noncomparative trial of women from Latin America and the U.S.

"Failure rates are lower in the U.S. cohort," he explained, "when viewed beside Latin America. The 6 month life-table rate for all users was 15.1 per 100 women, with a 95% confidence interval of 8.9 to 21.1."[1]

Improper use was cited as a factor in the majority of pregnancies that occurred among women in the study. According to Farr, "Overall, 76% of the 25 pregnancies that we report were attributed to user failure." The study defined user failure as "a pregnancy in which the subject had a history of product misuse at any time during her participation in the study."[1] Misuse included irregular use of the female condom or use of another method.

Farr concluded that "the overall interim 6 month life-table pregnancy rate is within acceptable levels and is comparable to other barrier methods."[1] The final study enrolled 377 women, of whom 353 were eligible to contribute data on efficacy. The findings were similar to preliminary results: the 6 month life-table probability of failure for the female condom was 15% (12% among U.S. women and 22% among Latin American women; the difference was not statistically significant).

Since the time of the FDA meeting, reanalyses of the clinical trial data suggested a lower estimated "perfect use" failure rate, which assumes the method is used correctly and consistently. Trussell et al estimate a 5.1% failure rate with perfect use.[4] Among typical users, the failure rate about equals that of the diaphragm, sponge and cervical cap. Thus far, there have been no comparable efficacy trials with the male condom. In late 1995, the FDA updated the labeling of the female condom, lowering the expected use failure rates and extending the shelf life of the product to 3 years (see box on the following page).

Disease Prevention

The ability of the female condom to protect against disease infection is seen as an important aspect given the current epidemic of STDs and the growing incidence of AIDS, especially among women. Women are reported to be far more susceptible to heterosexual transmission of human immunodeficiency virus (HIV) than men. One study suggested that women are up to 17 times more likely to be infected by an HIV-positive male partner than men are by an HIV-positive female partner (although this issue continues to be the subject of much investigation and debate).[5]

The number of AIDS cases in women is "relentlessly moving forward," explained Mary E. Guinan, MD, PhD, Special Assistant for Evaluation (HIV) at the Centers for Disease Control and Prevention, who testified at the FDA meeting. "In 1991, the total was 5,700 cases. ...The increase is approximately 17% in cases in women from 1990 to 1991." In 1994, 18% of AIDS cases in those ages 13 years and older occurred among

Female Condom Labeling Revisions

The FDA has changed the labeling of the female condom. On a yearly basis, the failure rate for the female condom is estimated to be 5% when used correctly and consistently (perfect use). Previous product labeling did not give a 12-month perfect-use failure rate. The new, 12-month failure rate with "typical use" (which includes incorrect or nonuse) is 21%, with a range of 18% to 25%; this is a drop from the 25% failure rate listed in the old labeling. In addition, the device now has a shelf life of 3 years, up from 2 years.

The female condom is now listed for Medicaid reimbursement or other similar programs in 36 states. The manufacturer, The Female Health Company, has established a toll-free number for clinicians with questions about the female condom or who wish to share clinical experiences.

Phone: (800) 635-0844 • Fax: (312) 280-9360

12-Month Failure Rates of Female Condom

	Typical Use*	Perfect Use**
Old Labeling	25%	None Given
New Labeling	21% (range = 18% to 25%)	5%

*Indicates the method may have been used inconsistently, not used with every act of intercourse, or may have failed during use.

**Perfect use means that the method was used correctly with every act of intercourse; failure is due to slippage or breakage.

women. This steadily increasing proportion represents a threefold increase from 1985 to 1994.[6] Regarding protection for women against infection, Dr. Guinan added, "I advocate condoms to protect against sexually transmitted diseases, but if they're not used, they're not effective. ...I believe that if we had something that was under the control of women, it would be much more utilized."

With regard to disease prevention, the FDA panel raised concerns over the material integrity of the device and requested further data on ripping and breakage. In terms of permeability, however, the polyurethane film used in the manufacture of the female condom is twice as thick as the latex rubber used in condoms, and laboratory tests conducted by Voeller et al have suggested the viral permeability of the material is less than that of latex.[7]

The permeability studies performed on the female condom included the use of gaseous tracers, such as helium and nitrogen, in addition to traditional aqueous dye and viral methods. The use of gases was described as a state-of-the-art method by Bruce Voeller, PhD, who attended the FDA meeting to discuss the findings of his research. "In contrast with aqueous methods," Dr. Voeller noted, "the gas method is not subjected to the problems of surface tension and hole wetting in the same ways. The aqueous dye and viral methods, however, are more kindred to the female condom's actual environment in sexual use."[1]

Dr. Voeller explained that "if gases and dyes, orders of magnitude smaller than STD agents, and a tiny virus could be blocked by the (female condom), it is reasonable to assume larger viruses and the much larger bacterial STDs will be blocked." He concluded by noting that "all of our studies, including the liquid ones simulating coitus, tested and found no leakage through any of the whole (female condoms) that we evaluated or the (individual polyurethane) sections."[1]

The manufacturer presented some data that suggest the device may help prevent vaginal trichomoniasis reinfection.[8] The study evaluated 104 women with documented vaginal trichomoniasis; 50 controls and 54 female condom users. Among users, 20 women were compliant, ie, they used the female condom correctly with every act of intercourse. Although the results were not statistically significant, the researchers found a 0% reinfection rate among the compliant users compared to a 14% and 15% reinfection rate for controls and noncompliant users, respectively.

Trussell et al estimate that with perfect use the device could afford 94% protection against HIV. The estimate applies to women having intercourse twice weekly with an infected partner.[4] More research is needed, however, before any definitive conclusions can be made regarding the female condom's effectiveness at preventing specific STDs.

Acceptability and Proper Use

Concerns were raised during the FDA meeting regarding method acceptability and whether the product would interfere with the user's sexual responsiveness. Although no data were presented on the specific topic of responsiveness, Mary Ann Leeper, PhD, head of the device's development team, addressed the general issue of product acceptability. Dr. Leeper told the FDA panel that motivation to use the product is an important aspect in its acceptability and affects the likelihood of its being used properly.

According to Dr. Leeper, "Women who are sexually active, concerned about sexually transmitted disease as well as unintended pregnancy, in general like using the female condom and tend to use it properly with no problems. Women who are married and in long-term, monogamous relationships—and generally only interested in a method to help protect against unintended pregnancy—find other methods, such as oral contraceptives, easier to use."[1]

To facilitate ease of use, guidelines established by the Obstetrics and Gynecology Devices Panel require that instructions accompanying products such as the female condom be understandable by users with a fifth- to sixth-grade education and include a pictorial for users who are illiterate. Concerns over potential language barriers were also expressed at the FDA meeting. "It is very important that the information about the condom be written in a language accessible to all women," noted Sabrina Sojourner of the Women of Color Partnership Program during a presentation to the panel. "If the information is not clear and not accessible, it impacts the entire community."[1]

Product Labeling

The FDA panel objected to inclusion of claims of protection against specific STDs in the labeling, noting that although the results of viral permeability tests were favorable, no conclusive data exist to verify the claims of protection against *individual* diseases. Having only presented data on one specific STD, trichomoniasis,[8] the manufacturer agreed to revise product labeling and reduce the claim of disease protection to the less-specific version carried by male condoms. The FDA ultimately required the company to state in its labeling: "Latex condoms for men are highly effective at preventing sexually transmitted diseases, including AIDS (HIV infection), if used properly. If your partner is not going to use a male latex condom, you can use [the female condom] to help protect you and your partner."

The FDA also required that pregnancy rate information be included in the product's labeling. FDA Reviewer Christine L. Brauer stated that "effectiveness information, including pregnancy rate information, should be included in the labeling of the device and presented in an appropriate manner for a consumer to make an informed decision about the use of the product."[1]

Conclusion

Although the female condom may not offer a lower pregnancy rate than the male condom, the device does provide women with a female-controlled contraceptive method that helps prevent STDs and AIDS. Women for whom pregnancy prevention and disease protection is a combined goal are currently advised to use condoms in combination with an effective method of fertility regulation, such as hormonal contraceptives. The availability of an additional disease prevention method—especially one that is controlled by the woman herself—represents an important step in the nationwide effort to stop the spread of HIV and other STDs.

References

1. Food and Drug Administration. Obstetrics and Gynecology Devices Panel: Forty-Eighth Meeting (meeting transcript). Washington, DC:U.S. Department of Health and Human Services; 1992.

2. Wisconsin Pharmacal Corporation. REALITY, The Female Condom (press release). January 1992.

3. Trussell J, Hatcher RA, Cates W Jr., et al. Contraceptive failure in the United States: an update. *Stud Fam Plann* 1990;21(1):51-54.

4. Trussell J, Sturgen K, Strickler J, et al. Comparative contraceptive efficacy of the female condom and other barrier methods. *Fam Plann Perspect* 1994;26:66-72.

5. Padian NS, Shiboski SC, Jewell NP. Female-to-male transmission of human immunodeficiency virus. *JAMA* 1991;266:1664-1667.

6. Centers for Disease Control and Prevention. Update: AIDS among women—United States, 1994. *MMWR* 1995;44:81-84.

7. Voeller B, Coulter SL, Mayhan KG. Gas, dye, and viral transport through polyurethane condoms. *JAMA* 1991;266:2986-2987. Letter.

8. Soper DE, Shoupe D, Shangold GA, et al. Prevention of vaginal trichomoniasis by compliant use of the female condom. *Sex Transm Dis* 1993;20:137-139.

5.2: Acceptability Issues

In August 1994, the female condom reached drugstore and supermarket shelves across the country. Although approved by the Food and Drug Administration in May 1993, the product had only been available in family planning and sexually transmitted disease (STD) clinics.

The Female Health Company (a division of Wisconsin Pharmacal) began marketing the product to consumers with an extensive print and educational campaign designed to familiarize women with the way the product looks and how to use it. The device is specifically aimed at a woman who wants to protect herself, especially against HIV infection, when her male partner refuses to use a latex condom. The primary advantage of the female condom is the woman's ability to control the method without relying on her partner. The product can be inserted prior to foreplay and intercourse, without interrupting the sexual encounter. Another advantage over male latex condoms is that individuals who are allergic to latex can safely use the method.

Because the device is visible and can be felt outside the vagina, however, the concern about men objecting to its use may still hold. Women who are concerned about a man's response or who are unable to negotiate the use of a male condom may not find it easier to negotiate the use of a female condom. On the other hand, men may be more willing to accept the female condom when the woman has already inserted it because they do not have to take any action themselves. In addition, use of the female condom does not interrupt the sexual encounter.

The aesthetics of the device have been its major drawback. Many initially find the device cumbersome. Educational pamphlets from the manufacturer acknowledge the initial strangeness—"If you think it looks funny...you're right. Remember, you never saw a female condom before"—and encourage women to practice inserting one before using it for the first time.

Getting women to use the female condom may take more than helping them become familiar with its looks, however. According to Denese O. Shervington, MD, MPH, a psychiatrist and Associate Director of Public Health for the Department of Obstetrics and Gynecology at Louisiana State University Medical Center, "The female condom seems to challenge our traditional gender roles and ideas about sexuality. I was surprised that a product with the potential to stem the spread of HIV wouldn't be greeted with more enthusiasm. But, it seems that the idea of women taking control of their sexuality stirs some deeply held beliefs. I don't think an advertising campaign will be able to overcome initial resistance. I believe education that addresses how women feel about themselves, their sexuality, and their relationships must take place in order to increase use and acceptance of the female condom."

Dr. Shervington conducted a pilot study among 18 African-American women.[1] Initially, most women and their partners did not like the way the female condom looked. After focus group discussions, all women decided to try the product. Even though some male partners made fun of the product initially, all agreed to give it a try.

"What I found," Dr. Shervington said, "was that as women personalized their own risk of HIV, they became willing to use the product. The focus group discussions were particularly important for uncovering how women felt about using a product that put them in control. We also talked about their relationships. Interestingly, even some married women realized that perhaps their relationships might be characterized as 'inconsistent' monogamy." One of Dr. Shervington's most important findings was that once the women got over their initial reservations about using the device, they felt they had more control over their sexual health.

Men may be concerned that the female condom will feel unpleasant and/or decrease sexual pleasure. Dr. Shervington found that some of the men and women stated they preferred the product over the male condom because they liked the feel of the polyurethane better than latex. Users also liked the fact that the male partner had more room in the larger size of the female condom. The device is not tight fitting and thus provides a different kind of sensation for the man than a male latex condom.

Family planning clinics in the United States have been offering female condoms since 1993. Sue Epler, RN, is Director of the Planned Parenthood Clinic in New York's Bronx borough, one clinic that has been carrying the device. According to Ms. Epler, "Before we began offering the female condom in our clinic, we asked the staff to try it and give us some feedback. What we found was that about half liked it. Like any contraceptive method, some people will like it and some won't. But, it's so important for women to have another option to protect against STDs—one that they can be in control of. Many men who are HIV-positive often have no intention of either telling their partners or using a male condom."

One survey of 52 women at a health clinic in Harlem, New York City, found that about two-thirds liked using the female condom.[2] The women were health care workers and patients recruited by word of mouth from a hospital infectious disease clinic. Group educational sessions provided women with a forum to broach concerns and questions about the method. The clinic distributed female condoms to the women, who returned at periodic intervals to obtain more condoms and fill out questionnaires regarding their experiences.

According to Erica Gollub, DrPH, who conducted the Harlem study and is an epidemiologist at the Philadelphia Department of Public Health, "The results are quite promising. About two-thirds of the women reported that they liked the female condom somewhat or very much. About three-fourths of the women and more than two-fifths of their partners reported liking the device more than the male condom. Some of the problems reported included invagination of the outer ring, the penis entering the vagina to the side of the condom and the device riding the penis (sticking to and moving with the penis rather than remaining in place in the vagina). These problems occurred in about 10% to 20% of participants and can usually be helped by adding extra lubricant to the inside of the device or penis.

"My feeling is that women are pleased about having another way to protect themselves. The three things women reported liking best were the feeling of protection, the feel of the condom and the sense of control. My experience has been that women have had a great response to the female condom because they're frustrated by the limited choices they have for STD protection and by having to ask the man to please wear a condom," she added.

Additional research is currently under way or soon to begin. One study at the Philadelphia Department of Public Health plans to measure the female condom's effectiveness as a barrier to gonorrhea, chlamydia, syphilis and other STDs. Another study will look at which method of protection women will use when given a choice and evaluate the effect of safer sex education efforts. An ongoing study funded by the National Institute of Child Health and Human Development at the University of Alabama at Birmingham's School of Public Health is evaluating the female condom's efficacy at preventing STDs as compared with the male condom.

References
1. Shervington D. Experiences of African American women with the use of the Reality® female condom. Presented in a poster at the X International Conference on AIDS, Yokohama, Japan, August 1994.
2. Gollub EL, Stein Z, El-Sadr W. Short-term acceptability of the female condom among staff and patients at a New York City hospital. *Fam Plann Perspect* 1995;27:155-158.

5.3: Patient Counseling

Your patients may ask you about the female condom.
Here are some questions and possible answers.

Q: *What does it feel like during sex?*

A: The material is polyurethane, a type of plastic that is stronger, thinner and softer than latex. The device should be comfortable for both partners. There is no way to tell exactly how it will feel for you or your partner until you try it.

Q: *How do I insert the device?*

A: The insertion is much like that of a tampon or diaphragm. Squeeze the inner ring (at the closed end of the pouch) and insert it up into the vagina to cover the cervix. It's a good idea to try inserting one before you use it for the first time. This will help you to become more comfortable with proper insertion while not under the pressure of a sexual encounter. Make sure to read the instructions carefully. Maximum pregnancy and STD protection depend upon correct use.

Q: *Is there more than one size?*

A: No, the female condom is designed to fit most women.

Q: *How much do they cost?*

A: The female condom costs about $2.75 to $3.00 per condom and is available in boxes of 3 ($8.99) and 6 ($16.99). Family planning clinics may be providing them at a lower cost. The product is available in drugstores and supermarkets around the country. The product is more costly than male condoms.

Q: *Do I need to use a spermicide?*

A: No, you do not need to use a spermicide, but you can if you wish. The female condoms are prelubricated and come with an extra bottle of lubricant. The lubricant does not contain spermicide.

Q: Can I use the female condom during my menstrual period?

A: Yes, but remove it soon after intercourse.

Q: Should the man wear a condom if the woman is using a female condom?

A: No.

Q: How does the device feel to a man?

A: Some men report liking the female condom better than male condoms. There may be two reasons for this. One, the polyurethane is a plastic that transmits heat well, giving a more natural sensation of body warmth during sexual intercourse. Two, the size of the female condom allows more room for the penis than the male condom, a sensation that may be more pleasurable.

Q: Can I use the female condom more than once?

A: No, use the female condom one time only. Take out the device after intercourse before standing up.

Q: When do I put it in?

A: A woman has many options about when to insert the device. You can insert the female condom up to 8 hours before sex, during foreplay or just prior to intercourse.

Addressing Patient Concerns

If she says...	*You might suggest...*
It's noisy (squeaks).	Add more lubricant to the device or penis.
It rides the penis (sticks to and moves with the penis instead of remaining in place in the vagina).	Add more lubricant to the device or penis.
My male partner feels the inner ring.	Review the instructions for insertion. Feeling the inner ring may be caused by not pushing the ring far enough into the vagina. Push the inner ring as far up into the vagina as it will go, behind the pubic bone and over the cervix. Or, check to see if the sheath is twisted.
The outer ring was pushed up into my vagina.	Use more lubricant.
The penis was inserted to the side of the device upon entering the vagina.	Have either partner guide the penis during entry.
Minor irritation or discomfort for either partner.	Review insertion instructions; use extra lubricant.

■6 Female Sterilization

Female sterilization has long been considered one of the most highly effective methods of contraception. During the past 2 decades, however, questions arose concerning whether tubal sterilization might alter menstrual patterns or result in more gynecological morbidity. Does a "post-tubal sterilization syndrome" exist? If so, what could be the causative biologic mechanism(s)? Does the type of procedure influence subsequent development of the syndrome? These and other questions are addressed in the first section of this chapter.

The second section covers the recently completed Collaborative Review of Sterilization (CREST). This long-term, prospective study of American women found some startling trends—among them, cumulative 10-year failure rates are higher than previously believed and place women at a greater risk of pregnancy than clinicians had realized. The section also takes a look at which women are most likely to regret their sterilization and provides a review of key counseling issues. A third section describes the Filshie clip, a tubal occlusion device recommended for approval in the United States in February 1996.

6.1: Post-Tubal Sterilization Syndrome

Although the existence of a "post-tubal sterilization syndrome" has been postulated since the 1950s, a clear, specific case definition is lacking. Moreover, the existence of such a syndrome has yet to be substantiated. Studies, to date, especially those done in the 1970s, have been methodologically flawed and have failed to yield consistent results. It appears that a large proportion of the changes in menstrual function after sterilization may be explained by the fact that many women choosing sterilization are discontinuing oral contraceptives (OCs). After sterilization, women may attribute altered menstrual patterns to the procedure rather than to the discontinuation of prior birth control methods.

Post-tubal sterilization syndrome is a loosely defined entity. Symptoms attributed to the syndrome include pelvic pain, change in sexual behavior, changes in mental health, alteration of the menstrual cycle, increased blood loss, exacerbation of premenstrual syndrome (PMS) and abnormal hormone levels. Concern remains because millions of women have selected sterilization as a means of birth control (Figure 1).[1,2] In the U.S., sterilization is the leading method of contraception used by married women.[2]

Further concern exists regarding the potential for menstrual dysfunction as a result of tubal sterilization. This morbidity might lead to subsequent hysterectomy.[3] Early studies suggested that 10% to 50% of patients reported menstrual disturbances 6 months to 10 years after tubal sterilization—which would place millions of women at long-term risk of the syndrome.[4]

Figure 1

Percentage of Women Using Contraception 15 to 44 Years of Age Who Relied on Female Sterilization: United States, 1982 and 1988

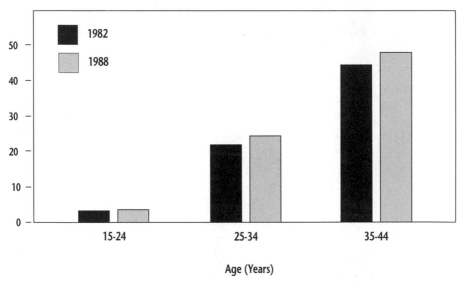

Age (Years)

Source: Mosher WD, et al, 1990 (see reference 1).

Other Explanations for Menstrual Changes

Stopping oral contraceptive use just prior to sterilization may also be a cause of menstrual irregularities after sterilization.[5] Women who discontinue this method of contraception will experience menstrual changes regardless of subsequent tubal surgery. Because OCs regulate menstrual cycles and frequently decrease duration and amount of blood flow, patients who discontinue pill use usually return to their former longer duration and heavier bleeding patterns. This must be considered when documenting menstrual change after sterilization. A woman's recollection of previous menstrual patterns may be vague, particularly if she has been using OCs for many years.

The signs and symptoms of post-tubal sterilization syndrome may, in fact, be related to the normal aging process or gynecological abnormalities. As a woman ages, menstrual cycles may change as hormonal patterns fluctuate. This is true particularly during the perimenopausal period. Lower back pain, irregular bleeding or dysmenorrhea can be related to endometriosis. Localized endometriosis after sterilization has been documented in a number of cases.[6] In addition, leiomyomas and neoplasms must be ruled out as underlying causes.

Study Findings and Limitations

A retrospective study by Williams et al in 1951 opened the controversy about post-tubal sterilization syndrome.[7] Williams described a possible relationship between tubal sterilization and subsequent abnormal uterine bleeding in 200 women. He compared the rate of abnormal uterine bleeding after sterilization (17%) in these 200 women to the rate found for 3,222 obstetrical cases (5%). He found that "The data...suggest that individuals who are subjected to sterilization procedures later develop a higher percentage of abnormal uterine bleeding than would be expected in a comparable number of unselected normal women. ...It seems most likely that this predisposition to abnormal bleeding is related to the underlying disease or condition for which the sterilization is performed rather than to any mechanical interference with ovarian or uterine function resulting from the operative procedure."[7] Despite Williams' conclusion, the issue of whether sterilization could cause subsequent menstrual irregularities had been raised.

The question of whether post-tubal sterilization syndrome exists remains unanswered largely because of inconsistencies in study design. The majority of studies conducted in the 1970s had serious methodological flaws. They were small, retrospective reviews, based on women's recall of menstrual patterns. Many of the studies ignored such factors as increasing age, number of years since the operative procedure, type of surgery, menstrual status of the patient before surgery and the cessation of OCs.

Over the past 2 decades, researchers have performed many investigations of post-tubal sterilization syndrome, yet the body of evidence offers no definitive support of the syndrome's existence.[8-20] The following short summaries of key studies shed light on the evidence for and against the post-tubal sterilization syndrome.

Kasonde and Bonnar, 1976, are the only group that measured blood loss to assess menstrual change.[8] Their study included 25 women. Blood loss was measured before sterilization and at 6 months and 12 months after sterilization. Researchers concluded that there was no change in blood loss in this group of women.

Radwanska et al, 1979, described endocrine changes in 40 women requesting sterilization reversal.[9] Progesterone levels during the midluteal phase (5 to 10 days before the next menstrual period) were measured, although no data were reported on whether multiple progesterone levels were done and averaged in each cycle. A significant decrease in the level of progesterone was detected in the sterilized women as compared to control women.

Corson et al, 1981, initiated a controlled study in 48 women with hysterectomies, or women sterilized by bipolar electrosurgery or an occlusive ring technique. Midluteal progesterone levels were measured. No significant difference was demonstrable when the four groups were compared.[10]

Donnez et al, 1981, used midluteal phase progesterone measurements and endometrial biopsy to measure luteal function in women with tubal sterilization and a control group.[11] A higher frequency of luteal defects (progesterone levels lower than 10 ng/mL or endometrial retardation) was seen in women receiving tubal ligation and electrocoagulation than in women sterilized using the clip technique. Other researchers have reached opposite conclusions with regard to the presence of luteal phase defects in sterilized women.[10,16,21]

Bhiwandiwala et al, 1983, conducted a noncontrolled, multicenter, prospective study involving 10,004 women.[12] They examined menstrual pattern changes following interval or postabortion laparoscopic sterilization. Cycle regularity, cycle length, flow duration, amount of flow, dysmenorrhea and intermenstrual bleeding were used to evaluate pattern changes. The women were evaluated at 6, 12 and 24 months. No changes, except a slight increase in pain among women who had unipolar electrosurgery, were seen in this large group of women.

Fortney et al, 1983, conducted a study of 1,555 sterilized women.[13] This study compared the effects of different methods of sterilization on menstrual patterns. A multiple regression analysis and a single additive score of menstrual change composed of cycle length, regularity, duration of bleeding and dysmenorrhea were used. The results indicated that tubal rings and clips were associated with less change than electrocoagulation or ligation.[13] However, use of an additive menstrual change score is a questionable methodology.

Vessey et al, 1983, used hospital records to study 2,243 sterilized women.[14] Women were evaluated up to 6 years after sterilization. A control group of 3,551 women whose husbands had vasectomies was used. Outcomes were measured by comparing hospital referrals or admissions for gynecological or menstrual disorders. These researchers found no significant differences between the two groups.

DeStefano et al, 1985, analyzed one of the more rigorous studies to date, the Walnut Creek Contraceptive Drug Study.[15] This group looked at long-term menstrual pattern changes in 719 women. The study used nonsterilized women as a control group and followed women for up to 87 months. The women in the tubal sterilization group were younger than controls. At 2 years, the tubal sterilization group was comparable to the control group, but in the following years, changes were noted. Abnormal cycles were three times more prevalent in the sterilized group at 49 to 87 months than in the control group. Women who had abnormal cycles prior to sterilization were at greatest risk. No increase of PMS was reported.

Alvarez et al, 1989, reported results from a small, prospective, longitudinal study of ovarian endocrine function in women receiving sterilization by the Pomeroy or Uchida technique.[16] Hormone levels were measured before the sterilization, at 2 months and at 6 months post-sterilization. Women sterilized by the Uchida technique experienced a slight change in plasma progesterone at the 2-month test interval; otherwise, there was no change.

Rulin et al, 1989, conducted a large multicenter, controlled, prospective trial using "before" and "after" interviews of sterilized and nonsterilized women.[17] Investigators interviewed 1,642 women rating menstrual cycles, duration of menstrual flow and bleeding between periods. No difference was seen between the sterilized group and the nonsterilized group for these parameters. However, the prevalence of dysmenorrhea increased in 11% of sterilized women, compared with 2% of the control group.[17]

Shain et al, 1989, prospectively compared menstrual data from 227 sterilized women against 219 nonsterilized women to determine the extent of change in the sterilized group.[4] Interviews questioning 16 variables were used to determine menstrual function. Results were analyzed by sterilization method. No adverse changes were seen in women banded with Falope rings. Cauterization and Pomeroy sterilization, however, resulted in heavier bleeding, a greater incidence of dysmenorrhea and abnormal cycle lengths when compared to controls.

Garza-Flores et al, 1991, reported no major changes in ovarian function in women sterilized by the Pomeroy ligation technique.[18] Garza-Flores prospectively evaluated

16 women at 3 and 12 months post-sterilization, and another group of 15 women, of whom six were evaluated at 1 year and nine at 5 years post-sterilization. Midluteal progesterone and estradiol serum levels were assessed by serial measurements. No major changes in menstrual patterns, associated symptoms or clinical manifestations of gynecological illness were observed.

Rojansky and Halbreich, 1991, conducted retrospective and prospective evaluations of women seeking treatment for premenstrual symptoms.[19] Twenty-five of the 78 participating women had undergone tubal sterilization from 2 to 23 years prior to the study. Premenstrual symptoms and hormone levels (estradiol, progesterone, testosterone, thyroid stimulating hormone and total thyroxine) were assayed during the midfollicular phase and again during the late luteal phase of the menstrual cycle. Premenstrual symptoms during the luteal phase were compared to those reported previously. No significant differences were noted in PMS symptoms between sterilized and nonsterilized women. There was no difference in the luteal phase hormone levels of these two groups. The authors concluded that PMS symptoms are not associated with tubal sterilization.

Wilcox et al, 1992, examined 5-year data from the CREST study, which involved 5,070 women.[3] This multicenter, prospective study examined changes in six menstrual variables and categorized results based on method of sterilization. Overall, no changes in menstrual patterns were seen at 2 years; however, changes were seen in subsequent years. The results showed more increases in menstrual pain, amount of bleeding and intermenstrual spotting, but decreases in days per cycle and days of bleeding per cycle after year 2. This study is limited by the subjective nature of event reporting and by the lack of a nonsterilized control group, which would have controlled for events related to the aging of the study population or other time-dependent variables.[3] Although 10-year data from the recently completed CREST study have not been fully analyzed, preliminary findings suggest no evidence of a post-tubal sterilization syndrome.[22]

Shy et al, 1992, used population-based hospital discharge data to investigate tubal sterilization and subsequent hospitalization for menstrual disorder.[20] A group of 7,253 sterilized women were compared with an age-matched group of 25,448 nonsterilized women and a nonmatched group of 5,283 women whose husbands chose vasectomies. The risk for hospitalization was 2.4 times greater after tubal sterilization; however, Shy found no biologically plausible explanation for this risk. A possible reason for the higher incidence in hospitalization was the difference in childbearing ability. Women expecting no additional children may have chosen such hospital-based treatments as hysterectomy to correct problems over other treatment options. Hysterectomy occurred in 59% of sterilized women versus 45% in the control group. The authors note "women who elect tubal sterilization for contraception are inherently greater users of elective gynecologic surgeries (eg, curettage, hysterectomy)."

Proposed Theoretical Explanations

Investigators have proposed that procedures that cause more tissue destruction (tubal ligation, electrosurgery) may cause more changes than the application of clips or rings.[23] Some researchers have proposed that this alteration in structure, especially within the vasculature, is responsible for post-tubal sterilization syndrome.[15,21]

Researchers also suggest that if the blood supply to the ovaries is changed, hormone levels may be altered. This may result in a decrease in ovulation due to a decrease in blood flow to the ovaries. A reduced arterial blood supply could reduce the amount of follicle-stimulating hormone (FSH) and the amount of luteinizing hormone (LH) delivered to the ovaries. Over a period of time, reduced estrogen and progesterone levels would then stimulate the production of FSH and LH, establishing a peri-menopausal condition. Proof for this theory is lacking and studies evaluating luteal phase defects after sterilization have been inconclusive.[11,21,24]

In 1977, Rioux determined that ovarian function and hormonal levels remain unaltered, even after hysterectomy; these findings contradict the theory of disruption of the utero-ovarian blood supply.[25] In addition, Alvarez (1989) found no difference between sterilization techniques that caused more pelvic structure damage versus less damaging techniques.[16]

Does Technique Matter?

Several investigators reported that menstrual changes or hormone levels differ by the method of tubal occlusion. That the lowest rate of menstrual disturbance occurs with methods that lead to less tissue destruction is a prevailing premise. Yet, the more recent studies by Wilcox and Shy argue against this hypothesis. Wilcox found more menstrual changes in women sterilized by the clip method than those treated by electrocoagulation. Shy found the risk of menstrual disturbance to be lowest among women treated by unipolar sterilization compared with the other sterilization methods. Furthermore, although Radwasanka et al found changes in progesterone levels, such results were not seen by others investigating hormone changes.[9,10,16,18,19,26,27]

Counseling

Women considering sterilization should be counseled prior to the procedure regarding the possible existence of the post-tubal sterilization syndrome. Proper counseling, which takes into consideration the woman's menstrual history, can do much to alleviate anxiety, especially if she has heard of the syndrome from the media.

It is important to tell patients that some studies suggest that a minority of women may experience menstrual changes after sterilization. These changes may be perceived either positively or negatively, depending upon the individual. Women going off the pill or discontinuing the use of IUDs should be made aware that their menstrual patterns are likely to return to those prior to using these methods of contraception. Patients should also be made aware that menstrual patterns often become more irregular as menopause approaches.

Those least likely to experience menstrual changes are women under 35 who had normal menstrual patterns before sterilization. Although women with abnormal menstrual patterns before surgery are at most risk for experiencing change, the majority of sterilized women experience no change in menstrual patterns after sterilization.

Summary

Whether menstrual disturbances experienced by a minority of women are a result of sterilization or are dependent upon sterilization technique remains to be confirmed. The many articles written on the subject have not satisfactorily answered questions about the nature and the extent of these changes or their etiology. Although earlier articles tend to report an increase in menstrual disturbance after sterilization, most of the studies have methodological shortcomings. These include failure to control for patient category, previous contraceptive use, age and parity, failure to use a control group, failure to report improvements in menstrual patterns, failure to look at more than one change at a time, and failure to define terms and quantify changes.[13]

Recent studies tend to report no change in menstrual patterns. These studies are typically prospective trials involving large groups of women. None of the trials support the hypothesis that reduced blood flow to the ovaries results in hormonal changes that could effect a menstrual change. In conclusion, the literature suggests that if post-tubal sterilization syndrome occurs at all, it affects few women.

References

1.   Mosher WD, Pratt WF. Contraceptive use in the United States, 1973-88. *Advance data from vital and health statistics; no 182.* Hyattsville, Maryland: National Center for Health Statistics, 1990.

2.   Mosher WD. Contraceptive practice in the US: 1982-1988. *Fam Plann Perspect* 1990;22:198.

3.   Wilcox LS, Martinez-Schnell B, Peterson HB, et al. Menstrual function after tubal sterilization. *Am J Epidemiol* 1992;135:1368-1381.

4.   Shain RN, Miller WB, Mitchell GW, et al. Menstrual pattern change 1 year after sterilization: results of a controlled, prospective study. *Fertil Steril* 1989;52:192-203.

5.   Rulin MC, Turner JH. Posttubal ligation syndrome - a misnomer. *Am J Obstet Gynecol* 1985;151:13-19.

6.   Rock JA, Parmley TH, King TM, et al. Endometriosis and the development of tuboperitoneal fistulas after tubal ligation. *Fertil Steril* 1981;35:16-20.

7.   Williams EL, Jones HE, Merrill RE. The subsequent course of patients sterilized by tubal ligation. *Am J Obstet Gynecol* 1951;61:423-426.

8.   Kasonde JM, Bonnar J. Effect of sterilization on menstrual blood loss. *Br J Obstet Gynaecol* 1976;69:926-928.

9.   Radwanska E, Berger GS, Hammond J. Luteal deficiency among women with normal menstrual cycles, requesting reversal of tubal sterilization. *Obstet Gynecol* 1979;54:189-192.

10.   Corson SL, Levinson CJ, Batzer FR, et al. Hormonal levels following sterilization and hysterectomy. *J Reprod Med* 1981;26:363-370.

11.   Donnez J, Wauters M, Thomas K. Luteal function after tubal sterilization. *Obstet Gynecol* 1981;57:65-68.

12.   Bhiwandiwala PP, Mumford SD, Feldblum PJ. Menstrual pattern changes following laparoscopic sterilization with different occlusion techniques. *Am J Obstet Gynecol* 1983;145:684-694.

13.   Fortney JA, Cole LP, Kennedy KI. A new approach to measuring menstrual pattern change after tubal sterilization. *Am J Obstet Gynecol* 1983;147:830-836.

14.   Vessey M, Huggins G, Lawless M, et al. Tubal sterilization findings in a large prospective study. *Br J Obstet Gynaecol* 1983;90:203-209.

15.   DeStefano F, Perlman JA, Peterson HB, et al. Long-term risk of menstrual disturbances after tubal sterilization. *Am J Obstet Gynecol* 1985;152:835-841.

16.   Alvarez F, Faundes A, Brache V, et al. Prospective study of the pituitary-ovarian function after tubal sterilization by the Pomeroy or Uchida techniques. *Fertil Steril* 1989;51:604-608.

17.   Rulin MC, Davidson AR, Philliber SG, et al. Changes in menstrual symptoms among sterilized and comparison women: a prospective study. *Obstet Gynaecol* 1989;74:149-154.

18. Garza-Flores J, Vazquez Estrada L, Reyes A, et al. Assessment of luteal function after surgical tubal sterilization. *Adv Contracept* 1991;7:371-377.

19. Rojansky N, Halbreich U. Prevalence and severity of premenstrual changes after tubal sterilization. *J Reprod Med* 1991;36:551-555.

20. Shy KK, Stergachis A, Grothaus LG, et al. Tubal sterilization and risk of subsequent hospital admission for menstrual disorders. *Am J Obstet Gynecol* 1992;166(6 Pt 1):1698-1705;discussion 1705-1706.

21. Hague WE, Maier DB, Schmidt CL, et al. An evaluation of late luteal phase endometrium in women requesting reversal of tubal ligation. *Obstet Gynecol* 1987;69:926-928.

22. Peterson HB, Xia Z, Hughes JM, et al. The risk of pregnancy after tubal sterilization: findings from the U.S. Collaborative Review of Sterilization. *Am J Obstet Gynecol* 1996;174:1161-1170.

23. Cattanach J. Oestrogen deficiency after tubal ligation. *Lancet* 1985;April 13:847-849.

24. El Mahgoub S, El Shounbogy M, El Zeniny A. Long-term luteal changes after tubal sterilization. *Contraception* 1984;30:125-131.

25. Rioux JE. Late complications of female sterilization: a review of the literature and a proposal for further research. *J Reprod Med* 1977;19:329-340.

26. Winston RML. Tubal anastomosis for reversal of sterilization in 45 women. In: Brosens I, Winston RML, eds. *Reversibility of Female Sterilization* London: Academic Press, 1978.

27. Gomel V. Profile of women requesting reversal of sterilization. *Fertil Steril* 1978;30:39.

6.2: Failure Rates, Counseling Issues and Post-Sterilization Regret

The recently published Collaborative Review of Sterilization (CREST) sheds new light on previously held concepts regarding female sterilization. This large prospective study, conducted by the Centers for Disease Control and Prevention (CDC), is the only U.S. study to assess long-term risks of various sterilization methods in a large cohort of women.

In a paper presented at the September 1995 Annual Meeting of the American Gynecological and Obstetrical Society, and published in the April 1996 issue of the American Journal of Obstetrics and Gynecology, *Herbert B. Peterson, MD, and colleagues reported the findings. The most notable is the risk of pregnancy after tubal sterilization is higher than generally believed. The investigators found an overall life-table cumulative failure rate, over a period of 10 years, of 18.5 failures per 1,000 sterilizations (1.9%), a risk that varies by timing and type of procedure as well as by the age of the woman when sterilized.*

Introduction

Sterilization is the most widely used method of contraception in the U.S. According to the National Survey of Family Growth, in 1990, 26% of all U.S. women relied on sterilization (18% female and 8% male) for contraception.[1] The largest numbers of women depending on sterilization were 35 to 44 years of age; 33% of these women used either female or male sterilization for birth control. Among women using contraception, the percentage relying on female sterilization increased consistently with increasing age: 33% of those ages 30 to 34, 45% of those ages 35 to 39 and 51% of those ages 40 to 44. About 600,000 to 700,000 female sterilizations occur yearly in this country.

U.S. statistics mirror international trends. According to a 1995 study of sterilization in Great Britain, based on data from the General Household Survey, among couples under age 50, sterilization is the primary method of contraception, with slightly more women than men being sterilized—a trend that has remained relatively constant in recent decades.[2] The British survey also documented that the resort to sterilization is much quicker after the birth of the third child than after the second.

Many studies suggest an additional noncontraceptive benefit of tubal steriliza-tion—a lower risk of ovarian cancer (Figure 1).[3-5] For example, the Nurses' Health Study, a prospective study of over 120,000 female nurses, found a strong inverse asso-ciation between tubal ligation and ovarian cancer. This protective effect persisted even after adjustment for age, oral contraceptive use, parity and other ovarian cancer risk factors (RR=0.33; 95% confidence interval [CI], 0.2-0.6).[4] The study also found a weaker inverse association between simple hysterectomy and ovarian cancer (RR=0.7; 95% CI, 0.5-1.0). Researchers continue to explore this finding, but have yet to determine a cause that explains the effect.

Figure 1

Relative Risks of Ovarian Cancer in Women with Tubal Sterilization: Summary of Results from Seven Studies

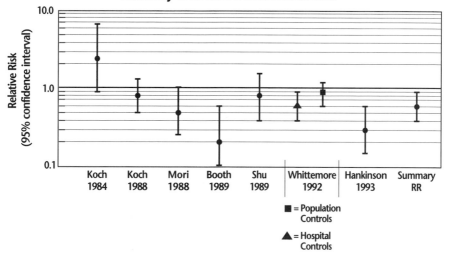

Source: Adapted from Hankinson SE, et al, 1993 (see reference 4).

The CREST Study

The CDC recently completed the CREST study—a landmark, 10-year look at female sterilization.[6] Researchers followed a group of 10,685 women for up to 14 years after their sterilizations. The procedures were performed between 1978 and 1986 at one of 16 medical centers in nine cities: Baltimore, Maryland; Buffalo, New York; Chapel Hill, North Carolina; Honolulu, Hawaii; Houston, Texas; Memphis, Tennessee; Sacramento, California; St. Louis, Missouri; and San Francisco, California.

Specially trained nurses interviewed women entering the study prior to steriliza-tion, by telephone at 1 month after sterilization and by telephone annually thereafter for 5 years. Additional telephone follow-up was conducted for those enrolled early enough in the study to have had 8 to 14 years elapse since their sterilizations.

CREST researchers documented 143 sterilization failures, which they were careful to classify as "true failures." Pregnancies that could possibly be classified as "luteal phase pregnancies" (a pregnancy identified after sterilization but having occurred prior to the procedure, n=34), a result of tubal anastomosis or *in vitro* fertilization (n=16), or were unclassifiable because of lack of information (n=5) were dropped from the failure group.

The CREST researchers classified sterilization procedures as follows: Partial salpingectomies included modified Pomeroy-type ligation, other types of partial salpingectomy, and total salpingectomy via laparotomy. Partial salpingectomies were then classified as to timing, ie, postpartum or interval. Laparoscopic approaches included unipolar and bipolar coagulation, spring clip application and silicone band application. Only women who had the same method of tubal occlusion on both tubes were included in the analysis.

The study sample differs in composition from the general U.S. population in race, but is similar in age. For example, the CREST sample contains slightly more black women than the general U.S. population and more patients from other minority groups as well. In an interview for this article, Herbert B. Peterson, MD, elaborated on the sample characteristics. Dr. Peterson is principal study investigator for CREST and Chief of the Women's Health and Fertility Branch of the Division of Reproductive Health, National Center for Chronic Disease Prevention and Health Promotion, at the CDC. "Although the CREST sample has proportionately more black women than the general population, it does, however, approximate the average age of women throughout the U.S. who have sterilization procedures each year." That demographic likeness is important because several of the study's most striking findings were age-related.

Dr. Peterson commented further on the make-up of the sample group. "The extent to which findings in our cohort are generalizable to all women having sterilizations is unclear," he said. "In addition, our sample is drawn exclusively from teaching institutions and we do not know whether our findings are generalizable to community hospital settings. Nevertheless, the study tells us much more about the long-term experience related to sterilization than was known previously," Dr. Peterson explained. "And, because of the complexity of carrying through a large, long-term follow-up study, we're unlikely to see similar studies in the U.S. in the near future."

Failure Rates

Overall failure rates

Failure rates are higher than previously believed. CREST reports an overall cumulative failure rate of 1.9%—more than double what has been accepted as the standard failure rate for tubal sterilization. This failure rate contrasts sharply with previous studies of common tubal occlusion techniques that cite figures lower than 1%. Until now, comparisons of contraceptive failure rates have reported the probability of failure during the first year after sterilization ranging between 0% and 0.4%.[7] These failure rates, however, have been based on investigations having only 1 or 2 years of follow-up.

Dr. Peterson advised that the overall failure rate needs to be viewed in context. He cautioned, "We shouldn't generalize this overall failure rate finding to the total U.S. population because it is an average of widely differing rates for specific methods—a method mix [in the CREST study] that is not the same as the proportional mix across all sterilizations performed in the U.S. The study's percentage of silicone band procedures, for instance, is much larger than its prevalence in the general population." In the CREST study, silicone band application was the most commonly performed method (31% of participants).

Failure rates by method

The relative risk of sterilization failure differed by method (Figure 2). For example, compared to postpartum partial salpingectomy, the highest relative risk of failure occurred with interval partial salpingectomy (RR=3.9; 95% CI, 1.4-10.6). Spring clip application had the second highest failure rate (RR=3.7; 95% CI, 1.5-8.9), followed, in decreasing order of risk, by bipolar coagulation, silicone band application and unipolar coagulation.

Dr. Peterson pointed out that the high failure rate for interval partial salpingectomy may have been skewed by steering higher risk women away from laparoscopic procedures and toward the interval laparotomy approach. According to Dr. Peterson, "Those

Figure 2

Overall Relative Risk of Sterilization Failure by Method of Sterilization

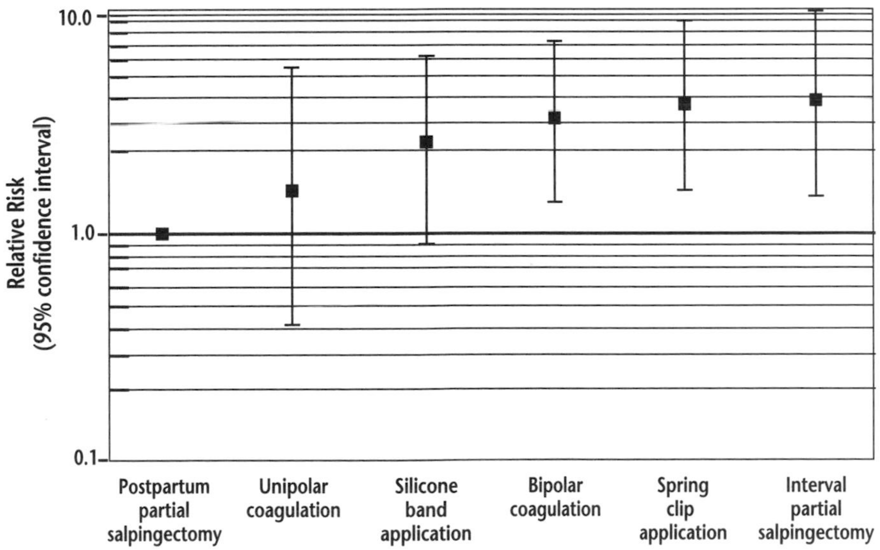

Source: Peterson HB, et al, 1996 (see reference 6).

Figure 3a

Life-Table Cumulative Probability of Pregnancy per 1,000 Procedures among Women Undergoing Tubal Sterilization by Method

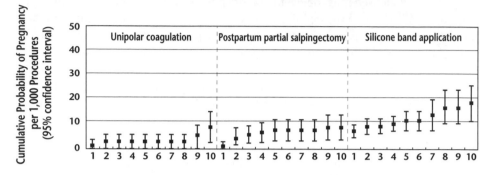

Number of Years Since Sterilization

Source: Peterson HB, et al, 1996 (see reference 6).

women who were sterilized by interval partial salpingectomy—which had a much higher 10-year failure rate (20.1 per 1,000 patients) than earlier studies would have led us to expect—were considered inappropriate candidates for the laparoscopic approach by their surgeons because they presented other risk factors, like prior abdominal or pelvic surgery or prior pelvic infections. We believe that steering women with other risk factors toward the interval laparotomy procedures contributed to its high failure rate."

CREST findings clearly indicate that failures are not exclusive to or more numerous during the first 2 years following the procedure. Failures do occur long after the procedure and the cumulative risk increases with time (see Figures 3a and 3b). The prevailing belief has been that the risk of failure is highest within the first year and then virtually disappears.[8,9] The CREST study ended after a 10-year follow-up, but its data indicate that failures may well continue to occur beyond 10 years after sterilization.

Of all methods, spring clip applications resulted in the highest first-year (1.8%) and 10-year failure rates (3.7%). The majority of spring clip failures occurred early, the rate rising from 18.2 to 23.8 per 1,000 between years 1 and 2. On the other hand, unipolar coagulation remained consistently effective for 8 years; the cumulative probability of pregnancy rose only in years 9 and 10. Postpartum partial salpingectomy also provided consistent protection against pregnancy during the full 10 years, although the cumulative probability of pregnancy increased between years 1 and 2. The cumulative probability of pregnancy with bipolar coagulation, and to a lesser extent with the silicone band, rose steadily each year throughout the 10-year period.

Cumulative 10-year failure rates

By gathering data over 10 years, CREST researchers have contributed to a new understanding and reassessment of long-term sterilization failure rates. The long-term

Figure 3b

Life-Table Cumulative Probability of Pregnancy per 1,000 Procedures among Women Undergoing Tubal Sterilization by Method

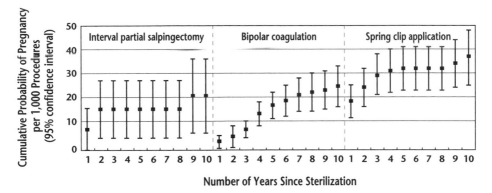

Number of Years Since Sterilization

Source: Peterson HB, et al, 1996 (see reference 6).

probabilities of failure were high for some methods. The highest cumulative 10-year probability of failure, 3.7%, is reported for the spring clip (36.5 per 1,000 procedures). Bipolar coagulation resulted in the second highest 10-year, cumulative risk of pregnancy, 2.5% (24.8 per 1,000 procedures). Postpartum partial salpingectomy and unipolar coagulation are the most effective methods, each having a 0.8% failure rate (7.5 per 1,000 procedures). According to Dr. Peterson, "because method failures continued to occur many years after sterilization, the concept of cumulative probability of failure is important, particularly for those women sterilized at a young age, who have many more years of potential fertility during which they could experience a sterilization failure."

Figure 4

Relative Risk of Failure by Age at Time of Sterilization

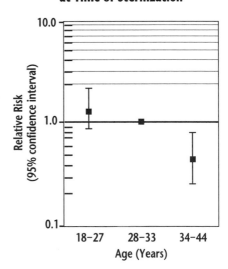

Source: Peterson HB, et al, 1996 (see reference 6).

Age and risk of failure

CREST data indicate that the risk of failure is greatest among women sterilized at a younger age (Figure 4). According to CREST authors, "In general, the younger a woman was at the time of sterilization, the more likely she was to have a sterilization failure. The older a woman was at the time of sterilization, the less likely the method

179

Figure 5a

Life-Table Cumulative Probability of Pregnancy per 1,000 Procedures among Women Ages 18 to 27 Years at the Time of Sterilization

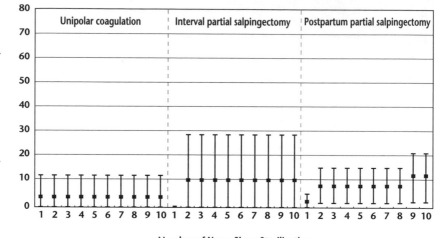

Number of Years Since Sterilization

Source: Peterson HB, et al, 1996 (see reference 6).

of sterilization was to affect the cumulative probability of failure." For example, the highest cumulative 10-year probability of failure was found for women ages 18 to 27 sterilized by bipolar coagulation; their risk of accidental pregnancy was a little over 5% (54 per 1,000 procedures). Among women ages 28 to 33 at the time of bipolar sterilization, however, the 10-year cumulative risk dropped to 2% (21 per 1,000 procedures); for women ages 34 to 44, the risk decreased still further to 0.6% (6 per 1,000 procedures).

Among the youngest women (ages 18 to 27 years at time of sterilization), failure rates varied by type of procedure. Unipolar coagulation, interval partial salpingectomy and postpartum partial salpingectomy all provided consistent protection over 10 years (Figure 5a). On the other hand, silicone band application, spring clip application and bipolar coagulation afforded less protection; failure rates increased consistently and often substantially over the 10-year period (Figure 5b).

Postpartum partial salpingectomy has one of the lowest failure rates when averaged across all age groups. For this method, however, like the others, the highest cumulative probability of pregnancy was found among the youngest group in the sample: 11.4 per 1,000 procedures for women ages 18 to 27; 5.6 for those ages 28 to 33; and 3.8 for those over 34 years of age. Among women 18- to 27-years-old at time of bipolar coagulation, 2.8% became pregnant 5 years after the operation. Failures of that method occurred with regularity throughout the 10-year follow-up, as did silicone band failures.

The numbers of young women choosing sterilization, however, may be declining. Amy Pollack, MD, MPH, president of AVSC International (Access to Voluntary and

Figure 5b

Life-Table Cumulative Probability of Pregnancy per 1,000 Procedures among Women Ages 18 to 27 Years at the Time of Sterilization

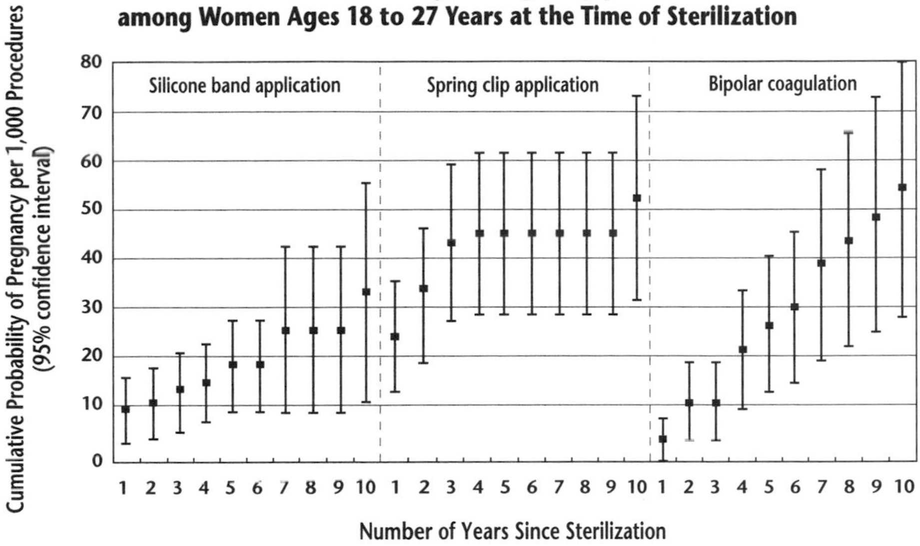

Source: Peterson HB, et al, 1996 (see reference 6).

Safe Contraception), believes that the percentage of women choosing sterilization may be decreasing, especially among younger women, for several reasons. In an interview for this article she said, "Women and their health care providers have more confidence in other forms of birth control, notably oral contraceptives. Data now support the use of oral contraceptives among healthy, nonsmoking women over age 35 years up until menopause," she explained. "Also women are marrying later and waiting longer after marriage to start families—all factors that raise the age at which a woman considers permanent contraception."

Ectopic Pregnancy

Many pregnancies that occur after sterilization are ectopic.[10,11] In CREST, ectopic pregnancies accounted for 33% of failures. Therefore, sterilized women who suspect they might be pregnant, even many years after the operation, should immediately be checked by their clinician—not only because of the longer-term failure risk, but also because the chance of ectopic pregnancy is high.

Bipolar sterilization failures, in particular, have been associated with a higher incidence of ectopic pregnancy. As many as 50% of bipolar coagulation failures are ectopic.[12,13] Future analyses of CREST data will evaluate whether the ectopic failure rate, like the overall failure rate, also varies by age and method.

Implications of the CREST Findings

The higher failure rates found in CREST have implications for those who consider female sterilization for birth control. First, vasectomy may now become a more attractive permanent option, since its failure rate is lower than that of tubal sterilization. Second, some long-term, reversible contraceptive options, such as the Copper T 380A intrauterine device (IUD) and subdermal implants, now rival sterilization in effectiveness, while remaining superior in safety. The Copper T 380A IUD, for example, is now approved for 10 years before needing replacement. Failure rates of this IUD are less than 1% at 1 year and about 2% at 8 years.[14] For some sterilization methods, particularly bipolar coagulation and the spring clip, the CREST cumulative failure rates are higher than that of this IUD. Similarly, subdermal implants have a 5-year lifespan and a reported 5-year failure rate of under 1%.[7] Injectable contraception is also another option that is highly effective and requires user compliance only once every 3 months.

Another important implication of the CREST study is that sterilization methods vary substantially in terms of effectiveness. The high failure rates for spring clip application and bipolar coagulation point to the need for skill on the part of the clinician in order to maximize effectiveness of these methods. One study, in fact, found that all the spring clip application failures in that study were attributable to misapplication.[15]

The high failure rate for bipolar coagulation, on the other hand, may not reflect the failure rate obtainable today. CREST sterilizations were performed up to a decade or more in the past. Since then, optimal bipolar coagulation technique has become more widely documented and employed.[16] Overall, comparisons between mechanical device methods and electrocautery have differed among studies.[17]

Moreover, it has been difficult to draw clear conclusions based on conflicting reports comparing the relative efficacy of postpartum and interval procedures.[18,19] CREST data suggest that postpartum procedures are more effective than interval procedures; however, this finding may be due, in part, to selection bias.

Postpartum Sterilization

In 1985, one in every 10 women hospitalized for childbirth chose to be sterilized before leaving the hospital.[20] Postpartum sterilization is convenient for both surgeon and patient. And, because the cost of performing the procedure at this time is lower, it may also make sterilization available to candidates who would otherwise find expense to be a deterrent.

The CREST data have shed some light on the efficacy of postpartum sterilizations. The long-term CREST findings indicate that unipolar coagulation and postpartum partial salpingectomy have the lowest cumulative failure rates of all the methods studied (both are 7.5 per 1,000 patients). Dr. Peterson explained that "many different procedures are lumped under the postpartum partial salpingectomy classification, although most were recorded as modified Pomeroy procedures."

Although CREST data are favorable for unipolar coagulation, this particular technique has been associated with a high risk of thermal bowel injury.[21] For this reason, unipolar coagulation, though effective, has been largely replaced in the U.S. by bipolar procedures. Bipolar coagulation procedures also destroy a smaller section of the tube, thereby increasing the probability of successful reversal.

A review of available literature on postpartum tubal sterilization suggests the following guidelines to help ensure the highest safety and efficacy possible[18,19]:

- Postpartum tubal sterilization via minilaparotomy is medically safe, whether performed while the woman is still on the delivery table or within 48 hours of delivery.

- The laparoscopic approach is generally not used postpartum because it is difficult and risky due to the large uterine fundus and vascular edematous adnexa.

- Among the three commonly used tubal occlusion techniques, the Pomeroy method or its modifications are probably more effective than rings or clips due to the dilated size of the tubes immediately postpartum. Unipolar and bipolar electrocautery are also associated with high efficacy; however, unipolar coagulation has been associated with serious risks, most notably thermal bowel injury. Both electrocautery methods may lower the probability of successful reversal since they damage a larger section of the tube than mechanical device applications.

- Whether the delivery is vaginal or cesarean, only patients with no complications and who have delivered a healthy baby should be considered as candidates for any sterilization procedure. Not only is this medically safer, it also diminishes the risk of post-sterilization regret.

Regret after Sterilization

Some women will regret having been sterilized.[22] Reversal is far from sure, nor is it an option for every patient. A 5-year interim report from CREST found that about 6% of the women interviewed said they had spoken with a health care provider regarding a possible reversal at some time during the 5 years following their sterilizations.[23]

A successful reversal depends on many factors. Although several popular methods (Pomeroy techniques, clips and rings) have reported successful reversal rates of between 70% and 80%, operative success depends not only on the skill of the surgeon but also on patient characteristics and the condition of the remaining tube. The ideal candidate for tubal reanastomosis is younger than 43 years of age, of average body weight, has documented ovulation and at least 4 cm of healthy tube remaining.[24,25]

Indicators of post-sterilization regret

The characteristic most often associated with post-sterilization regret is the young age of the patient. Women under 30 are twice as likely to regret their decision as those who are older than 30 at the time of sterilization.[22] In the 5-year CREST analysis, young age was the strongest predictor of regret; among women 20 to 24 years of age at sterilization, an average of 4.3% reported regret over the follow-up period.[22] This percentage dropped to 2.4% among women ages 30 to 34 years. The timing of the operation is also an indicator of future regret—women undergoing postpartum sterilization are more likely to regret their decision than those who undergo interval sterilization.

In the 5-year CREST data, a significantly higher correlation with later regret was found among those sterilized at the time of cesarean delivery. This factor had also surfaced in other reports, one of which indicated that women sterilized at a repeat cesarean were more likely to seek tubal reversal than those sterilized at their first. Nevertheless, even among those women having both age-related and postpartum risk factors, fewer than 10% regretted their decisions.[22]

Regret has also been linked to changes in marital status, death of a child, socioeconomic status, emotional factors and forces at work in the couple's relationship.[26,27] Although it is impossible to predict future events that will affect regret, the variety of factors that may influence regret after sterilization further emphasize the need for thorough patient education and counseling prior to the procedure.[27] In addition to assessing obvious indicators of potential regret such as age and parity, clinicians should explore the patient's motivation carefully and include the partner in patient education discussions.

Making the Decision

Sterilization usually ends childbearing; however, childless patients may also be interested in this contraceptive option. Little is known about childless women who select sterilization as a method of contraception. One study that sought to examine factors influencing post-sterilization regret in women with children and those without children found little difference between the two groups.[28] Although the study was small—35 women, half of whom were childless—its findings were consistent with a review of the literature on regret, and the study's interviews illuminate counseling issues for childless women.

Interviewers examined the decision-making process that led patients to voluntary sterilization, and their findings paint a picture of careful consideration. For all the women in this study, the decision to be sterilized preceded surgery by at least a year. For most, the decision was a long-standing one. Interestingly, 29% of the childless women had made the decision 4 or more years prior to the operation, and several reported that they had not had the procedure earlier because they had been unable to find a physician who was willing to sterilize a childless woman.

Most of the women in the study had based their decision on several considerations of varying importance. Childless women were mainly concerned about side effects of other forms of contraception. Childless women also frequently mentioned reasons of age, career and lack of interest in childrearing. This study followed its subjects for 5 years, and in that time, only three expressed "any regret," and none requested a reversal. These study participants are presently approaching menopause and the researchers plan a 14-year follow-up evaluation comparing them with a control sample using reversible methods of birth control.[28]

How Often Do Patients Request Sterilization Reversal?

In the 5-year interim analysis of CREST, many more women requested information about tubal sterilization reversal than actually sought the operation.[22] Women younger than 30 at the time of sterilization were twice as likely to seek such information as women ages 30 to 34. Women who had experienced changes in marital status were 2.8 times more likely to seek information as those whose status had not changed. Only 0.2% of the sterilized women chose to attempt reversal. The study does suggest, however, that requests for reversals may increase over time, and it is likely that new reports drawing on the long-term CREST data will explore the issue further. Other factors identified with seeking reversal include the intensity and persistence of regret, perceived ability to conceive, perceptions regarding the potential for success and accessibility of the reversal procedure.[26]

Patient Counseling

Although still an effective method of contraception, sterilization is less effective than previously believed. Counseling should be adjusted to take the latest CREST data into consideration. Clinicians should discuss the new failure rates associated with different methods, emphasizing that failures, although infrequent, can occur 10 years or more after the procedure. Ectopic pregnancy should be explained, and women should be urged to contact a physician at any sign of possible pregnancy, even many years after their sterilization.

The following counseling guidelines for health care providers have been adapted from Pollack and Soderstrom[29]:

- Pre-sterilization discussions and decision-making should take place well in advance of the operation, and consent forms should be signed prior to admission for the procedure, especially if sterilization is to be performed in conjunction with childbirth or abortion.

- Emphasize that sterilization should be regarded as permanent. Despite what the patient may have heard about reversals, the data show that reanasto-mosis is infrequently pursued, expensive and not always successful (70% to 80% success rates are associated with ideal reanastomosis conditions, ie, supportive patient characteristics and at least 4 cm of undamaged tube). In addition, the prospects for reversal depend upon the condition of the tube, which is influenced by the type of sterilization procedure.

- Involve both partners in the decision and discuss both male and female sterilization. Vasectomy is a safer, less expensive, simpler operation and is highly effective.

- Discuss sterilization in conjunction with a full explanation of all contraceptive methods, especially of long-term, reversible methods. Even if a woman has specifically requested sterilization, she may not be aware of the latest information about implants, injectables and IUDs.

- Inform the patient of failure rates associated with sterilization and the risk of ectopic pregnancy. Let the woman know that failures may occur long after the procedure; suspected pregnancy should be ruled out as soon as possible.

- Emphasize that sterilization provides no protection against sexually transmitted disease or AIDS.

- Screen candidates for indicators of post-sterilization regret. Any of the following characteristics makes a woman more at risk for regret:

- sterilization at the time of abortion

- sterilization at the time of delivery

- young age of the patient

- Discuss methods appropriate for the patient, including side effects, failure rates and recovery. If some methods are not appropriate, they too should be discussed and the clinician's choice should be explained. Explain the following to the patient:

  - surgical procedure

  - preoperative instructions

  - the surgical site

  - timing of the procedure

  - type of anesthesia

  - length of recovery

- Describe all medical benefits and risks:

  - general surgical risks

  - risk of failure to complete the procedure with the chosen technique

  - the possibility of unrelated changes in menstruation due to age or to change in contraceptive method

- Answer all questions, including one that is often left unexpressed, "What happens to the egg released from the ovary?"

- Discuss the possible effect on sexuality. There is no evidence of detrimental effects to sexuality after sterilization. In fact, some studies have indicated that sexuality may improve because couples don't worry about unwanted pregnancy.

- Provide printed patient education materials that the woman and her partner can review privately.

Conclusion

The choice of permanent contraception involves many factors, only one of which is effectiveness. Patients must make sterilization choices based on a range of factors, and relative efficacy is just one consideration. "Choice of a contraceptive method is a personal decision that the clinician and patient reach together after reviewing all the options and their attendant risks and benefits. The CREST data give patients and clinicians more information about those choices," said Dr. Peterson.

References

1. Peterson LS. Contraceptive use in the United States: 1982-90. *Advance Data from Vital and Health Statistics* February 1995;260:1-8.

2. Murphy M. Sterilisation as a method of contraception: recent trends in Great Britain and their implications. *J Biosoc Sci* 1995;27:31-46.

3. Irwin KL, Weiss NS, Lee NC, et al. Tubal sterilization, hysterectomy and the subsequent occurrence of epithelial ovarian cancer. *Am J Epidemiol* 1991;134:362-369.

4. Hankinson SE, Hunter DJ, Colditz GA, et al. Tubal ligation, hysterectomy, and the risk of ovarian cancer. *JAMA* 1993;270:2813-2818.

5. Whittemore AS, Harris R, Itnyre J, and the Collaborative Ovarian Cancer Group. Characteristics relating to ovarian cancer risk: collaborative analysis of 12 US case-control studies. II: Invasive epithelial ovarian cancers in white women. *Am J Epidemiol* 1992;136:1184-1203.

6. Peterson HB, Xia Z, Hughes JM, et al. The risk of pregnancy after tubal sterilization: findings from the U.S. Collaborative Review of Sterilization. *Am J Obstet Gynecol* 1996;174:1161-1170.

7. Trussell J, Hatcher RA, Cates W Jr., et al. Contraceptive failure in the United States: an update. *Stud Fam Plann* 1990;21:51-54.

8. Vessey M, Huggins G, Lawless M, et al. Tubal sterilization: findings in a large, prospective study. *Br J Obstet Gynaecol* 1983;90:203-209.

9. Trussell J, Leveque JA, Koenig JD, et al. The economic value of contraception: a comparison of 15 methods. *Am J Public Health* 1995;85:494-503.

10. Zhuomin Z, Liju W, Zhiyan Z, et al. An epidemiological study on the relationship of ectopic pregnancy and the use of contraceptives in Beijing—the incidence of ectopic pregnancy in the Beijing area. *Contraception* 1994;50:253-262.

11. Holt VL, Chu J, Daling JR, et al. Tubal sterilization and subsequent ectopic pregnancy. *JAMA* 1991;266:242-246.

12. Kjer JJ, Knudsen LB. Ectopic pregnancy subsequent to laparoscopic sterilization. *Am J Obstet Gynecol* 1989;160:202-204.

13. McCausland A. High rate of ectopic pregnancy following laparoscopic tubal coagulation failures. Incidence and etiology. *Am J Obstet Gynecol* 1980;136:97-101.

14. Schmidt F, Sivin I, Waldman S. The copper T380 IUD. In: Bardin CW, Mishell DR Jr, eds. *Proceedings from the Fourth International Conference on IUDs*. Boston: Butterworth-Heinemann, 1994; 298-307.

15. Stovall TG, Ling FW, Henry GM, et al. Method failures of laparoscopic tubal sterilization in a residency training program. A comparison of the tubal ring and spring-loaded clip. *J Reprod Med* 1991;36;283-286.

16. Soderstrom RM, Levy BS, Engel T. Reducing bipolar sterilization failures. *Obstet Gynecol* 1989;74:60-63.

17. Trussell J, Kost K. Contraceptive failure in the United States: a critical review of the literature. *Stud Fam Plann* 1987;18(5):237-283.

18. Chi I-C, Gates D, Thapa S. Performing tubal sterilization during women's post-partum hospitalization: a review of the United States and international experiences. *Obstet Gynecol Survey* 1992;47:71-79.

19. Chi I-C, Petta CA, McPheeters M. A review of safety, efficacy, pros and cons, and issues of puerperal tubal sterilization—an update. *Adv Contraception* 1995;11:187-206.

20. Taffel SM, Placek PJ. The rise in postpartum sterilization in cesarean and vaginal deliveries: U.S. 1970-85. Presented at the 115th Annual Meeting of the American Public Health Association annual meeting. New Orleans, Oct. 19, 1987.

21. American College of Obstetricians and Gynecologists. Sterilization. *ACOG Technical Bulletin* April 1996;Number 222.

22. Wilcox LS, Chu SY, Eaker ED, et al. Risk factors for regret after tubal sterilization: 5 years of follow-up in a prospective study. *Fertil Steril* 1991;55:927-933.

23. Wilcox LS, Chu SY, Peterson HB. Characteristics of women who considered or obtained tubal reanastomosis: results from a prospective study of tubal sterilization. *Obstet Gynecol* 1990;75:661-665.

24. Hogdall CK, Nielsen J, Ovlisen B. Reversal of female sterilization using macro technique. *Acta Obstet Gynecol Scand* 1989;68:737-742.

25. Siegler AM, Hulka JF, Peretz A. Reversibility of female sterilizations. *Fertil Steril* 1985;43:499-510.

26. Chi I-C, Jones DB. Incidence, risk factors, and prevention of poststerilization regret in women: an updated international review from an epidemiological perspective. *Obstet Gynecol Surv* 1994;49:722-732.

27. Miller WB, Shain RN, Pasta DJ. The pre- and poststerilization predictors of poststerilization regret in husbands and wives. *J Nerv Ment Dis* 1991;179:602-608.

28. Smith EM, Friedrich E, Pribor EF. Psychosocial consequences of sterilization: a review of the literature and preliminary findings. *Comprehensive Psychiatry* 1994;35:157-163.

29. Pollack AE, Soderstrom RM. Female tubal sterilization. In: Corson SL, Derman RJ, Tyrer LB, eds. *Fertility Control*. 2nd ed. London, Ontario;Goldin Publishers, 1994:295-296.

6.3: The Filshie Clip

In February 1996, an advisory panel of the U.S. Food and Drug Administration (FDA) recommended approval of the Filshie clip for use in this country. Associate Editor of The Contraception Report, *Elizabeth Connell, MD, chaired the panel. The Filshie clip, a tubal occlusion device, is widely used in Canada, Australia and the United Kingdom, where it is manufactured by Femcare, Inc.*

Description and Application

The device is smaller than a penny and designed to occlude the tube with minimal destruction. It is made of titanium with a silicone rubber lining, which expands to keep the tube compressed as it flattens. Using a customized applicator, the surgeon half closes the upper jaw to insert the applicator and clip through a cannula or operating laparoscope. When the surgeon releases the finger bar, the applicator and clip reopen and can be used as soft-nosed forceps to pick up the tube and examine the placement site. Once satisfied that the clip is positioned correctly, the surgeon squeezes the finger bar to its full limit. The clip is released automatically from the applicator and locked onto the tube. Ideally, the clip is applied across the isthmus, leaving an equal amount of tube on either side.

The remaining tube is considered to be adequate for successful reanastomosis. Albert Yuzpe, MD, Professor Emeritus of Obstetrics and Gynecology at the University of West Ontario in London, Ontario, Canada, spoke about the results of Canadian studies that had successful reversal rates after Filshie clip sterilization of 90%. Dr. Yuzpe characterized the application technique as easy to learn and having few complications, primarily because the surgeon can be sure of correctly seating the clip before it is locked into place.

Safety and Efficacy

The panel considered safety and efficacy data from studies conducted by Family Health International (FHI). In total, FHI conducted 11 studies of the Filshie clip at 43 sites in 10 countries. Over 6,000 women were sterilized with Filshie clips and almost 4,000 were sterilized with other methods, including the tubal ring and the Wolf clip.

Four of the studies were designated pivotal evaluations: all were prospective, comparative, randomized and multicenter investigations of interval sterilizations. The studies compared the tubal ring and Wolf clip to the Filshie clip, with over 400 women in each of the two comparison groups. In the two studies comparing the Filshie and Wolf clips, the pooled analysis yielded a 12-month cumulative pregnancy rate of 0.1 per 100 women for the Filshie clip group and 0.7 per 100 women for the Wolf clip group. In the two studies comparing the Filshie clip and the tubal ring, the pooled analysis yielded the same 12-month cumulative pregnancy rate for both methods—0.2 per 100 women.

A subset of women from each of these studies was followed for 24 months after sterilization. In the Wolf clip comparison, the Filshie clip group had two pregnancies in 24 months, a cumulative rate of 0.7 per 100 women; the Wolf clip group had six pregnancies, a cumulative rate of 2.8 per 100 women. In the 24-month follow-up of the tubal ring comparison groups, the Filshie clip sample again had two pregnancies, a cumulative rate of 0.7 per 100 women; the tubal ring sample had one pregnancy, a 24-month cumulative rate of 0.3 per 100 women.

The panel also had requested data from the single postpartum study conducted by FHI. In that prospective study, the pregnancy rate for women who received the Filshie clip sterilization was significantly higher than those sterilized by the Pomeroy method: at 24 months, the Filshie clip rate was 1.7, and the Pomeroy method rate was 0.4 per 100 women. This study indicates that the Filshie clip may be less effective when used postpartum than when applied during interval sterilizations. It should be noted that all these efficacy data are based on 1 and 2 years of follow-up; long-term data, such as those obtained by CREST, are not available.

In safety studies, the Filshie clip compared positively with other devices—the surgical injury rate was a low 1.6 for the entire population. The most common injury was a tubal mesosalpingeal injury, caused more often by the tubal ring than the Filshie clip. Only one ectopic pregnancy was reported among the more than 5,000 Filshie clip sterilizations in the overall population.

In five cases, the Filshie clip had migrated (was found in a place other than attached to the fallopian tube). The researchers explained that after necrosis of the occluded tube, the clip may drop into the abdominal cavity. In these five migrations, the tube was completely occluded and the clip was still closed when discovered. In two cases, the Filshie clip had provoked a foreign body reaction. The other three migrations were incidental findings and had caused no reactions or discomfort to the patient.

Filshie Clip Device and Applicator

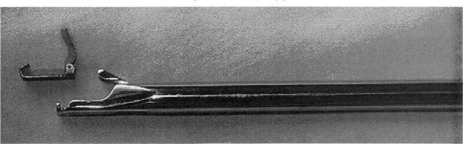

FDA Recommends Approval with Conditions

The panel's recommendation to approve had a short list of conditions: that the manufacturer clarify reuse guidelines for the device applicator and provide final results of toxicology testing, information on magnetic resonance compatibility and further information about the timing of the postpartum study procedures. The panel also wished to review labeling prior to final approval, expressing particular interest in discussion of "migration" and its causes, and of the higher failure rates associated with postpartum versus interval applications of the Filshie clip.

Male Sterilization

Vasectomy is a highly effective, safe, and popular means of surgical contraception. Those who are interested in learning more about vasectomy may wish to refer to the following reviews:

1. Peterson HB, Huber DH, Belker AM. Vasectomy: an appraisal for the obstetrician-gynecologist. *Obstet Gynecol* 1990;76:568-572.

2. Haws JM, Feigin J. Vasectomy counseling. *Am Fam Physician* 1995;52:1395-1399.

3. Liskin L, Benoit E, Blackburn R. Vasectomy: new opportunities. *Population Reports* Series D, Number 5;March 1992:1-23.

7 Contraception for Adolescents

Adolescents represent a population with special contraceptive needs. Teens may experience pressure to begin sexual activity early, yet often do not use contraception and underestimate the risks of unprotected intercourse. In addition, many adolescents are at high risk of sexually transmitted diseases (STDs). Teens may also be ignorant of where to get birth control and how to use it; often, they are afraid their parents will find out and may be reluctant to speak with a clinician unless they can be assured of confidentiality. The pressures on teens are complex and need to be taken into consideration when counseling them about contraception.

Over the course of several years, The Contraception Report *covered many professional meetings devoted to adolescent reproductive health. This chapter represents a compilation of material from the 1993 and 1995 conferences of the North American Society for Pediatric and Adolescent Gynecology (NASPAG) and from a symposium given at the American Academy of Family Physicians' 1991 Scientific Assembly.*

How can clinicians better meet the needs of sexually active young people? How can they better communicate with teens and their parents? What are the specific advantages and disadvantages of various birth control methods for adolescents? How can clinicians encourage teens to protect themselves against STDs? This chapter provides the answers to these questions through discussions with many experts in the field.

Introduction

Teens should be encouraged to delay sexual intercourse. In fact, one innovative program uses peers to counsel teens and promote abstinence.[1] "Postponing Sexual Involvement" is one component of a teen sexuality education program offered through Grady Memorial Hospital in cooperation with Emory University School of Medicine in Atlanta, Georgia. This program helps teens role-play responses to pressures to have sex and emphasizes the benefits of postponing sexual intercourse, but at the same time, provides information about contraception. Another program, "Reducing the Risk," is a high school sex education effort. The curriculum emphasizes avoiding unprotected sex through abstinence or using contraception.[2] The program has been successful at helping teens to learn more about abstinence and contraception and to delay the initiation of intercourse. Other programs take a long-term, holistic approach, following teens for many years and offering incentives, such as financial assistance with college, for postponing childbearing. Despite some promising results,

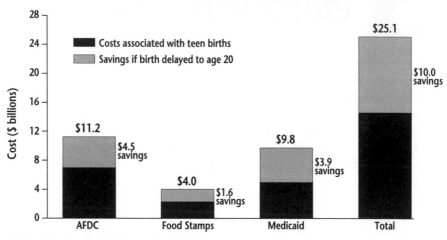

Figure 1

Single-Year Public Cost for All Families Started by a Teen Birth and Potential Savings Associated with Delaying These Births (in $ Billions)

AFDC = Aid to Families with Dependent Children

Source: Center for Population Options, 1992 (see reference 4).

however, data from the Youth Risk Behavior Survey show that by the 12th grade, two-thirds of young American men and women have had sexual intercourse at least once.[3] Thus, many teens need facts about pregnancy and STD prevention.

Costs of Teenage Pregnancies

The impact of unplanned teen pregnancies in terms of social and economic costs to our society is staggering. A cost study by the Center for Population Options measured the societal cost of teenage childbearing in 1990 by using data from Aid to Families with Dependent Children (AFDC), food stamps and Medicaid (Figure 1).[4] National single-year public costs for all families started by a teen birth were $25 billion. The study estimated, however, that if these births could have been delayed until the teen reached age 20, an annual savings of $10 billion could have been realized. Helping teens postpone initiation of sexual intercourse and improving access to and use of birth control among sexually active teens are some important steps to reduce these economic costs.

Adolescent Sexual Behavior and Pregnancy Trends

Wendy Baldwin, PhD, discussed adolescent sexual behavior, pregnancy and birth trends in the United States during the ninth annual NASPAG meeting held in Toronto, Canada, in April 1995. She emphasized that the problem of adolescent pregnancy should be considered not only from a clinical or caseload perspective, but also in relation to the overall picture. Dr. Baldwin, Deputy Director for Extramural Research at the National Institutes of Health, explained that adolescent pregnancy is not a problem unique to homeless and disadvantaged youth. "Very few pregnant teens are homeless. This group represents only one segment of the broader picture," she said.

Sexual activity among U.S. adolescents has increased dramatically over the last 3 decades.[5] Today, most adolescents initiate intercourse during their middle to late teenage years.[3,5]

"Despite these trends," Dr. Baldwin continued, "teenagers generally do not initiate sexual intercourse as early as most adults believe. Nor do all teenagers have sex. Although the likelihood of having intercourse increases steadily with age, nearly 20% of adolescents do not have intercourse at all during their adolescence." Early initiation of intercourse (age 13 or 14) is infrequent. Furthermore, many teenagers who had intercourse during their early teens report that they were forced to do so.[5]

Although levels of sexual activity are high, the U.S. adolescent pregnancy rate remains relatively stable. According to Dr. Baldwin, "Pregnancy rates among sexually experienced teenagers (those who have ever had sex) have actually declined 19% over the last 2 decades, but because the proportion of adolescents who have had intercourse has grown, the overall teenage pregnancy rate has increased by 23% (Figure 2)."[5]

Furthermore, the majority of teenage pregnancies (approximately 85%) are unintended.[5] In contrast, among older women, about 55% of pregnancies are unintended. Despite the fact that teens have a high proportion of unintended pregnancies, adolescents account for only about one-quarter of the total number of unintended pregnancies in the U.S.

Figure 2

Comparison of Pregnancy Rates between All Women and Sexually Experienced Women 15 to 19 Years of Age, United States, 1972 to 1990

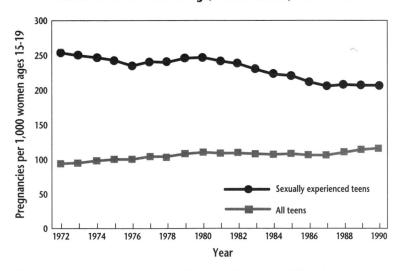

Source: The Alan Guttmacher Institute. Sex and America's Teenagers, 1994;41.
Reproduced with permission of the publisher, The Alan Guttmacher Institute, New York.

"Half of unintended pregnancies occur within the first 6 months of exposure to sexual activity," said Dr. Baldwin. "The younger the teen is when initiating intercourse, the longer she'll take to adopt a method of contraception. We need to reach adolescents before they're sexually active and emphasize the need to use contraception. Teens need to understand that the first time they have intercourse they are at risk for unintended pregnancy, regardless of whether they think they'll have sex again or not," said Dr. Baldwin.

In 1990, about 1 million births occurred among teenage women.[5] While the birth rate for all teens 15 to 19 years of age rose by about 13% between 1980 and 1990, for sexually experienced teens the birth rate declined slightly during the same period.[6] In addition, pregnancy and abortion rates for sexually experienced teens declined by about 8% and 14%, respectively. In contrast, however, among the youngest teens (ages 13 and 14), the birth rate increased 15%.

While the overall teen birth rate has remained relatively stable among sexually experienced teens, nonmarital births have increased. From the early 1960s to the late 1980s, nonmarital births to adolescents ages 15 to 17 years rose from 33% to 81%.[5] This increase represents a change in the context of adolescent sexual activity and pregnancy. "Understanding the context of sexual activity is critical to understanding any of the other trends that we've observed for adolescents," said Dr. Baldwin.

The percentage of nonmarital births that occur among teens as compared to women ages 20 years or older, however, has declined over time. In 1990, among all women, teens accounted for less then one-third (31%) of nonmarital births.[5]

The trend of increasing prevalence of sex among unmarried adolescents partly reflects a trend in later marriages. Compared to the 1950s, a smaller proportion of young people are marrying. As a result, the majority of teenagers who have intercourse are unmarried when they first have sex.

The U.S. has approximately the same rates of teenage sexual activity as industrialized European nations, yet its teen pregnancy rate is substantially higher.[7] As a result, U.S. teens have a greater number of abortions, nonmarital births and marital births. According to S. Jean Emans, MD, Associate Editor of *The Contraception Report*, "Many other Western democracies are trying to combat the issue of teenage pregnancy. We (Americans) are trying to combat primarily teenage sexual activity. I would like to see less teenage sexual activity, as well, but our lack of focus on providing affordable contraceptive services results in many teenagers having inadequate access to services when they do become sexually active." A comparative study of adolescent pregnancy and childbearing in developed countries found that industrialized nations, such as The Netherlands, Sweden and France, which have much lower rates of teenage pregnancy than the U.S., also have government policies that strongly support easily accessible and affordable contraceptives for sexually active teens.[7] Strong government support of contraception and sexuality education are some of the reasons why teenage pregnancy rates are lower in these countries.

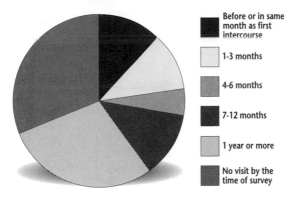

Figure 3

Delay in Seeking Medical Contraception after Initiation of Intercourse among U.S. Women Ages 15 to 19 Years, 1988

Before or in same month as first intercourse

1-3 months

4-6 months

7-12 months

1 year or more

No visit by the time of survey

Source: The Alan Guttmacher Institute. Sex and America's Teenagers, 1994;33. Reproduced with permission of the publisher, The Alan Guttmacher Institute.

Contraceptive Use among Adolescents

Contraceptive use at first intercourse has increased since the early 1980s.[8] However, in spite of this increase, only two-thirds of adolescents use some method of birth control, usually the male condom, the first time they have intercourse.

The majority of adolescents delay seeking medical contraceptive services until after they initiate sexual intercourse. Only about 40% of adolescents seek medical contraceptive services within the first year of becoming sexually active (Figure 3).[5]

Delay may occur for several reasons. For example, adolescents who do not perceive themselves at risk for an unintended pregnancy may delay seeking medical services. Other reasons for delay include the fear of a pelvic exam or the fear that parents will find out that the adolescent is sexually active.

One study found that the perception of birth control as dangerous contributes to delay.[9] The study of junior and senior high school students ages 11 to 18 years explored the reasons teenagers had for delay in obtaining contraceptive services. The researchers found participants' perceptions regarding birth control were more important than cost or ignorance of a source of contraception. Among sexually active teens, whether or not they used the contraceptive services available, the most important reasons given at baseline for not accessing services were: (1) fear that contraception is dangerous, cited by 40%; (2) fear of parental discovery, cited by 31%; and (3) awaiting "closer" partner relationships, cited by 31%. A fourth reason teens delayed accessing services was the fear of the physical examination. As many as 23% of the young women gave this reason for not obtaining contraception. These reasons were so compelling that even after exposure to an intensive program offering medical and educational contraceptive counseling services, the sexually active young women who still had not sought contraceptive assistance continued to give these reasons as prime explanations for their delay.

This study lends support to the belief that unwarranted fear of contraception, often inadvertently fostered by the media, can have an impact on the choice of whether or not to practice birth control. Teenagers are constantly being exposed to sexual issues through the media. Although adept at portraying a glamorized representation of sex, the media are reluctant to run ads about birth control, STDs and acquired immunodeficiency syndrome (AIDS) prevention. This makes it particularly important to counsel teenagers (and all women) about the comparative risks of each method, emphasizing the health benefits that may be conferred by the method and the importance of protecting oneself against unwanted pregnancy and STDs.

A delay in obtaining and using contraception exposes teens to unwanted pregnancy, the consequences of which are substantial. According to Dr. Emans, "The implications of teenage parenthood are quite considerable. Often, a young mother is caught in a continuing cycle of poverty, has lower earning potential, needs long-term public support, interrupts or forfeits her educational goals and is more socially isolated. This is particularly true of our poorest segment of the population. There are also a number of health risks for the offspring of these teenagers, as well, including perinatal mortality and morbidity, low birth weight and slow development. In addition, problems with parenting occur, particularly among the youngest teenage mothers."

In a study by Dr. Emans that looked at adolescents treated in a suburban private-practice setting and an inner-city adolescent clinic, significant differences in prior contraceptive use were observed between the two populations. For example, the suburban teens had a higher likelihood of prior use of some contraceptive, whereas the inner-city teens were four times as likely to have *never* used any method of birth control (Figure 4).[10] Furthermore, the suburban teens were more than twice as likely to have *always* used a method before coming in for their initial contraceptive visit (38% vs 15%). Dr. Emans commented, "Inner-city young people are much more likely to have never used a method before coming into the clinic. That has tremendous implications when they discontinue the pill because they have nothing to fall back on in terms of barrier methods. It is incredibly important, when clinicians prescribe oral contraceptives (OCs) for inner-city teens, to educate them about barrier methods for pregnancy and STD protection so they can have something to fall back on if they discontinue the pill."

Figure 4

Prior Use of Contraception

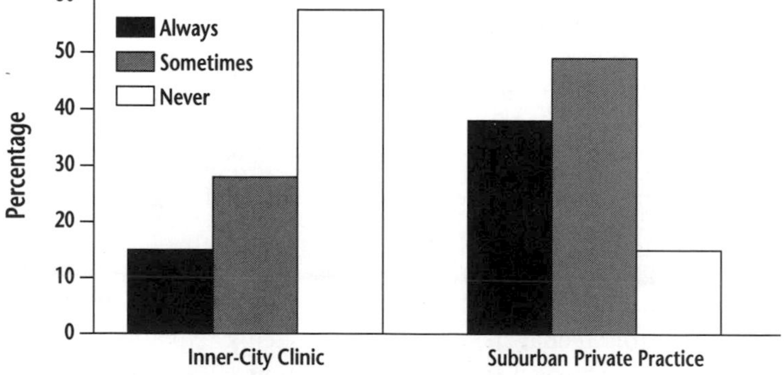

Source: Emans SJ, et al, 1987 (see reference 10).

Factors Identified with Adolescents Seeking Contraceptives

Factors have been identified that are associated with an adolescent being more likely to seek contraception. In particular, the perception that pregnancy is a negative outcome is important. According to Dr. Emans, "As one might guess, the suburban patient who is headed to college is going to perceive pregnancy as more of a negative outcome than the young person living in the inner city with a poor school system, who has very few options. So, we can see that much of the unwanted pregnancy problem is related to the environment in which the young person lives. Older age is also associated with teens coming in and telling you directly that they need contraception." Some of the other reasons a teen might be likely to seek contraception include: a pregnancy scare; having taken a sex education course; influence of family, friends or clinician; and the perceived risk of HIV (human immunodeficiency virus) infection.

In fact, a negative pregnancy test is an opportunity for intervention, since many of these adolescents will become pregnant in the next year. At least two recent studies support the need for such intervention. Stevens-Simon et al reviewed medical records of 71 teens in two urban clinics 18 to 24 months after a negative pregnancy test result.[11] These researchers found that two-thirds of the adolescents who returned to the clinics during the study period had conceived. In addition, of the 30 young women who were given a contraceptive method, 87% subsequently conceived.

Similarly, Zabin et al performed a cross-sectional study of young women presenting to clinics for pregnancy tests.[12] Self-administered questionnaires inquired about prior pregnancy tests, pregnancies, sexual and contraceptive histories and childbearing attitudes. A total of 2,926 patients ages 17 years or younger from 52 clinics participated. From this sample, the researchers estimated that almost three out of five patients in this age group had a negative pregnancy test result at a clinic before their first conception. The authors suggest that these women be identified routinely by health care providers for more intensive contraceptive counseling.

The Hidden Agenda

With teens, it is also important to be aware that they may visit the practitioner with contraception in mind, but not come right out and say what they want. "It's very important to be aware of the possible 'hidden agenda.' Many young people will come in with menstrual cramps when they really want oral contraceptive pills because they heard that their best friend came to see you and had cramps and received a prescription for oral contraceptives," Dr. Emans stated.

Contraceptive Choices

During the ninth annual NASPAG meeting, Paula J.A. Hillard, MD, gave a presentation concerning contraceptive choices for the adolescent. Dr. Hillard, Associate Editor of *The Contraception Report*, discussed the range of contraceptive choices for teens, compliance issues associated with each method and counseling suggestions to improve compliance and method continuation rates.

"Adolescents choose a particular contraceptive method based on several factors," she began. "Popularity of a method, accessibility and knowledge or fear of side effects are all factors that influence contraceptive choice. In addition, there are trends and fads in terms of popularity of contraception for adolescents. Teenagers often choose a method based on what their friends are using or by what they hear in the media. Negative stories, in particular, may frighten young women and lead to a fear of contraception."

Oral Contraceptives

The latest data from the 1995 Youth Risk Behavior Survey indicate that the percentage of female high school students who used the pill before their last intercourse was 20%.[3] Among female high school seniors, one-quarter reported using the pill before last intercourse.

When used correctly, the expected failure rate for combined oral contraceptives is less than 1%. The failure rate among typical users is 3%. Unfortunately, among typical adolescent users, the failure rate ranges from 5% to 15%.[13] "The higher failure rate for adolescents does not mean that the pill is metabolized differently by adolescents," Dr. Hillard explained. "What it does mean is that some problems exist with consistent and correct use."

Compliance with OCs — Since compliance with OCs greatly impacts efficacy, accurate information about the pill is essential. "Many adolescents and adult women believe there are substantial risks associated with oral contraceptive use. Misperceptions and concerns about possible side effects may act as a deterrent to OC use and a contributing factor in noncompliance and OC discontinuation. For example, there is a myth among many pill takers that the pill lasts longer than you're actually taking it. Teens may stop taking the pill, but still believe they're protected for a few months. I think that myth is very, very widespread," said Dr. Hillard.

One of the best ways to help ensure compliance is through patient counseling. Dr. Hillard asks new patients what they've heard about the pill and what fears they have about taking it. "If you don't address those fears, whether they tell you about them or not, then you're missing an opportunity to encourage consistent pill use. Patients need to know that side effects are transitory and they need to know whom to call if they have questions. It's important to be sensitive and responsive to their fears and concerns," said Dr. Hillard. (See Chapter 1 for further discussion about misinformation about the pill and counseling strategies.)

Lack of understanding about correct use of OCs also affects compliance. "The first step in patient counseling," Dr. Hillard explained, "is to be sure the patient knows how to take her OC correctly. This includes showing the teen the pill package and the order in which to take the pills. Patients also need to know what to do if they miss one or more pills. Scheduling frequent follow-up visits is another strategy that can improve compliance with OCs. We need to be sure that we are accessible to our patients.

"Emphasizing the noncontraceptive health benefits of OCs may also influence adolescents to continue taking the pill consistently," Dr. Hillard suggested. "For example, one study found that adolescents who experienced relief of dysmenorrhea were the most likely to use the pill in a consistent, ongoing manner.[14] Reminding her [the patient] that she will get some relief from her dysmenorrhea and will have lighter, easier and more predictable periods makes a difference. This is one way to help avoid the on-again, off-again cycle of taking the pill that can occur in adolescents," added Dr. Hillard.

Anticipatory Counseling about Side Effects

Dr. Emans also stressed the need to anticipate concerns about side effects and give appropriate guidance. She stated, "Minor side effects can have very major consequences in terms of a high pregnancy rate for teens. Teens who do experience breakthrough bleeding or amenorrhea are more concerned than those who don't. They sometimes lose confidence in the pill and say, 'No pill works for me,' and sometimes this is made worse by the fact that they've had multiple shifts of pills. Breakthrough bleeding may lead to increased anxiety, disruption of sexual relations and, obviously, having to use more tampons or pads, which can be relevant for teens in high school, where they have 5 minutes to change classes and run to the bathroom. So, periods can be a big deal for teenage girls."

Dr. Emans continued, "In our study of adolescents seen in different practice settings, we have been very interested in oral contraceptive compliance. We have found that teens have many concerns about oral contraceptives. It is interesting to note that weight gain is number one, but others, such as infertility and birth defects, are not concerns of the medical profession at all, yet are of concern to teens."

The concern expressed regarding these side effects varies in terms of the population (Figure 5). Suburban teens are overwhelmingly concerned about weight gain, an issue which needs to be addressed with the teen from the very first time oral contraceptives are discussed. Inner-city teens are concerned about weight gain, too, but also have fears about blood clots, birth defects and infertility. Knowing that these fears may be

Figure 5

Concerns Expressed about Oral Contraceptives by Teens in an Adolescent Clinic (n=61) and in Private Practice (n=49)

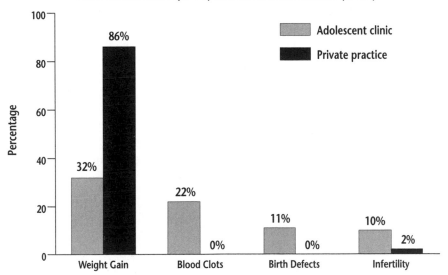

Concerns about Oral Contraceptives

Source: Emans SJ, et al, 1987 (see reference 10).

present in the minds of young women, practitioners should make an attempt to dispel misconceptions regarding the pill to help improve compliance.

"I would suggest, also" Dr. Emans cautioned, "that there should be no set schedule of appointments for adolescents who are at high risk for teen pregnancy. Teens in your practice who have school failure or who are the siblings of parenting teens are at greater risk of noncompliance. If your patient has a teenage sister who's either pregnant and carrying to term or a parenting teen, that teenager is at high risk of an unplanned pregnancy. It's very important to reach out and make sure that youngster is in for frequent visits. Young people who have sexually transmitted diseases, who have multiple (or serial) partners or who are involved in substance abuse also need to be seen frequently, not every 6 months or every year."

In addition, Dr. Emans emphasized the need for discussion of pill use instructions with teens. "Written and verbal instructions need to be given. Usually, we review our written instructions with teens and do a question-and-answer session. Some teens accidentally lose their written instructions; others purposely lose them because they don't want the instructions to be found at home. In fact, only 11 of 209 patients (approximately 5%) in our study of adolescents had read their instruction sheets (created by the study team) prior to the 3-month follow-up and all had experienced breakthrough bleeding or amenorrhea.

"Our study also suggested that it does not matter whether the pill is monophasic or triphasic. We observed that adolescents can equally follow the directions of triphasics as monophasics, so we don't have to say, 'Well, they're not smart enough to follow triphasic directions,' because clearly they do as well."

Mothers' Perceptions of the Pill

Another aspect to the problem of misperceptions about the pill is that mothers of teens may also have negative attitudes about oral contraception. "In one Canadian study," Dr. Hillard explained, "mothers were the source of contraceptive information for 15% of teens.[15] The mothers of many teenagers today are familiar with the pills that were available in the '60s and '70s—pills that were high-dose and caused more nuisance side effects, such as nausea. During the '70s, there was a lot of negative media coverage about the pill. So, mothers of today's teens may be giving their daughters obsolete information."

Dr. Hillard also discussed methods of contraception requiring less patient compliance. She stressed that while implants, injectables and the intrauterine device (IUD) differ from OCs with regard to compliance issues, patient counseling is equally important.

Injectables

Injectable contraception provides another useful option for patients who have had problems with compliance. As with implants, menstrual changes with injectables warrant thorough counseling. "It is helpful to discuss with the patient how she and her partner will handle irregular bleeding. Counseling is also important to ensure that the adolescent returns every 12 weeks for her shot," Dr. Hillard stated. Patients also need to be aware that although injectables cause irregular bleeding early in use, eventually, many women experience amenorrhea. Patients may perceive amenorrhea as a benefit if they understand that it is not harmful, can be expected with long-term use and does not necessarily mean they are pregnant. Amenorrhea may also be a substantial benefit for adolescents with cognitive or physical problems that make menstrual hygiene difficult.

Other counseling issues include the possibility of weight gain and the potential effect of depot medroxyprogesterone acetate (DMPA) on bone density. Teens frequently fear weight gain and need careful monitoring at each visit, coupled with dietary counseling. Issues concerning the impact of DMPA on bone density need further study because early adolescence is the time of the greatest acquisition of bone mass. One small study of adolescents using subdermal implants, OCs or DMPA found that DMPA use was associated with bone loss.[16] (For further discussion of counseling issues and bone density with DMPA, see Chapter 2.)

Injectables can also be used prior to insertion of implants. Dr. Hillard suggested that for patients considering implants, injectables offer a short-term opportunity to decide whether they can tolerate the menstrual changes and other side effects that are likely to occur with implants.

IUDs

Dr. Hillard mentioned IUDs briefly. "There are some clinical situations where the IUD may be appropriate for an adolescent. Particularly with adolescent mothers who may have been unsuccessful with other methods of contraception, the IUD may be appropriate." IUDs are not a good choice for adolescents with multiple sexual partners who are at risk for STDs.

Subdermal Implants

Subdermal implants represent a highly effective contraceptive method that does not depend upon compliance. One study of subdermal implants in adolescent mothers found that among the reasons adolescents gave for choosing implants, difficulty remembering to take pills and ease of use of implants were important factors in their decision.[17]

Nuisance side effects, such as irregular bleeding, make preinsertion counseling especially important to enhance continuation with the method. "Success with implants depends critically on counseling. The best way to deal with side effects is to tell young women what side effects they should expect. It is also helpful to discuss, beforehand, how the teen will manage side effects like breakthrough bleeding," said Dr. Hillard.

During the 1995 NASPAG conference, Barbara O'Connell, MD, Assistant Professor of Obstetrics and Gynecology at the University of Wisconsin Medical School in Madison, Wisconsin, presented final data from a 3-year study of the use of subdermal implants in an adolescent population.[18]

The study, a collaborative NASPAG project begun in 1992 and coordinated by Dr. Emans, determined factors that influence teens to choose subdermal implants and the impact of side effects on satisfaction and continuation rates. Researchers also evaluated the effect of implants on condom use.

A total of 197 patients from five centers completed the initial form and 112 returned for follow-up (mean duration 13 months). The mean age of the initial study population was 17 years. The majority of participants (95%) came from metropolitan areas and were enrolled in Medicaid (75%). Nearly three-quarters of patients were in school; 12% had dropped out. Of all study participants, 74% had used oral contraceptives and 58% had used condoms at last intercourse. The majority had had a previous pregnancy.

Condom use was similar before and after insertion of implants. Eighteen percent of patients who used condoms prior to implants continued using them after receiving implants. Some who had never used condoms began to use them; however, 19% of patients who used condoms before having implants inserted discontinued condom use after receiving the implants. "This is the group that we are most concerned about," Dr. O'Connell said. "There is also a large percentage (54%) of patients who reported not using condoms *before or after* implants. In general, condom use remains low in the adolescent population. As health care providers, we need to emphasize, both among patients seeking implants as well as all sexually active adolescents, the importance of condom use for preventing disease," said Dr. O'Connell.

The only statistically significant finding concerned weight gain. A small, but significant, mean increase in weight of 1.3 kg occurred (p=0.0003). Analysis of implant users followed between 1 and 23 months showed the weight gain was gradual and stabilized at 18 months. The majority of patients had no change in headaches, acne or depression.

Data revealed that the majority of patients were very satisfied with the method. Only a small percentage of patients requested removal (Figure 6).

Adolescents gave various reasons for requesting removal, including irregular bleeding, headaches, depression, acne and desired pregnancy. More than half of those patients requesting removal gave "other" reasons for wanting their implants out. The reasons this "other" group gave for removal included hair loss and partner wanting the method removed. "It is interesting that although the headaches, acne and depression remained similar before and after insertion of implants, teens cite these as the reasons they're having their implants out," said Dr. O'Connell.

Figure 6

Satisfaction Rates with Subdermal Implants among Adolescents

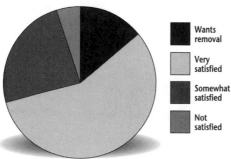

Wants removal

Very satisfied

Somewhat satisfied

Not satisfied

Source: *Adapted from O'Connell BJ, et al, 1995 (see reference 18).*

Continuation Rates among Adolescents and Adults

A study of continuation with subdermal implants by Levine et al found similar rates in adolescents and adults for up to 50 months of use.[19]

About 1,800 patients received implants and 1,688 of these patients have been followed. Forty percent of the patients were adolescents. The cumulative removal rate for teens was

Table 1

Subdermal Implant Continuation Rates in Adults and Adolescents

Duration of Use	Adults (age ≥20 years)	Adolescents (age <20 years)
12 months	98.8% (n=974)	99.7% (n=635)
24 months	96.5% (n=883)	97.1% (n=547)
36 months	92.1% (n=542)	95.7% (n=278)
48 months	91.1% (n=97)	86.6% (n=45)
Overall	91.1	93.6

Source: Levine AS, Holmes MM, Haseldon C, et al. Subdermal contraceptive implant (Norplant) continuation rates among adolescents and adults in a family planning clinic. J Pediatr Adolesc Gynecol 1996;9:67-70. Reproduced with permission of Rapid Science Publishers.

about 6%, compared to 9% for adults (Table 1).

Patients who requested implants received thorough education and counseling about the method prior to insertion. This included watching video-tapes of insertion and removal, and graphic depiction of some of the possible side effects. In addition, patients received a 30- to 60-minute counseling session with a health care worker. Following insertion of the implants, patients received personal counseling by a multidiscipli-nary team for any concerns or complications.

Patients can call 24 hours a day, 7 days a week, and all calls are immediately answered. During business hours, a family planning clinic staff person speaks with the patient. The other calls are answered by a resident on call. These patients are generally brought into the family planning clinic within 24 or 48 hours of a contact. All contacts are addressed immediately in the clinic. And when someone goes home after a clinic visit, they usually get a phone call 1 or 2 weeks after that visit to make sure all is going well.

The study authors emphasize that an important message for patients is that something can be done. The patient can be seen in the clinic and reassured, or treatment can be initiated. The high continuation rates are likely the result of a combination of thorough education, intensive surveillance and the open-door policy for problems related to use of implants.

Use in Adolescent Mothers

A study conducted at the Hospital of the University of Pennsylvania between September 1991 and July 1992 investigated the use of implants among adolescent mothers.[17]

Investigators followed prospectively 98 postpartum adolescents who chose lev-onorgestrel implants or oral contraceptives. Continuation rates among the implant group were high. The investigators reported that at follow-up (mean duration 15 months), 95% of the implant group, but only 33% of those in the oral contraceptive group, continued using the method they had chosen.

The investigators also compared pregnancy rates between the two groups. Signifi-cant differences occurred: 38% of adolescents who chose OCs became pregnant, compared to 2% of implant users (p<0.001).

Reasons given for choosing the contraceptive method varied. Among the reasons women in the implant group gave for choosing implants were: difficulty remembering to take pills (71%), side effects of oral contraceptives (38%), fear of pregnancy (57%), ease of use of implants (48%) and encouragement from others (34%). Oral contraceptive users, on the other hand, cited fear of insertion (55%), concern about irregular bleeding (24%), concern about other side effects (15%) and the fear that the implants would be visible (9%) as reasons for choosing the pill.

Barrier Methods

Dr. Hillard continued her discussion of contraceptive choices for adolescents by highlighting advantages and disadvantages of barrier methods.

Condoms — "Many barrier methods, such as condoms, have the advantage for adolescents of being available without a prescription," said Dr. Hillard. Recent data indicate that adolescent condom use is increasing. One study found that among sexually active 17- to 19-year-old males living in metropolitan areas, rates of reported condom use at most recent intercourse more than doubled between 1979 and 1988, from 21% to 58%.[20] The Youth Risk Behavior Survey also found an increase in condom use among both male and female high school students. Between 1991 and 1995, use of the condom at last intercourse increased from 38% to 50% among young women and from 55% to 60% among young men.[3,21]

In addition, condom use at *first* intercourse has increased since the early 1980s. The rate of condom use at first intercourse reported by young women increased from 23% in 1982 to 48% in 1988.[8]

The female condom provides young women with another contraceptive option. Because the method is relatively new on the market, there are insufficient data on the use of the female condom among adolescents. Its efficacy in STD prevention is also not well documented. "The primary advantage of the female condom is the fact that it is a 'female-controlled' method, which allows a woman to gain some measure of protection when her partner is unwilling to use a male condom," Dr. Hillard said.

Other Barrier Methods — Other barrier methods include the diaphragm and cervical cap. Unlike condoms, the diaphragm and cervical cap require a clinic visit for fitting and instruction. Neither the diaphragm nor the cap is widely used among adolescents. As of January 1995, the contraceptive sponge, which was available without a prescription, is no longer being manufactured and distributed in the U.S.

Strategies for STD Protection

During a symposium held at the American Academy of Family Physicians' Scientific Assembly in late 1991, Dr. Emans elaborated on the use of barrier methods, specifically the condom, for disease prevention among teens. Dr. Emans began by acknowledging that STDs are widespread among teens and emphasized that condom use needs to be discussed with adolescents, particularly young women who are choosing to use the pill or other hormonal methods.

"I think it is very important to acknowledge that many teens will stop using condoms when they start using OCs," she said. "Teens are at high risk for infection with chlamydia, HPV (human papillomavirus), gonorrhea, herpes, HIV, etc. It's important that we emphasize strategies for STD protection. We need to work with teens and say, 'How could you get your boyfriend to use a condom? What have you tried before? What do you know about condoms?' Of course, every time I prescribe pills, I give condoms with those pills in order to make it clear to the young person that I believe it's important for them to protect themselves from STDs."

Dr. Emans pointed out, "Although studies suggest condom use among young people is increasing, less than half who recently used a condom always do. So, we have to emphasize that teens need to use a condom *always* because a lot of kids say, 'Well, I do most of the time.' Particularly with HIV infection becoming more widespread, we need to tell them that 'most of the time' is not enough."

Dr. Emans continued, "One of the surveys I'd really like to emphasize, because it underscores the importance of physicians doing AIDS counseling rather than just relying on the mass media and schools, is a survey done by telephone of teenagers in Massachusetts in 1986 and 1988.[22] Positive changes were observed in terms of increased AIDS education in the schools and more youngsters adopting condoms, although the percentage *always* using condoms was still quite low. The point I'd like to stress is that 80% of these youngsters had seen a physician, but only 13% reported that they had been counseled about AIDS.

"The study investigators also looked at what made teens more likely to use condoms.[23] A logistic regression analysis identified the beliefs and behaviors associated with consistent condom use. Sexually active teens in the survey were three times more likely than other survey respondents to use condoms if they believed condoms could prevent AIDS or HIV infection; 2.7 times more likely if they carried condoms; 2.4 times more likely if they would not be embarrassed to use a condom; and 1.8 times more likely if they worried that they could get AIDS. Importantly, *if they had discussed AIDS with a physician*, they were 1.7 times more likely to be condom users. So, there's a real role for physicians to increase the education of the individual patient. It can be particularly useful to try to decrease the embarrassment of teens regarding condoms and to talk about their risk behaviors, one of which is not using a condom.

"In summary, we have to address the issue of saving lives. Many of us feel that teens will be the next wave of the population infected with HIV. So, it is essential to talk with teens about abstinence, delaying sexual involvement, contraception and, at the same time, emphasize the use of condoms for STD protection."

Contraception and Chronic Disease

At the 1993 seventh annual NASPAG conference, a contraception workshop dealing with chronic disease and teens was co-moderated by Susan M. Coupey, MD, Associate Professor of Pediatrics at Yeshiva University's Albert Einstein College of Medicine in New York, and Dr. Hillard. The workshop addressed some of the special counseling and compliance concerns with this population and outlined appropriate contraceptive methods for teens with selected chronic illnesses.

Definition

Dr. Coupey began by defining chronic disease: "We define chronic illness as a serious ongoing health condition that has lasted or is expected to last for at least 1 year, and produces or is likely to produce one or more of the following sequelae: shortened life expectancy, disability, disfigurement, limitation of function, a medical care requirement that is greater than usual for age, surgical intervention required, special ongoing treatments required, dependency on medication or special diet, and dependency on technology. When you define chronic illness in this way, many of these kids are not what we consider 'sick'—they're not ill. This definition would include, for instance, a teen with mild mental retardation who required someone to help her with schoolwork and so on."

Incidence

According to Dr. Coupey, "About 6% of the adolescent population has some form of chronic health condition with limitation of function. Asthma is probably the most common chronic medical condition in adolescents. Mental retardation and other mental health problems are also quite common." She added that "the prevalence of chronic illness is higher in the lower socioeconomic groups."

Dr. Coupey pointed out that the relatively high prevalence of chronic illness in the adolescent population is a fairly recent phenomenon. "It's a phenomenon of better medical care and has only occurred over the last 30 years," she explained. "The reason is not because the incidence of chronic illness is changing, it's because the survival rate is getting so much better. More and more adolescents with chronic diseases are living longer and, because of the better medical care, are growing and developing more normally. They're beginning to behave much more like adolescents who don't have chronic illness, and are therefore engaging in many sexual risk behaviors. Studies have shown that most adolescents who have a chronic illness, who are not severely disabled or severely mentally retarded, have sexual behavior that is very similar to that of other adolescents."

Contraceptive Choice

Regarding the impact of compliance issues on choosing appropriate contraception for young teens with chronic illness, Dr. Coupey explained that contraceptive choice may change as the adolescent reaches higher levels of maturity: "I would stress to you that the kind of adolescent who comes into your clinic, who is having sexual intercourse at a relatively young age—at 13, 14 or 15—and who also has a chronic illness is really a very, very high-risk person. I would urge you, with these early and middle adolescents with chronic illness who are sexually active, to think that perhaps the contraceptive method you would choose for their lifetime may not be the method that's appropriate for right now. You may have to go with a higher-risk method for a couple of years until they mature enough to be able to comply better with other methods."

Dr. Hillard agreed with Dr. Coupey concerning contraceptive choice. She further explained that in patients with chronic illness, "We should weigh not only the risks and benefits of various methods of contraception, but also the risks of various medical conditions related to pregnancy. We need to think about the effects of pregnancy on the course of the patient's disease. Is there an effect of the disease or the disease treatment on the fetus? What about the effect of the disease on the patient's ability to parent? These are the things we need to consider."

Dr. Hillard addressed the use of oral contraceptives in teens with chronic illness. She expressed concern that some physicians not specifically trained in reproductive health might be relying upon older data when making clinical decisions. "I think it's really important that we have a consultation with the physician who is managing the chronic illness or disease," advised Dr. Hillard. "One of the things I find as an Ob/Gyn is that sometimes my colleagues, particularly in internal medicine and subspecialty pediatrics, are not very familiar with the latest data and information. For example, they may be giving misinformation about oral contraceptives based on data from 20 years ago that do not apply to today's low-dose pills."

Depending upon the individual case, Dr. Hillard explained that OCs may be appropriate for patients not usually considered candidates because of their medical condition. She explained, for example, that "an individual with diabetes may well be able to use oral contraceptives as her effective method of contraception." Dr. Hillard added, "Even given some of the so-called 'absolute' contraindications, in an individual clinical situation it may be that oral contraceptives are the only method of contraception that an individual can use effectively.

"What about hypertension and low-dose pills?" Dr. Hillard continued. "There are studies that show small increases in blood pressure with OC use; however, in general, these increases are very small and probably not clinically significant. Low-dose pills may be an option for a period of time if the blood pressure is well-controlled, appropriate follow-up is maintained, and age and other risk factors are considered.

"One special group that needs to be taken into consideration is teenage girls who are taking isotretinoin. Individuals who are taking this medication for severe cystic acne need to avoid conception during that time, so you need to think about a very effective, reliable method of contraception."

Another aspect of treating adolescents with chronic illness is the potential for allergy to latex. A large volume of cases of allergy to latex have been reported among individuals with myelodysplasia or congenital urinary abnormalities.[24] Symptoms of latex allergy may include urticaria, wheezing or even potentially fatal anaphylaxis. It is important for clinicians to use nonlatex gloves for doing pelvic examinations and surgery on young women with myelodysplasia. It is also possible that young women will develop allergies to latex condoms or the diaphragm.

Practitioners should be aware of the potential for latex allergy when counseling patients. A nonlatex, polyurethane male condom is now available in the western United States and is expected to be available nationwide in 1997. Another option for those allergic to latex is the polyurethane female condom.

Contraceptive Counseling and Adolescents

The important, practical issue of how to communicate with and counsel adolescent patients was addressed at the 1993 NASPAG conference in a workshop by Trina Menden Anglin, MD, PhD, Associate Professor of Pediatrics at the University of Colorado School of Medicine in Denver, and Estherann Grace, MD, Assistant Clinical Professor of Pediatrics at Harvard Medical School in Boston. The workshop provided strategies for effective interviewing of adolescent patients—and their parents—as well as educational approaches designed to enhance compliance with contraceptive regimens.[25,26]

The Initial Interview

Dr. Anglin began the workshop session by explaining the importance of collecting psychosocial information from the adolescent during the initial interview. She acknowledged that "many physicians—in particular, those who haven't gone through residency more recently—may see collecting psychosocial information as time consuming, and they are not really sure what ends it serves." Dr. Anglin explained, however, "If you want to enhance compliance with contraception, you need to know more about the teenager, the teenager's family, how that teenager is doing as a person and how that teenager is functioning in her environment."

Stressing the importance of starting slowly and gaining the patient's trust, Dr. Anglin offered this practical advice: "As a basic rule of interviewing, you should begin with less-sensitive areas—chat a little bit about what's going on at school or what she enjoys doing in her leisure time. This will help you develop a relationship with the teen, and hopefully enhance her trust and confidence in you. You can then move on to domains like the patient's reproductive health history and sexual behavior."

Parental Involvement

The question of parental involvement in adolescent interviewing was addressed in the workshop. Dr. Grace explained, "If you're going to get any accurate information, you need to have time alone with your patient." Dr. Anglin agreed, offering some tips on dealing with parents who are reluctant to leave the patient's side: "I introduce myself primarily to the young woman and then secondarily to the mother. Sometimes, I'll have the teenager introduce her mom to me. I explain that we're going to spend a few minutes chatting together, but that I'm going to spend most of the time with the daughter by herself."

Confidentiality

The issue of confidentiality was also addressed in the NASPAG workshop. This issue is a very important one for adolescent patients, according to a survey published in *JAMA*.[27] The study reported that 58% of adolescents had health concerns they did not want shared with their parents. Moreover, a quarter of the adolescents surveyed reported that they would not seek health services in some situations if their parents might be informed (Figure 7). The study concluded that "interventions to address confidentiality issues are thus crucial to effective adolescent health care." Another survey of high school students in Massachusetts also found that adolescents who know that their doctors provide confidential care are about three times more likely to discuss sexuality-related issues than teens who don't believe their care is confidential.[28]

With regard to confidentiality, Dr. Grace stated, "I handle it proactively: I tell the mother straight out as soon as I meet her, 'I will provide your daughter's reproductive needs confidentially—all sexual issues are confidential.'" On the other hand, Dr.

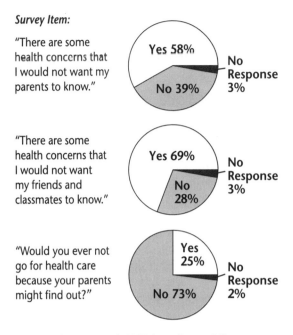

Figure 7

Perceptions of Adolescents Regarding Confidentiality Issues

Survey Item:

"There are some health concerns that I would not want my parents to know."

Yes 58%
No 39%
No Response 3%

"There are some health concerns that I would not want my friends and classmates to know."

Yes 69%
No 28%
No Response 3%

"Would you ever not go for health care because your parents might find out?"

Yes 25%
No 73%
No Response 2%

Source: Cheng TL, et al, 1993 (see reference 27).

Anglin reminded the group, "It's your decision; it's not the patient's decision. Sometimes, you can negotiate with the patient about what the parent should be told and how the parent should be told. If I believe it's important for a parent to be told, then I say, 'I think this is something that is really important for us to discuss with your mom, and how would you like us to do that?' So, I'm giving her a sense of control over the strategy, but not over the decision to do it."

Contraceptive Compliance

Dr. Grace agreed that parents should not be left out of the process entirely. In fact, parental knowledge may actually enhance compliance with contraception. Dr. Grace explained, "In dealing with compliance, the policy statement that's put out by the American Academy of Pediatrics says to involve the parents when possible. Those of us who work with adolescents might feel we want to keep the parents out. Studies on parental involvement and compliance have yielded conflicting results. Our OC study showed improved compliance in adolescents whose mothers were not aware of OC use, but this may be a reflection of the age or sociodemographics of the population Dr. Emans and I studied. Compliance may be improved for a young teen, however, if her mother can be supportive."

Drs. Anglin and Grace offered practical advice on counseling techniques designed to enhance patient compliance. Dr. Grace warned that health practitioners should "never give an adolescent more than three things to remember. If you give them more than three things, they're not going to get it. With the pill, you really only have to tell them two things to remember: (1) when to start it—first day or Sunday start—and (2) that they have to take it every day at the same time. And, I literally say to them, 'There are only two things you have to remember.' The third thing I tell them is, 'If you have any questions, call me. Don't ask your friends, don't ask others you know who are taking the pill—call me.' The fact that you are available will increase your patients' compliance. And this works, regardless of their socioeconomic status. It's a question of communicating with your patient. There is absolutely no substitute for the bonding between patient and doctor."

Interactive Communication

On the topic of written versus verbal oral contraceptive instructions, Dr. Grace explained, "Printed material is prudent, but don't rely on that alone. I'm a great believer in communicating the instructions to the patient." Dr. Anglin agreed, stressing the importance of communicating interactively with the patient: "I think a lot of us are used to just talking at patients, just giving them a whole rundown of all the facts we'd like them to hear. It doesn't work. It's much more effective to engage your patient in an interactive way." Dr. Anglin suggested first asking a patient what she knows about a particular topic—STDs, for example—instead of simply reciting a prepared monologue.

Dr. Grace stressed the importance of condom use by patients taking OCs—especially adolescents, whose sexual behavior patterns often place them at increased risk for STDs. With regard to adolescent pill users, she explained, "I tell them that they may not wish to tell their partners that they're taking the pill so that their partners will continue using condoms. We're doing a study looking at people who used condoms prior to starting the pill. Many stop using them once they go on the pill, and that's the thing that concerns me most of all."

Dr. Grace also stressed the importance of incorporating the noncontraceptive health benefits of OCs into a contraceptive counseling session. "I very strongly emphasize the positive benefits of the pill, right off the top," she said. With regard to potential side effects, Dr. Grace added, "I say to the patient, 'I do not anticipate you having any problems. If you do, I need to hear from you immediately and we'll change the pill. We will keep looking for a pill that you do not know you're taking.' That, to me, is the ideal pill for your patient."

References

1. Howard M, McCabe JB. Helping teenagers postpone sexual involvement. *Fam Plann Perspect* 1990;22:21-26.

2. Centers for Disease Control and Prevention. Youth Risk Behavior Surveillance—United States, 1995. *MMWR* 1996;45:i-85.

3. Kirby D, Barth R, Leland N, et al. Reducing the risk: a new curriculum to prevent sexual risk-taking. *Fam Plann Perspect* 1991;23:253-263.

4. Center for Population Options. *Teenage Pregnancy and Too-Early Childbearing: Public Costs, Personal Consequences.* 6th ed. Washington, DC:1992.

5. The Alan Guttmacher Institute. *Sex and America's Teenagers.* New York, NY: The Alan Guttmacher Institute;1994.

6. Spitz AM, Velebil P, Koonin LM, et al. Pregnancy, abortion, and birth rates among US adolescents—1980, 1985, and 1990. *JAMA* 1996;275:989-994.

7. Jones EF, Forrest JD, Goldman N, et al. Teenage pregnancy in developed countries: determinants and policy implications. *Fam Plann Perspect* 1985;17:53-63.

8. Forrest JD, Singh S. The sexual and reproductive behavior of American women, 1982-1988. *Fam Plann Perspect* 1990;22:206-214.

9. Zabin LS, Stark HA, Emerson MR. Reasons for delay in contraceptive clinic utilization. *J Adolesc Health* 1991;12:225-232.

10. Emans SJ, Grace E, Woods ER, et al. Adolescents' compliance with the use of oral contraceptives. *JAMA* 1987;257:3377-3381.

11. Stevens-Simon C, Beach R, Eagar R. Conception after a negative pregnancy test during adolescence. *Adolesc Pediatr Gynecol* 1993;6:83-85.

12. Zabin LS, Emerson MR, Ringers PA, et al. Adolescents with negative pregnancy test results. An accessible at-risk group. *JAMA* 1996;275:113-117.

13. Forrest JD, Jones EF. Contraceptive failure in the U.S.: revised estimates from the 1982 National Survey of Family Growth. *Fam Plann Perspect* 1989;21:103-109.

14. Robinson JC, Plichta S, Weisman CS, et al. Dysmenorrhea and use of oral contraceptives in adolescent women attending a family planning clinic. *Am J Obstet Gynecol* 1992;166:578-583.

15. Herold ES, Goodwin MS. Perceived side effects of oral contraceptives among adolescent girls. *Can Med Assoc J* 1980;123:1022-1026.

16. Cromer BA, Blair JM, Mahan JD, et al. A prospective comparison of bone density in adolescent girls receiving depot medroxyprogesterone acetate (Depo-Provera), levonorgestrel (Norplant), or oral contraceptives. *J Pediatr* 1996;129:671-676.

17. Polaneczky M, Slap G, Forke C, et al. The use of levonorgestrel implants (NORPLANT) for contraception in adolescent mothers. *N Engl J Med* 1994;331:1201-1206.

18. O'Connell BJ, Bacon J, Klein-Havens K, et al. Norplant contraceptive use in the adolescent population. Presented at NASPAG ninth annual meeting, April 21-23, 1995; Toronto, Canada.

19. Levine AS, Holmes MM, Haseldon C, et al. Subdermal contraceptive implant (NORPLANT) continuation rates among adolescents and adults in a family planning clinic. *J Pediatr Adolesc Gynecol* 1996;9:67-70.

20. Sonenstein FL, Pleck JH, Ku LC. Sexual activity, condom use and AIDS awareness among adolescent males. *Fam Plann Perspect* 1989;21:152-158.

21. Centers for Disease Control and Prevention. Trends in sexual risk behavior among high school students—United States, 1990, 1991, and 1993. *MMWR* 1995;44:124-125,131.

22. Hingson R, Strunin L, Berlin B. Acquired immunodeficiency syndrome transmission: changes in knowledge and behaviors among teenagers. Massachusetts statewide surveys, 1986 to 1988. *Pediatrics* 1990;85:24-29.

23. Hingson RW, Strunin L, Berlin BM, et al. Beliefs about AIDS, use of alcohol and drugs, and unprotected sex among Massachusetts adolescents. *Am J Public Health* 1990;80:295-299.

24. Emans JB. Current Concepts Review. Allergy to latex in patients who have myelodysplasia. *J Bone Joint Surg* 1992;74-A:1103-1109.

25. Goldenring JM, Cohen E. Getting into adolescent heads. *Contemp Pediatr* 1988;5:75-90.

26. Neinstein LS. The office visit and interview techniques. In: *Adolescent Health Care: A Practical Guide.* Baltimore, MD: Williams & Wilkins;1991.

27. Cheng TL, Savageau JA, Sattler AL, et al. Confidentiality in health care: a survey of knowledge, perceptions, and attitudes among high school students. *JAMA* 1993;269:1404-1407.

28. Thrall JS, McCloskey L, Rothstein E, et al. Perception of confidentiality and adolescents' use of health care services and information. Poster presentation. *Society for Adolescent Medicine Annual Meeting;* March 7, 1997, San Francisco, CA.

8 Sexually Transmitted Diseases

Sexually transmitted diseases (STDs) are widespread in the United States. Compared to other industrialized nations, the U.S. has the highest overall rates of STDs. Unfortunately, the newest STD, acquired immunodeficiency syndrome (AIDS), is highly fatal and can be spread by heterosexual, as well as homosexual, behaviors and intravenous drug use. While other STDs may not be fatal, many seriously injure women and their fetuses. Young people are at high risk. These facts make it imperative for clinicians to help patients understand how to protect themselves.

The fields of contraception and STD prevention are interrelated, yet questions remain. What are the most effective contraceptive methods to help prevent the spread of disease? How effective is the condom at preventing human immunodeficiency virus (HIV) transmission? Do spermicides increase or decrease the risk of HIV transmission? What factors influence infectivity? These questions are addressed in this chapter, which provides an overview of the current STD epidemic, contraceptive methods and their impact on disease prevention, and counseling strategies.

8.1: Contraception and the STD Epidemic

The United States is currently in the midst of an STD epidemic. Although anxiety over the spread of the deadly AIDS virus often overshadows the epidemic proportions of less life-threatening STDs, there is cause for concern here, as well. In fact, genital ulcers caused by certain STDs can increase the likelihood that HIV exposure will result in infection with the virus.[1] STDs can also lead to a number of serious complications, such as pelvic inflammatory disease (PID), infertility, ectopic pregnancy, adverse pregnancy outcome, infant pneumonia, infant death, mental retardation and neoplasia.[2]

In an effort to prevent a rise in the number of STD infections, family planning clinics across the nation are recommending that clients use two contraceptive methods together—the "belt-and-suspenders" approach. Oral contraceptives (OCs), injectables or implants are usually recommended as highly effective means of preventing pregnancy, while the simultaneous use of a barrier method—usually the male condom—is recommended to prevent disease.[3]

The STD Epidemic

STDs have long been a major public health concern in the U.S. In the early part of the 20th century, much of this concern focused on syphilis and gonorrhea, leading to the discovery near the close of World War II that penicillin was an effective treatment for both diseases. Incidence of new infections fell considerably and a decade later, it appeared that modern medicine had defeated these once-serious STDs. In response to this success, public health programs were curtailed in the mid-1950s.[1]

The success, however, was short-lived. In the 1970s, syphilis was again on the rise—rapidly among certain population groups—and penicillin-resistant strains of gonorrhea had emerged. Many of the lesser-known STDs also showed increasing incidence rates—including such viral infections as herpes, for which there was no cure. These trends continued into the 1980s, when, in July 1981, acquired immunodeficiency syndrome was identified.

As the scope of the AIDS epidemic became known, prevention of the spread of HIV became this country's foremost public health priority, dominating the STD field—and the media—during the past decade.[2] Meanwhile, the epidemic among non-HIV-related STDs has continued—often in relative obscurity. As a result, the number of reported STD cases has reached an estimated 12 million annually.[4] Young people are particularly at risk: two-thirds of new STD cases occur in individuals under the age of 25.[2] These figures, however, represent only those individuals infected with *symptomatic* STDs. Since many STDs do not always cause noticeable symptoms, the extent of the epidemic is believed to be even greater than the statistics indicate.[1]

Syphilis — According to the Centers for Disease Control and Prevention (CDC), syphilis reached its highest incidence in over 40 years in 1990, when more than 50,000 new cases of the disease were reported.[4] Although the incidence of primary and secondary syphilis had been slowly rising since 1950, the number of new cases soared 75% from 1985 to 1990. In contrast, between 1991 and 1994 the number of syphilis cases dropped each year, reaching the fewest number of cases reported since 1977.

The dramatic increase in the syphilis epidemic between 1985 and 1990 has been linked to the use of illicit drugs. The common practice of exchanging sex for drugs, especially among users of crack cocaine, enables the disease to spread rapidly among this population. Cocaine use has also been associated with the concurrent increase in the incidence of congenital syphilis, which has paralleled the rise and fall of syphilis in women.[2] Cocaine users are less likely to seek prenatal care and thus less likely to receive treatment for STDs, such as syphilis, prior to delivery.

The decline in syphilis cases between 1991 and 1994 occurred among all racial and ethnic groups and in all geographic regions of the U.S.[4] Despite the decline, minorities continue to be affected disproportionately. In 1994, for example, blacks accounted for about 87% of all reported cases of primary and secondary syphilis. This represents a 60-fold greater number of cases among blacks than among non-Hispanic whites (Figure 1).

Primary and Secondary Syphilis — Rates by Race and Ethnicity: United States, 1981-1994 and the Year 2000 Objective

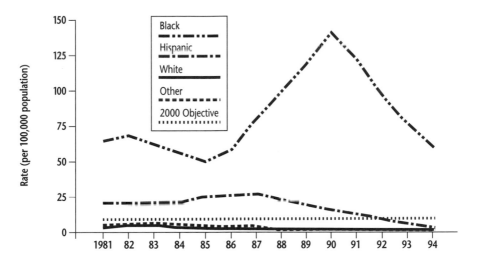

Note: "Other" includes Asian/Pacific Islander and American Indian/Alaska Native populations.
Source: Centers for Disease Control and Prevention, 1994 (see reference 4).

Furthermore, the rate varies by geographic location. The South has the highest rate per 100,000 population and it appears that additional efforts to combat this disease are needed in this region.

Gonorrhea — The CDC documented nearly 420,000 reported cases of gonorrhea in 1994.[4] The number of cases of gonorrhea reached peaks of over 1 million in the mid-1970s and has been dropping steadily ever since (Figure 2). Although the total number of new cases has been decreasing, antibiotic-resistant gonorrhea cases continue to be of concern. For example, about 30% of gonococcal isolates collected by the CDC's Gonococcal Isolate Surveillance Project were found to be resistant to penicillin, tetracycline or both. As a result, penicillin/ampicillin treatment is no longer recommended therapy for the STD.[5] Many of the new therapies are considerably more costly—a major concern for publicly funded clinics. The per case cost of treating the disease has reportedly risen from less than $1 to several dollars since more expensive antibiotics are now recommended, eg, cefixime or ofloxacin.[3]

Both the cost and morbidity implications of gonorrhea extend far beyond the disease itself—especially for women. Gonorrhea can lead to PID, one of the principal causes of female infertility.[1] PID is also believed to be responsible for about 50% of all ectopic pregnancies, and the number of ectopic pregnancies has quadrupled in the past 2 decades.[2,6] The estimated cost of PID and its consequences (including infertility and ectopic pregnancy) was over $4.2 billion in 1990.[7]

Figure 2

Gonorrhea — Reported Rates: United States, 1970-1994 and the Year 2000 Objective

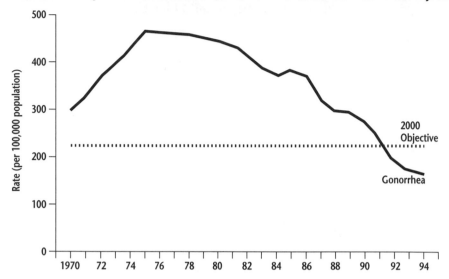

Note: *Georgia has been excluded for 1994.*
Source: *Centers for Disease Control and Prevention, 1994 (see reference 4).*

Chlamydia — In 1994, infection with *Chlamydia trachomatis* became a nationally reportable condition. The disease is prevalent among sexually active individuals of all socioeconomic levels and has emerged as the nation's most common bacterial STD. According to the CDC, "Despite the absence of chlamydia data from several states in 1994, this was the first year in which the reported number of cases of chlamydia infection...exceeded the reported number of cases of gonorrhea. ...This occurred amid growth in chlamydia control programs nationwide, together with continuing commitments to sustain gonorrhea prevention programs that began in the 1970s."[4]

Women are often asymptomatic, but account for the large majority of identified cases. "In 1994, for every chlamydia case detected and reported in males, more than five cases were detected in females (Figure 3). The discrepancy is attributable to screening strategies that focus on women because they are asymptomatic in the majority of cases.

"From 1984 through 1994, reported rates of chlamydia increased dramatically, from three cases per 100,000 population to 188. Trends continue primarily to reflect increased screening, recognition of asymptomatic infection (mainly in women), and improved reporting capacity rather than true trends in disease incidence.

"...The ability of large-scale screening programs to reduce chlamydia prevalence in women has been documented in areas where this intervention has been in place for several years. For example, the screening programs in federal Region X (Alaska, Idaho, Oregon and Washington) family planning clinics have demonstrated steady declines in chlamydia prevalence since 1988."

Figure 3

Chlamydia — Rates by Gender: United States, 1984-1994

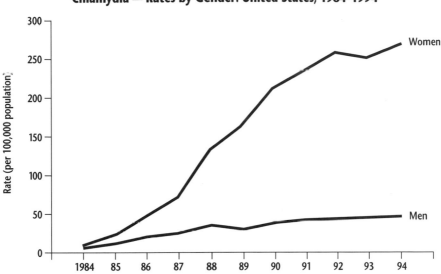

Source: *Centers for Disease Control and Prevention, 1994 (see reference 4).*

Like gonorrhea, chlamydia is a major cause of PID. Since the STD is asymptomatic in as many as 75% of women infected in the cervix, screening for chlamydia must be performed regularly if consequences such as PID are to be avoided.[2]

New protocols that include single-dose therapy options have improved the likelihood of successful treatment. Until recently, conventional treatment regimens required multiple daily doses for 7 to 10 days (for example, doxycycline 100 mg orally twice per day for 7 days as first-line therapy) and, thus, considerable commitment from patients who are often asymptomatic.[8]

This regimen is especially problematic in urban clinics, where patient follow-up is often suboptimal for determining compliance and success of therapy. The need for a simpler regimen in the treatment of chlamydia has prompted evaluation of such drugs as azithromycin, a single-dose azalide antibiotic. The CDC, in its *1993 STD Treatment Guidelines*, added single-dose azithromycin 1 g orally as an additional first-line therapy.[5] Cost, however, remains a barrier to use in many clinics.

Other STDs — Other STDs that are a notable part of the STD epidemic include human papillomavirus (HPV), herpes simplex virus (HSV) and trichomoniasis. Although comprehensive surveillance data are not available for viral STDs, estimates suggest that, with the possible exception of genital HSV, the number of cases has stabilized or declined.[4]

The estimated incidence of HPV or genital warts rose about sixfold between the mid-1960s and mid-1980s (Figure 4). Although the number of new cases has declined

Figure 4

Human Papillomavirus (Genital Warts) — Initial Visits to Physicians' Offices: United States, 1966-1993

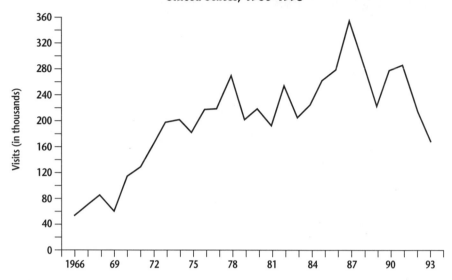

Source: Centers for Disease Control and Prevention, 1994 (see reference 4).

in recent years, HPV still infects up to 1 million individuals annually.[2] The disease has been associated with anogenital cancers, is difficult and expensive to treat, and commonly recurs in the infected individual.[1-3]

One in six Americans is infected with the genital herpes virus (HSV-2), and as many as 500,000 new cases occur each year.[2] Oral acyclovir, valcyclovir and similar antiviral agents are effective in symptomatic treatment—the infection itself is presently not curable. Studies of initial visits to physicians' offices for herpes treatment reveal a sevenfold increase in the past 2 decades.[4] A decline in the number of initial visits to physicians for this viral STD occurred between 1990 and 1992, but increased again in 1993.

Trichomoniasis affects an estimated 3 million individuals each year. The recommended treatment in the U.S. is the oral drug metronidazole; however, rare strains resistant to the drug continue to be documented. Although men can carry the infection, women predominantly suffer the symptoms of trichomoniasis, and evidence suggests an association between infection and premature birth.[2]

AIDS

The AIDS epidemic has been described by the CDC as the most devastating health problem of this century.[2] By the close of 1990, the total number of documented AIDS cases in the U.S. exceeded 161,000—over 40,000 in 1990 alone.[9] By the end of October 1995, the number of AIDS cases in the U.S. topped the half-million mark.[10] Almost 50% of these cases occurred between 1993 and October 1995. In addition to the rising number of AIDS cases, over 1 million Americans are estimated to be infected with HIV.[2] Once AIDS is diagnosed in HIV-infected individuals, the case-fatality rate has approached 100% within 5 years.[11] New antiviral therapy has lowered fatality rates in New York and elsewhere, however.

More than 300,000 people in the U.S. have died from AIDS since the disease was first identified.[10] During the 1980s, AIDS rapidly became one of the leading causes of death among young adults in this country. In 1993, HIV infection became the most common cause of death among people ages 25 to 44 years.[12] Among men ages 25 to 44 years, HIV infection/AIDS has surpassed heart disease, cancer, suicide, homicide and unintentional injuries to become the leading cause of death (Figure 5). Among women in the same age group, the disease ranks third.[12]

Although AIDS has predominantly affected the male population, the fastest rate of growth in HIV infection is now among women and minorities, particularly among the young.[13] In 1994, 18% of AIDS cases in those ages 13 years or older occurred among women. This steadily increasing proportion represents a threefold increase from 1985 to 1994 (Figure 6).[14] Furthermore, according to the CDC, "The AIDS epidemic among women continues to disproportionately affect racial/ethnic minorities, primarily in the Northeast and South. AIDS among women was primarily associated with two modes of HIV transmission: injecting drug use and heterosexual contact with an at-risk partner. …[However,] heterosexual contact is the most rapidly increasing transmission category for women."[14]

This is at least partly because women are believed to be more susceptible to heterosexual transmission of HIV than men. One study suggested that women are up to 17 times more likely to be infected by an HIV-positive male partner than men are by an HIV-positive female partner.[15] The risk of HIV transmission between the sexes seems to be equalized, however, when either partner has an STD. Many studies suggest that the presence of an STD, particularly ulcerative disease, greatly enhances the risk of virus transmission, and at least one study found this was true whether the direction of infection occurred from male-to-female or female-to-male.[16-18]

What about the risk for the fetuses of HIV-infected pregnant women? The U.S. Public Health Service recommends zidovudine to lower the risk of maternal-infant HIV transmission. Two reports published in 1994 found a significant reduction in risk of vertical transmission (from mother to fetus) with the use of zidovudine (see section 8.4 in this chapter for further discussion).

Prevention of STDs/HIV

The advent of the AIDS epidemic resulted in widespread campaigns promoting "safer-sex" practices throughout the past decade. Recommendations have centered on behavioral changes, such as postponing onset of coitus, practicing abstinence, using condoms consistently, decreasing the number of sexual partners, decreasing high-risk sexual behaviors, and decreasing intravenous and other illicit drug use. These strategies are useful for reducing the risk of both STD and HIV infection. Public campaigns aimed at reducing the spread of STDs and AIDS have also centered on the protective effects provided by barrier methods of contraception.

Figure 5

Leading Causes of Death among Men and Women 25 to 44 Years of Age: United States, 1982-1994

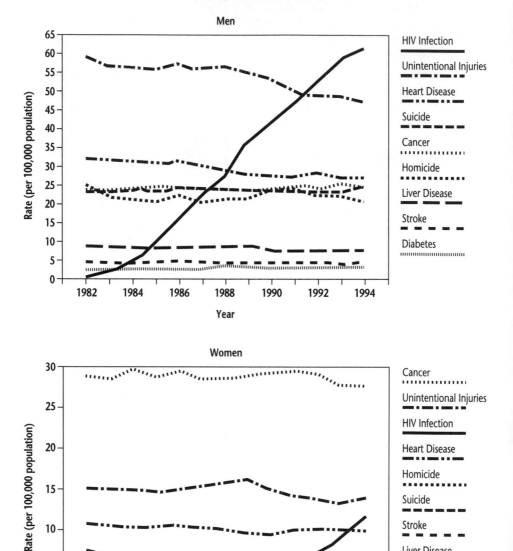

Source: *Centers for Disease Control and Prevention, 1994 (see reference 12).*

Figure 6

Number and Percentage of AIDS Cases among Women Aged ≥13 Years — United States, 1985-1994

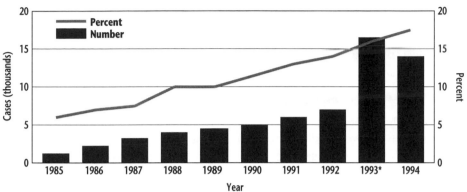

The AIDS surveillance case definition was expanded in 1993.
Source: Centers for Disease Control and Prevention, 1995 (see reference 14).

Diaphragm, Cervical Cap and Spermicides

Female barrier contraceptives protect women against some types of STDs, but increase the risk of other types of infections.[19-21] In general, barrier methods decrease the risk of acute diseases, such as chlamydial infection and gonorrhea, while also lessening the risk of long-term complications, such as PID, cervical neoplasia and ectopic pregnancy. On the other hand, diaphragm use has been associated with an increased risk of urinary tract infection, bacterial vaginosis and candidiasis.

While diaphragms and caps appear to reduce a woman's risk of developing PID, the degree of protection afforded by the device alone is not certain since most women use spermicides in conjunction with these methods. According to both laboratory and clinical studies, vaginal spermicides themselves decrease the likelihood of a woman acquiring STDs—most notably chlamydia and gonorrhea.[22]

Of the female barrier methods, spermicides perhaps have the most potential to help stem the spread of STDs, yet continuing controversy exists concerning whether currently available spermicides increase or decrease the risk of HIV infection. Some data suggest spermicides might enhance the risk of HIV transmission, while other data suggest a protective effect.[19,21,23,24] Enhancement of HIV transmission is postulated to occur because nonoxynol-9 has a detergent effect on the vaginal epithelium and can cause inflammation and disruption of cell membrane integrity—frequent use or use of high doses could increase susceptibility to HIV. On the other hand, laboratory findings suggest nonoxynol-9 is effective against HIV *in vitro*, and some data suggest that regular use of spermicides helps to decrease the risk of HIV transmission.[23,24] Available data are too limited to draw any definite conclusions.[25,26]

The Female Condom

The FDA approved another barrier method for women, the female polyurethane condom, in early 1992. Although one purpose of the female condom is to help provide protection against STDs, so far, researchers have gathered only limited data. (For further discussion of the female condom, see Chapter 5.)

Although these female controlled barrier methods offer a certain amount of protection against STDs and possibly HIV, the focus of most research and publicity in recent years has been the male condom.

Condoms and Disease Protection

Condoms have been used for centuries for protection against unwanted pregnancy and disease. Penile sheaths were fashioned predominantly from animal intestines until the mid-1840s, when development of the vulcanization process heralded mass production of synthetic condoms—the colloquial "rubber." Current worldwide condom production totals about 5 billion annually.[27]

One percent of condoms manufactured today continue to be made from the caecum of lambs. Although these natural membrane or "skin" condoms are popularly believed to provide greater sensation than latex, their effectiveness in preventing the spread of HIV and certain STDs is questionable. Both HIV and the hepatitis B virus have penetrated the porous surface of lambskin condoms in laboratory tests.[28] In cities such as San Francisco, concern over the inadequacies of lambskin condoms has prompted legislation—retail outlets selling the natural membrane products must post signs advising consumers that latex condoms offer greater protection against disease.[29]

The severity of the AIDS epidemic and the public endorsement of condom use for disease prevention by figures such as former Surgeon General C. Everett Koop, MD, ScD, have coincided with a dramatic increase in condom sales and use in this country. The 1988 National Survey of Adolescent Males found that levels of condom use among young men ages 17 to 19 and living in metropolitan areas had nearly tripled compared to 1979 levels—21% versus 58%.[30] A similar study reported the doubling of condom use among unmarried women between 1982 and 1987.[31]

Condom sales in this country rose more than 60% between 1986 and 1989.[32] Contributing to the rise in U.S. sales is the increasing proportion of women purchasing condoms. Some manufacturers have promoted this trend by developing condom lines marketed exclusively to women, while others have packaged their products in discreet plastic containers that resemble make-up compacts. Condoms have become so widely accepted in female society that women account for 40% to 50% of U.S. sales—up from 10% a few years ago.[32] Unfortunately, market reports from February 1994 through February 1995 indicate that sales of condoms have declined among young people 18 to 24 years of age.[33]

Used consistently and correctly, condoms provide a high degree of protection against the transmission and acquisition of most STDs and help decrease the risk of HIV infection.[18,34] The addition of a spermicide has been shown to improve the protective effect against both STDs and HIV.[35] The CDC recommends the use of spermicidal condoms for the prevention of HSV, gonorrhea, trichomoniasis, hepatitis B, syphilis, chlamydial infection and HIV.[28] A plastic (polyurethane) male condom is available in the United States. FDA labeling cites its usefulness for persons with allergy to latex, but does not advise use for protection against STDs because of a lack of human clinical trial data.

Unfortunately, condom use does not offer protection for the perineal area, where infections such as HPV can be transmitted. This drawback has been addressed in the design of the female condom.

Advice for Clinicians

Clinicians should be aware that as a contraceptive device, the condom is only moderately effective; first-year failure rates average about 12% among typical users (presumably due in large part to inconsistent use).[36] Hence, condoms can be used primarily to decrease STD risk in conjunction with a highly effective form of fertility regulation, such as oral contraceptives.

Dispensing condoms to patients without counseling, however, is not likely to result in effective disease prevention. Modification of behavior rarely occurs without specific and skillful intervention.[37] Providers of contraceptive care must therefore take an active role in risk assessment and patient counseling.

According to Michele Shedlin, PhD, a medical anthropologist in AIDS prevention research, practitioners need to be able to speak comfortably with their patients about specific sexual behaviors. Notes Dr. Shedlin, "When we help to design an educational outreach program, I talk with the people who will be working on it and ask them whether *they* will be comfortable talking about penises, vaginas, anal intercourse and oral sex. As a society, we have not been particularly comfortable with sexuality and *specifics* of sexual behavior. Now, with the advent of AIDS, we must learn to talk more openly about behavior." The ability to speak openly with patients about specific behaviors and an awareness of cultural factors that may inhibit such communication will aid in the taking of a comprehensive sexual history, enabling the practitioner to assess the individual's risk of infection with STDs and HIV.

Trust is an often overlooked but important risk factor for STDs and AIDS. Explains Dr. Shedlin, "'Know your partner' seems like excellent advice, but when you examine this idea further, it leaves a lot to chance. Getting to know your partner makes an assumption that your partner is being completely honest." A recent study examining the effectiveness of partner notification in cases of HIV infection supports this observation. Among partners of infected patients, only 7% were found to have been notified by the infected patient of his or her serologic status.[38] Providers must be aware of this risk factor and express to patients the potential hazards of unfounded trust.

When counseling patients who are at high risk for STD and HIV infection yet appear to be unconcerned about their own safety, Dr. Shedlin offers this advice: "AIDS prevention messages must address people's priorities, and suggested strategies must be perceived as realistic. For example, we work with women who are drug addicted and prostituting—women who have been exposed to lives of violence and abuse. These women may seem to have given up on their own futures, but the need to be there for their children gives them reason to survive. Thus, we may be able to reach them as mothers, not as prostitutes. Motivation to act on prevention information, as well as an understanding of the information, needs to be considered if we want to achieve behavior change with HIV/AIDS prevention education."

Patients who intend to use condoms to protect themselves from the threat of STDs and AIDS must be aware of the proper techniques of use. Practitioners should discuss the appropriate ways to put on and remove a condom, and the various "dos and don'ts" associated with condom use. Providers should also discuss potential partner responses to condom use with the patient. These responses should be anticipated and acted out in a role-playing fashion with the patient to ensure she has the confidence and interpersonal skills necessary to overcome potential partner resistance to condom use. (For specific patient counseling ideas, see section 8.2 in this chapter.)

Conclusion

The current STD epidemic, coupled with the threat of AIDS, requires that persons at risk of infection take appropriate precautions. The use of condoms in addition to another hormonal method of contraception is recommended for individuals seeking to prevent both pregnancy and disease. The contraceptive provider can play a crucial role in prevention through open and thorough patient counseling that will result in effective disease prevention practices by the patient.

References

1. Althaus FA. An ounce of prevention...STDs and women's health. *Fam Plann Perspect* 1991; 23:173-177.

2. Division of STD/HIV Prevention. *1990 Division of STD/HIV Prevention Annual Report.* U.S. Department of Health and Human Services, Public Health Service. Atlanta: Centers for Disease Control, 1991.

3. Donovan P. Family planning clinics: facing higher costs and sicker patients. *Fam Plann Perspect* 1991;23:198-203.

4. Division of STD/HIV Prevention. *Sexually Transmitted Disease Surveillance, 1994.* U.S. Department of Health and Human Services, Public Health Service. Atlanta: Centers for Disease Control, September 1995.

5. Centers for Disease Control and Prevention. 1993 sexually transmitted diseases treatment guidelines. *MMWR* 1993;42:i-102.

6. Expert Committee on Pelvic Inflammatory Disease. Pelvic inflammatory disease: research directions in the 1990s. *Sex Transm Dis* 1991;18:46-64.

7. Washington AE, Katz P. Costs of and payment sources for pelvic inflammatory disease: trends and projections, 1983-2000. *JAMA* 1991;226:2565-2569.

8. Stamm WE. Azithromycin in the treatment of uncomplicated genital chlamydial infections. *Am J Med* 1991;91:19-22.

9. Centers for Disease Control and Prevention. Update: acquired immunodeficiency syndrome—United States, 1981-1990. *MMWR* 1991;40:358-369.

10. Centers for Disease Control and Prevention. First 500,000 AIDS cases—United States, 1995. *MMWR* 1995;44:849-853.

11. Centers for Disease Control and Prevention. AIDS and human immunodeficiency virus infection in the United States: 1988 update. *MMWR* 1989;38(S-4):1-38.

12. Centers for Disease Control and Prevention. Update: Mortality attributable to HIV infection among persons ages 25-44 years—United States, 1994. *MMWR* 1996;45:121-125.

13. Centers for Disease Control and Prevention. *HIV/AIDS Surveillance Report* 1995;7:1-40.

14. Centers for Disease Control and Prevention. Update: AIDS among women—United States, 1994. *MMWR* 1995;44:81-84.

15. Padian NS, Shiboski SC, Jewell NP. Female-to-male transmission of human immunodeficiency virus. *JAMA* 1991;266:1664-1667.

16. Plummer FA, Simonsen JN, Cameron DW, et al. Cofactors in male-female sexual transmission of human immunodeficiency virus type 1. *J Infect Dis* 1991;163:233-239.

17. Rodrigues JJ, Mehendale SM, Shepherd ME, et al. Risk factors for HIV infection in people attending clinics for sexually transmitted diseases in India. *BMJ* 1995;311:283-286.

18. De Vincenzi I for the European Study Group on Heterosexual Transmission of HIV. A longitudinal study of human immunodeficiency virus transmission by heterosexual partners. *N Engl J Med* 1994;331:341-346.

19. Cates W Jr., Stone KM. Family planning, sexually transmitted diseases and contraceptive choice: a literature update—part I. *Fam Plann Perspect* 1992;24:75-84.

20. Rosenberg MJ, Davidson AJ, Chen J-H, et al. Barrier contraceptives and sexually transmitted diseases in women: a comparison of female-dependent methods and condoms. *Am J Public Health* 1992;82:669-674.

21. Stewart FH. Vaginal barrier contraceptives and infection risk. In: Mauck CK, Cordero M, Gabelnick HL, et al, eds. *Barrier Contraceptives. Current Status and Future Prospects.* New York: Wiley-Liss, Inc. 1994:105-122.

22. Washington AE, Cates W Jr., Wasserheit JN. Preventing pelvic inflammatory disease. *JAMA* 1991;266:2574-2580.

23. Feldblum PJ, Hira S, Godwin S, et al. Efficacy of spermicide use and condom use by HIV-discordant couples in Zambia. Presented at the International Conference on AIDS; July 19-24, 1992. Abstract WeC 1085.

24. Zekeng L, Feldblum PJ, Oliver RM, et al. Barrier contraceptive use and HIV infection among high-risk women in Cameroon. *AIDS* 1993;7:725-731.

25. Cates W Jr., Stewart FH, Trussell J. Commentary: the quest for women's prophylactic methods—hopes vs. science. *Am J Public Health* 1992;82:1479-1482.

26. Daly CC, Helling-Giese GE, Mati JK, et al. Contraceptive methods and the transmission of HIV: implications for family planning. *Genitourin Med* 1994;70:110-117.

27. Goldsmith MF. Sex in the age of AIDS calls for common sense and "condom sense." *JAMA* 1987;257(17):2261-2264.

28. Centers for Disease Control and Prevention. Condoms for prevention of sexually transmitted diseases. *MMWR* 1988;37(9):133-137.

29. Gebhart F. Warning of possible hazards of lambskin condoms spreads. *Drug Topics* 1991;135(21):96.

30. Sonenstein FL, Pleck JH, Ku LC. Sexual activity, condom use and AIDS awareness among adolescent males. *Fam Plann Perspect* 1989;21:152-158.

31. Forrest JD, Fordyce RR. U.S. women's contraceptive attitudes and practices: how have they changed in the 1980's? *Fam Plann Perspect* 1988;20:112-118.

32. Consumers Union. Can you rely on condoms? *Consumer Reports* 1989;March:135-142.

33. Condom suppliers aim to boost business. *Chain Drug Review* 1995;17:35.

34. Stone KM, Grimes DA, Magder LS. Personal protection against sexually transmitted diseases. *Am J Obstet Gynecol* 1986;155(1):180-188.

35. Kestelman P, Trussell J. Efficacy of the simultaneous use of condoms and spermicides. *Fam Plann Perspect* 1991;23:226-232.

36. Trussell J, Hatcher RA, Cates W Jr., et al. Contraceptive failure in the United States: an update. *Stud Fam Plann* 1990;21(1):51-54.

37. Grieco A. Cutting the risks for STDs. *Medical Aspects of Human Sexuality* 1987;March:70-84.

38. Landis SE, Schoenbach VJ, Weber DJ, et al. Results of a randomized trial of partner notification in cases of HIV infection in North Carolina. *N Engl J Med* 1992;326:101-106.

8.2: Patient Counseling

Patients may need help to come up with appropriate and comfortable ways to bring up the subject of condoms with their sexual partners. They also need specific advice about what to say to overcome partner resistance to condom use. The following provides some suggestions for both situations.

Icebreakers: Bringing Up the Subject of Condoms

It may be difficult to know what to say when bringing up the subject of condoms with a sexual partner. Men and women are often reluctant to mention condoms because of a concern about how they will be perceived. (Will my partner think I have AIDS [acquired immunodeficiency syndrome]? Will he/she think I'm promiscuous or be offended?) Patients may also fear rejection.

Here are some suggestions to make it easier. Advise patients to:

- Bring up the subject *before* initiating sexual activity. Condom use and the threat of sexually transmitted diseases (STDs) may not seem important in the middle of sexual play and arousal.

- Have condoms available—condoms only work when used. Women can keep them in their purses.

Here are some suggested "icebreakers":

- "I need to talk to you about something that's important to our relationship."

- "I see so much on television about AIDS and other sexually transmitted diseases that I'm concerned about protecting my health. Have you ever used condoms?"

- "My doctor says I should always use condoms during sex to protect myself and my partner."

Talking about Condoms: What Do I Say If My Partner Says... ?

"Wearing a condom (rubber) is no fun. I can't feel anything with one on."
"Sex may feel a little bit different, but a condom can also make intercourse last longer and feel better in the long run."

"Sex with condoms just doesn't feel as good."
"Sex may not feel the same as without a condom, but men can still have an orgasm while using a condom so it can't be that unpleasant. If we use condoms, I'll feel safer and more relaxed, and that will make sex more enjoyable for both of us."

"I don't like to stop in the middle of sex. It's a turn-off."
"We don't have to stop. I can help you put the condom on. Besides, seeing a doctor for a sexually transmitted disease or pregnancy is really a turn-off. Let's try to work this out."

"I don't shoot drugs," or "I'm not gay."

"I believe you, but we may not know everything about our past partners or their partners. Besides, many diseases don't have symptoms. Let's make sure we keep ourselves protected."

"I will not use a condom."

"I'm sorry you feel that way. I will not allow myself to take the chance of getting AIDS, herpes, gonorrhea or any other sexually transmitted disease. Perhaps, we shouldn't have sex until we can work out our differences. Or, we could give each other pleasure in other ways."

"If you really loved me, you wouldn't ask me to use a condom."

"Love isn't the issue—getting a sexually transmitted disease is. I think if you loved me, you would be more concerned about protecting us both."

"Don't you trust me?"

"We may both believe we're disease free and trust each other, but people can have the AIDS virus and not know it. Other diseases are like that, too. We may not be able to trust our past partners. I trust that using a condom will protect us both."

"Just this once."

"Once is all it can take to get pregnant or infected. I don't want to risk my life and health for 'just this once.'"

"I've been tested for all the diseases and I don't have any."

"Doctors usually only test you for two or three, but there are many more. My doctor told me I should always use a condom to protect myself."

8.3: Contraception, STDs and Risk-Taking Behavior

On May 20-22, 1994, the Association of Reproductive Health Professionals (ARHP) held a clinical conference on sexually transmitted diseases (STDs) in McLean, Virginia. "STD Update '94" focused on the interrelated issues of STDs, contraception and risk-taking behavior, as well as diagnosis and treatment of disease.

Infectivity Factors

Amy E. Pollack, MD, MPH, President of the AVSC (Access to Voluntary and Safe Contraception) in New York City, presented a session at the ARHP conference, entitled "STDs/HIV, Contraception and the Vagina." Dr. Pollack began by discussing some of the factors that influence STD infectivity in women.

According to Dr. Pollack, the cervix is thought to be the site in a woman's reproductive tract most vulnerable to human immunodeficiency virus (HIV) transmission. Because of this, she said, "protecting the cervix with a physical barrier probably does provide some general protection" against HIV infection; however, Dr. Pollack added that HIV infection can occur through the vaginal epithelium, as well. "We now have studies that show that when you do a hysterectomy or remove the cervix from animal models and then expose the animal model to a viral load, the virus still transgresses vaginal epithelium," although probably at a reduced rate. "It's not just the cervix—even though that's a more vulnerable area—where that transgression occurs."

Dr. Pollack explained that while HIV has been known to transgress normal, healthy vaginal epithelium, lesions and inflammation caused by other STDs can increase the risk. "We know that ulcerative lesions—lesions like those caused by herpes, syphilis and chancroid—increase the risk of HIV transmission," she said, noting that the ulcerated surface provides more direct access to the bloodstream. "Chlamydia, gonorrhea and trichomoniasis, which are the inflammatory infections, also increase the risk of transmission, although they increase that risk less than lesional disease.

"One of the other things that has an impact on infectivity," continued Dr. Pollack, "either to or from a partner, is the presence of menstrual blood. The presence of menstrual blood not only increases the free virus and the cellular fraction of virus, but also has a direct impact on the pH of the vagina—changing it from a more acid environment, which is normal, to a more neutral environment," which is more hospitable to HIV. "We know that virus viability is very dependent on the pH that it's exposed to." Dr. Pollack added that research on vaginal microbicides is focusing partly on how to acidify the vaginal environment.

Condoms and Disease Prevention

Dr. Pollack also discussed various methods of contraception and their role in preventing the spread of sexually transmitted diseases. She began with the male condom. Dr. Pollack explained that condoms provide highly effective protection against a variety of STDs. However, she stressed that this protection was dependent upon correct and consistent use of the method.

"When talking about STDs and HIV," said Dr. Pollack, "we need to look at condom users or nonusers, not condom 'sometimes-users.' Individuals who use condoms only sometimes have the same random chance of infection during episodes of nonuse as individuals who never use condoms. The rates [of infection] with sometimes-users are equivalent to the rates of never-users," she explained. On the other hand, added Dr. Pollack, "If you use a condom all the time, you're not likely to get infected—and that's been shown in multiple studies."[1-5]

In a separate presentation at the ARHP conference, Katherine M. Stone, MD, a medical epidemiologist with the Division of STD/HIV Prevention at the Centers for Disease Control and Prevention (CDC) in Atlanta, illustrated just how widespread the problem of inconsistent condom use is. Despite CDC's heavy promotion of condom use, Stone explained, "people are not using them *consistently*. If you look at 'always' versus 'most of the time'—and consistency of use is very important—only 16% of women are *always* using condoms. This is a problem because it's easier for women to get STDs from men than vice versa."

Dr. Pollack acknowledged that part of the problem may be the discomfort or lack of sensitivity that some condom users report. Because of this, she said, condom designers and manufacturers are "trying to be more creative with condom comfort issues. ...Researchers at Family Health International, for example, are trying to develop a condom that's tighter on the bottom so that it stays put and holds the semen in the condom. But, it gets baggier as you go up so that the plastic moves up and down," improving stimulation. "They've had a really good response—men seem to prefer that to a completely tight-fitting condom."

Female Condom

With regard to the female condom, Dr. Pollack said the device has potential in the effort to stem the spread of STDs and HIV, but that little clinical evidence exists in support of the female condom's disease prevention potential. "There are a few studies getting ready to examine HIV protection," she said. "There aren't really any studies looking at STD protection on a large scale. There was a small study looking at trichomoniasis reinfection that found a reduced incidence, but it wasn't a statistically significant reduction."

Spermicides

Dr. Pollack explained that spermicides, such as nonoxynol-9, may offer some protection against HIV infection and certain other STDs. She added that "one of the problems with spermicides is that we're not clear about how much needs to be used to have a contraceptive impact—let alone an impact on organisms. The various spermicides that are available have a wide range of doses associated with them." She added that "nonoxynol-9 and octoxynol-9 don't penetrate cervical mucus. So, one of the problems is getting enough of a load of a microbicide or a spermicide so that it actually covers the cervix."

With regard to developing new spermicidal/microbicidal agents, Dr. Pollack explained that the task can be complicated "because the environment—the vaginal ecology—has many different variables that come into play when you're trying to develop a spermicide. ...There are two factors that we're talking about, in general. One is the microbicidal and spermicidal potential—they're very hard to separate. We'd like to have a microbicide that wasn't spermicidal, but we're a long way away from that." The other factor, according to Dr. Pollack, is being able to "coat the vaginal mucosa, which is very difficult to do. And, that's where the vehicle that you're using to introduce it comes into play. In the future, we will see people working on vehicles that are better than what we work with now, that actually spread themselves evenly across the vaginal mucosa."

Diaphragm and Cervical Cap

With regard to other female-controlled barrier methods, such as the diaphragm and cervical cap, Dr. Pollack explained that correct, consistent use is essential to their effectiveness. "The studies that look at contraceptive efficacy rates and infection protection rates in diaphragm and cap users clearly indicate that their effectiveness rate is based on user effectiveness rates. In Brazil, there are studies that show that women who use the diaphragm all of the time have significantly lower rates of everything, including infection, because they use it reliably."

Dr. Stone noted, however, that "the diaphragm hasn't been studied in the same type of design as some of the other contraceptives. We really don't have a clue what it does to HIV. Some studies suggest a decrease in gonorrhea and chlamydia; other STDs we don't know about."

Withdrawal

Should withdrawal be considered a protective method against STD infection? "Withdrawal is interesting," Dr. Pollack explained, "because it's a commonly used method of contraception both here and overseas—and also a rarely talked about method of contraception, although the efficacy can be quite high if it's used properly." She noted, however, that the 19% typical failure rate indicates that withdrawal is often *not* used effectively.[6]

As for protection against infection, she continued, "Women who are using withdrawal should know that the preejaculate does have infective agents, such as HIV, in it." However, Dr. Pollack explained that "the viral load in preejaculate is much less than in semen, so exposure is decreased. People shouldn't be told that withdrawal will protect them from infection," she summarized, "although withdrawal is better than nothing."

STDs and Risk Taking

Deborah Reed, CRNP, President and CEO of Planned Parenthood of the Capital Region in Harrisburg, Pennsylvania, addressed the topic of risk taking at the ARHP conference. One of the key factors contributing to risk-taking behavior is the general lack of knowledge or concern among Americans about contracting an STD, Reed said, citing a February 1994 survey commissioned by the American Medical Women's Association.[7] "Sexually transmitted diseases are among the most common infectious diseases in the United States today, despite the fact that many of them can be cured. At current rates, it is estimated that at least one in four—perhaps, one in two—Americans will contract an STD at some point in their lives. Yet, this survey showed that most women do not believe that sexually transmitted diseases can happen to them.

"Despite recent public education efforts around HIV/AIDS, most American women —73% of them—are not concerned about getting HIV disease. They are even less worried about getting an STD: as many as 85% of women do not think they will get an STD. This suggests that most women do not understand that they could be at risk.

"The fact that most women are not worried about contracting STDs is a serious problem. As long as women do not believe it can happen to them, they will be less likely to take action or to encourage others, including their partners or friends, to behave in ways to help prevent the spread of sexually transmitted diseases.

"As health care professionals," she explained, "we need to be educated, ourselves, and encouraged to take a more active role in raising our patients' consciousness and awareness about the risks of STDs. During every opportunity that we have with a client, we need to educate them. ...We need to constantly reinforce—not just rely on a one-time counseling session."

Reed explained that patients should always be advised of the "risk-free option"—abstinence. Beyond that, she said, the emphasis should be placed on remaining in a mutually monogamous relationship. "The other thing that we need to emphasize is using the barrier methods of protection," Reed explained, adding that patients need to be taught necessary skills, not just told what to do. "Don't just *tell them* to use condoms," she said, "but *show them* how to use condoms. Don't tell them to use a female condom, but show them how to use it. Don't tell them to use spermicide, but show them."

Reed also stressed the importance of sensitivity when dealing with the emotionally charged issue of STDs. "We are dealing with diseases and conditions and behaviors that stir our most powerful emotions—the emotions of fear, anger, shame, denial and rejection. Remember that awareness, concern and lack of stigma promote risk-reducing behavior for our clients. You, yourself, as a health care professional, must work through your own fears, your own biases and your own concerns; otherwise, you cannot be effective. Counseling skills are essential to the effective delivery of STD prevention messages, but you must do it with respect, compassion and a nonjudgmental attitude," Reed concluded.

References

1. Centers for Disease Control and Prevention. Update: barrier protection against HIV infection and other sexually transmitted diseases. *MMWR* 1993;42:589-591,597.

2. Cates W, Stone KM. Family planning, sexually transmitted disease, and contraceptive choice: a literature update. *Fam Plann Perspect* 1992;24:75-84.

3. Weller SC. A meta-analysis of condom effectiveness in reducing sexually transmitted HIV. *Soc Sci Med* 1993;1635-1644.

4. DeVincenzi I, European Study Group on Heterosexual Transmission of HIV. Heterosexual transmission of HIV in a European cohort of couples [Abstract no. WS-CO2-1]. Vol 1. IXth International Conference on AIDS/IVth STD World Congress. Berlin, June 9, 1993:83.

5. Saracco A, Musicco M, Nicolosi A, et al. Man-to-woman sexual transmission of HIV: longitudinal study of 343 steady partners of infected men. *J Acquir Immune Defic Syndr* 1993;6:497-502.

6. Trussell J, Hatcher RA, Cates W Jr, et al. Contraceptive failure in the United States: an update. *Stud Fam Plann* 1990;21:1-5.

7. American Medical Women's Association. Women and sexually transmitted diseases: the dangers of denial. EDK Associates, Inc., New York, NY; February 1994.

8.4: Lowering the Risk of Maternal-Infant HIV Transmission

Two reports published in 1994 suggest that zidovudine (also known as AZT) may help to lower the risk of human immunodeficiency virus (HIV) transmission from mother to newborn.[1,2] The first report described interim findings from the AIDS Clinical Trials Group (ACTG) Protocol 076, sponsored by the National Institute of Allergy and Infectious Diseases and the National Institute of Child Health and Human Development.[1]

The randomized, double-blind ACTG study administered zidovudine to both mothers and newborns. Zidovudine was given orally to pregnant HIV-infected women starting at 14 to 34 weeks' gestation for the remainder of the pregnancy, intravenously to women during labor and orally to newborns for the first 6 weeks of life. Eligibility criteria included no previous antiretroviral treatment during the current pregnancy, no clinical indications for antiretroviral therapy antepartum and a CD4+ T-lymphocyte count >200/µL at initial assessment.

The risk of HIV transmission from mother to infant fell 68% in the group treated with zidovudine. Rates of HIV transmission were three times as high for the children in the control group (26%; 95% confidence interval [CI], 18%-34%) as compared to those in the zidovudine-treated group (8%; 95% CI, 4%-14%). An independent safety monitoring board recommended early termination of the study in order to offer the treatment to women in the control group.

Although results are promising, they may not apply to women with CD4+ T-lymphocyte counts ≤200 cells/µL or those treated previously with zidovudine for extended periods, who may have resistant strains of the virus. The trial also could not assess the relative value of the timing of the medication—ie, antepartum, during delivery or during the first 6 weeks of life. In addition, no data could be gathered on the efficacy of zidovudine given during the first trimester and any long-term side effects.

The second report, a nonrandomized, prospective cohort study at a university medical center and two general hospitals, found zidovudine therapy given during pregnancy and/or labor and delivery was associated with a significant reduction in maternal-fetal HIV transmission.[2] Of 26 mothers treated with zidovudine, only one (4%) had an infant that was infected, compared to 12 of 42 (29%) mothers not treated with zidovudine (p=0.01).

The study also assessed other maternal risk factors potentially influencing vertical transmission. These risk factors included maternal CD4 cell count, presence of immune complex dissociated (ICD) p24 antigen, complications of pregnancy and obstetric events during labor and delivery. An increased risk was associated with ICD p24 antigenemia at delivery (p=0.02) and with intrapartum events that increased fetal exposure to maternal blood (p=0.02). With respect to CD4 lymphocyte counts, zidovudine treatment afforded a significant protective effect, even in women with low CD4 cell counts. No substantial toxicity occurred in the 26 mother-infant pairs.

Public Health Service Recommendations

- All health care workers providing care to pregnant women and women of childbearing age should be made aware of the results of the ACTG study.

- HIV-infected pregnant women meeting the protocol eligibility criteria should be informed of the potential benefits, but unknown long-term risks, of zidovudine treatment as administered in Protocol 076.

- Patients should be informed that the ACTG Protocol 076 substantially reduced, but did not eliminate, the risk of HIV transmission.

- Until the potential for teratogenicity can be assessed, zidovudine therapy solely for the purpose of reducing the risk of maternal-fetal transmission should not be initiated earlier than 14 weeks' gestation.

Zidovudine Regimen Given to HIV-Infected Pregnant Women and Their Infants in ACTG Protocol 076

- Oral administration of 100 mg zidovudine five times daily, initiated at 14 to 34 weeks' gestation and continued for the remainder of the pregnancy.

- During labor, intravenous administration of zidovudine in a loading dose of 2 mg per kg body weight given over 1 hour, followed by continuous infusion of 1 mg per kg body weight per hour until delivery.

- Oral administration of zidovudine to the newborn (zidovudine syrup at 2 mg per kg body weight per dose given every 6 hours) for the first 6 weeks of life, beginning 8 to 12 hours after birth.

Unlike the ACTG study, zidovudine was not given to infants shortly after birth. In addition, mothers with lower CD4 lymphocyte counts were treated. According to the authors, "These data suggest that the beneficial effect of zidovudine therapy in reducing maternal-fetal HIV-1 transmission recently found in Protocol 076 of the placebo-controlled Acquired Immunodeficiency Syndrome Clinical Trials Group Study may extend to women with lower CD4 cell counts and suggest that prolonged treatment of infants may not be necessary."[2]

Two years later, further data from 402 mother-infant pairs entered into Protocol 076 confirmed the earlier report that treatment with zidovudine significantly reduced HIV-1 transmission from mother to infant. In addition, the researchers showed that maternal viral load is a risk factor for transmitting HIV-1 from mother to infant.[3] According to the authors, "In the placebo group, a large viral burden at entry or delivery or a positive culture was associated with an increased risk of transmission (the transmission rate was greater than 40% in the highest quartile of the RNA level)." The researchers recommend that women be given zidovudine to help prevent HIV-1 transmission to their infants regardless of the maternal plasma level of HIV-1 RNA or the CD4 cell count.

References

1. Centers for Disease Control and Prevention. Zidovudine for the prevention of HIV transmission from mother to infant. *MMWR* 1994;43(16):285-287.

2. Boyer PJ, Dillon M, Navaie M, et al. Factors predictive of maternal-fetal transmission of HIV-1. Preliminary analysis of zidovudine given during pregnancy and/or delivery. *JAMA* 1994;271:1925-1930.

3. Sperling RS, Shapiro DE, Coombs RW, et al. Maternal viral load, zidovudine treatment, and the risk of transmission of human immunodeficiency virus type 1 from mother to infant. *N Engl J Med* 1996;335:1621-1629.

Note to Clinicians

An International Antiretroviral Pregnancy Registry has been established by manufacturers of zidovudine and dideoxycytidine (ddC) to collect observational, nonexperimental data on exposure to these drugs during pregnancy. Practitioners wishing to enroll patients should call: (800) 722-9292, extension 8465; facsimile (919) 315-8981.

8.5: HIV/AIDS Educational Services

The Health Resources and Services Administration (HRSA) has established special services to help educate health care professionals about human immunodeficiency virus/acquired immunodeficiency syndrome (HIV/AIDS) via the telephone.[1] The first links health care workers around the world for live, interactive, toll-free audio teleconferences with internationally renowned clinical experts. The second, the national HIV Telephone Consulting Service, provides quick answers to clinical questions and operates out of San Francisco General Hospital. Because treatment of HIV-infected individuals changes rapidly, clinicians should check with local infectious disease experts, as well.

International State-of-the-Art HIV Clinical Conference Call Series

The program represents a collaborative effort between HRSA and several other federal and private agencies. Conference calls are held quarterly. The agencies canvass thousands of primary care providers to determine specific questions to be addressed. Before the program, a collated final list of questions is faxed to the panelists and all registered participants. Electronic polling and other new technologies allow participants to interact with panelists and ask on-line follow-up questions. The calls are accredited for continuing medical education. For further information and registration forms for future State-of-the-Art HIV Clinical Conference Calls, **fax** correspondence to Abe M. Macher, MD, at HRSA at (202) 690-7560 or (202) 690-6584.

National HIV Telephone Consulting Service

Primary care providers with HIV-related clinical management questions can reach expert consultants by calling the toll-free number from 10:30 AM to 8:00 PM EST, Monday through Friday. Call: (800) 933-3413. After hours, callers may leave a recorded question and a consultant will return the call. Ronald Goldschmidt, MD, of the Department of Family and Community Medicine at the University of California-San Francisco School of Medicine, directs the multidisciplinary consulting team of physicians, nurse practitioners and clinical pharmacists on hand to answer inquiries.

Reference
1. Sumaya CV, Macher AM, Bowen GS, et al. From the Health Resources and Services Administration. *JAMA* 1994;272:1242.

9 Issues in Reproductive Health

In a society bombarded by media messages every day, the media's impact on women's perceptions and use of birth control warrants attention. The pill, the intrauterine device (IUD) and, most recently, subdermal implants, have borne the brunt of many highly publicized stories—most of which emphasize risks and almost never mention benefits. These stories scare women and their clinicians and impede access to contraception.

Other reproductive health issues include helping women who breastfeed choose a contraceptive method. Can breastfeeding alone provide contraceptive protection? Which methods have the least impact on nursing mothers and infants? Are combination oral contraceptives (OCs) ever appropriate? While breastfeeding provides some natural protection against pregnancy in the early postpartum period, and may be highly desirable in developing countries, most women in the United States do not sustain breastfeeding patterns sufficient to maintain contraceptive efficacy and will need an alternative method at least by the sixth week postpartum.

In addition, concern exists over what to do for women with medical disorders who need contraception. Will the method exacerbate the illness? Are the risks associated with the birth control method outweighed by the possibility of a high-risk pregnancy? The third section of this chapter contains a risk benefit algorithm to help clinicians and patients decide.

The fourth section briefly covers suggestions to help your patients stop smoking. Smoking is dangerous no matter which contraceptive method is chosen; however, it is well known that the cardiovascular risks associated with OCs, for example, increase significantly among smokers. Women should be urged to stop smoking rather than to stop the pill.

9.1: How Media Undermine Contraception

Misperceptions about contraceptives are common among women in the United States. This problem is due primarily to unbalanced reporting in the mass media—the principal source of contraceptive information for most women in this country.

David A. Grimes, MD, Executive Editor of *The Contraception Report*, elaborated on the role of the media during a 1992 symposium held at the American Academy of Family Physicians' Scientific Assembly in San Diego. The symposium addressed patient concerns with oral contraception. Dr. Grimes discussed how the mass media influence attitudes toward contraception, the kinds of messages that patients receive, the relationship between those messages and contraceptive choice, and offered pragmatic suggestions for remedying this problem.

Dr. Grimes began by showing the audience an example of a spermicide advertisement, which directed three subliminal messages at patients. According to Dr. Grimes, "The first message contained in the advertisement is that this product contains no hormones and, hence, it's inherently better. The implication is that hormones are dangerous and 'bad for you.' Second, the advertisement states this woman's doctor told her to get off the pill, so women readers get a powerful, authoritative suggestion about discontinuing the pill. The third message is that the woman's body needed a 'rest.' She was just exhausted from taking all those birth control pills. In my experience, when you take a birth control rest, you get a pregnancy-induced rest, and from what I've seen of that process, it's not particularly restful."

In addition to subtle, and not-so-subtle, negative messages about hormones, the media stress "bad news" and often focus on the putative relationship between OCs and breast cancer. Dr. Grimes commented, "We are today in a birth control bind largely caused by media preoccupation with bad news. For example, the May 7, 1989 *London Sunday Times* ran an enormous headline announcing a report from the United Kingdom (U.K.) of a case-control study showing an increased risk of breast cancer among women below the age of 36 who had used the pill. Each of these letters measured 37 mm in height. By comparison, the other headline of the day, which announced the cancellation at the 11th hour of a nationwide strike by all family physicians in the U.K., was much smaller. Here in the U.S., we generally reserve headlines of this size for declarations of war or presidential assassinations, rarely for single studies of epidemiology."

Another example of how the breast cancer issue received lopsided media coverage occurred in October of 1983, when two articles linking pill use with breast cancer appeared in the same issue of *Lancet*. "A firestorm of controversy was touched off around the world, and the newspapers were quick to pick up on it. Coverage in the U.K. in the 3 months following publication was heavy—34 articles describing this adverse effect appeared in the national press and a total of 161 reports appeared in the local press. At about the same time, a report was published in the literature suggesting a protective effect against breast cancer. This generated one report in the national press and none in the local press. So, that is the balance of coverage that is typical regarding the health risks and benefits associated with OCs," explained Dr. Grimes.

The recent controversy over the possible increase in risk of venous thromboembolic events with pills containing the progestins gestodene and desogestrel is the latest example of how media impact contraception. British media announced the warning *before* clinicians were made aware of it, scaring many women and health care providers in the process. Early reports suggest that many women discontinued the pill on their own, with a concomitant rise in the number of elective abortions.

Reporting about contraception on television also leans toward the negative (Figure 1). "We know that television is the major source of information in this country," Dr. Grimes continued, "so I went to the *Television News Index and Abstracts* from Vanderbilt University, which catalogs the evening news on the three major networks every day, and has done so for many years. I tracked all the stories about contraception in 1977 and 1987.

In 1977, there was a 13-to-1 ratio of bad news to good news about contraception on the evening news programs. In 1987, it was a much more balanced ratio of 3 to 2. Nonetheless, because of this type of advertising and news coverage, women today are grossly misinformed about both the efficacy and safety of modern birth control methods, such as oral contraceptives, IUDs and implants."

Consequences of Unbalanced Media Coverage

Unbalanced media coverage in newspapers, magazines and television has created public perceptions of the birth control pill, the IUD and implants that are unwarranted. "Partly as a result of the blitz of negative media coverage, particularly with regard to the pill and breast cancer, but also with regard to implants and IUDs, many women and their physicians lost confidence in these methods. This decline in confidence leads to an increase in unintended pregnancy and unnecessary abortions, as women choose less-effective methods and often no method at all. Furthermore, media

Figure 1

Number and Content of Stories on Birth Control, Evening News, ABC, CBS and NBC Television Networks, United States, 1977 and 1987

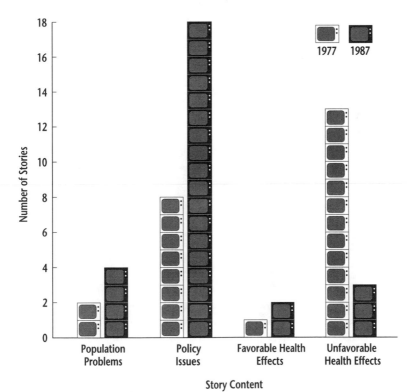

Source: *Adapted from Grimes DA. Breast cancer, the pill and the press. In: Mann RD, ed.* Oral Contraceptives and Breast Cancer. *Parthenon Publishing Group, Inc., 1989;309-318. Reproduced with permission of Parthenon Publishing Group, Inc., Pearl River, New York.*

preoccupation with bad news has resulted in a poor outlook for new products due to the hostile climate (ie, burdensome legal, insurance and malpractice concerns) and lack of funding for contraceptive research," Dr. Grimes stated.

Two recent surveys suggest that, although some misperceptions have declined in recent years, women continue to overestimate health risks of OCs and are largely unaware of the pill's noncontraceptive health benefits.[1,2] In early 1994, the American College of Obstetricians and Gynecologists (ACOG) announced the results of a Gallup poll on women's attitudes toward contraception, a long-awaited update to a similar 1985 survey. While the study showed a decline in the percentage of women who believe there are substantial health risks associated with pill use (76% to 54%), the proportion who cited cancer as the chief risk remained constant at approximately 30% (Figure 2). Regarding health benefits of pill use, only 6% of respondents were aware of the protective effect against cancer and 42% said OCs provided no health benefits other than prevention of pregnancy.[1]

A similar 1993 study of women coming to the Yale University Health Services' department of Obstetrics and Gynecology (including students, faculty, employees and their families) produced comparable results, suggesting that educational status has little effect on misperceptions about OCs.[3] In this study, 49% of women believed there were substantial risks to using the pill. Between 80% and 95% of respondents were

Figure 2

Comparison of Selected Results from the ACOG/Gallup Poll on Attitudes Toward Contraception, 1985 and 1994

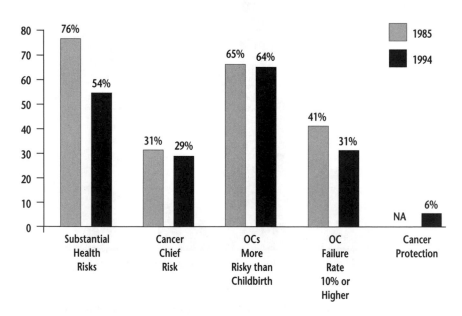

Sources: American College of Obstetricians and Gynecologists, 1985 and 1994 (see references 1 and 2).

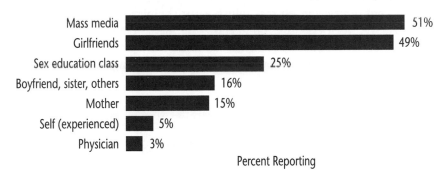

Figure 3

Sources of Contraceptive Information

Mass media	51%
Girlfriends	49%
Sex education class	25%
Boyfriend, sister, others	16%
Mother	15%
Self (experienced)	5%
Physician	3%

Percent Reporting

Source: Herold ES, et al, 1980 (see reference 4).

unaware of health benefits associated with OC use. The findings from these studies indicate that patients seeking OCs are likely to harbor myths, fears and misperceptions about the method.

A Canadian study of adolescent women found that 51% stated they had received most of their information concerning OCs from the media—as opposed to only 3% receiving OC information from a physician (Figure 3).[4]

The Canadian study also found that mothers were the source of contraceptive information for 15% of the adolescents. Mothers may also have negative attitudes about oral contraception. The mothers of many teenagers today are familiar with the pills that were available in the 1960s and '70s—pills that were high-dose and caused more nuisance side effects, such as nausea. During the '70s, the media often highlighted negative stories about the pill (eg, the Nelson Congressional pill hearings in 1970). Thus, mothers of today's teens may be giving their daughters obsolete information about the pill.

Misperceptions about oral contraceptives also exist in developing countries.[5] Family Health International conducted a survey of women of reproductive age in Thailand, Sri Lanka, Egypt, Senegal, Nigeria, Mexico, Costa Rica and Chile. About 50% to 75% of the women believed OCs carry substantial health risks. Among the non-African women, over 40% thought that taking the pill is more dangerous than childbearing. Similar to the ACOG and Yale reports, the researchers also found that the health benefits of OCs were virtually unknown.

Strategies for Addressing Media and Patient Misperceptions

Dr. Grimes described several strategies to address media and patient misperceptions about contraception. First, physicians and other reproductive health care providers can become involved with the local press and television. "We have to work hard to see if we can provide some balance. I would encourage those of you who are in a city that has a television station to call your local television news department and let them know you're interested in the issues so when these reports do appear on the wire services, they can call you for comment. I assure you, you can reach far more patients in 30 seconds on the evening news than you may in a lifetime of medical practice."

Because broadcast media often require brevity, complex epidemiologic findings can be shortchanged. A lack of background knowledge or desire for simplicity may prompt reporters to oversimplify or bias their discussions of epidemiologic findings. The following are other suggestions for dealing with the media (whether local or national):

- Describe the strengths, weaknesses and potential biases of a study. Caution against oversimplification.

- Place findings in a historical context; although scientists are trained not to make policy decisions on the basis of a single study, some reporters (and governments) lack similar constraints.

- Emphasize established benefits and put risks in perspective. For example, OCs provide protection against ovarian and endometrial cancers, pelvic inflammatory disease and ectopic pregnancy. Modern IUDs have been shown to be safe and highly effective. In addition, despite a spate of negative publicity, implants also remain a highly safe and effective contraceptive option.

"From a clinical point of view," Dr. Grimes concluded, "we need to counsel our patients very carefully as to the risks and benefits of the pill and other methods, listening to fears they may have and providing them with correct information. Simply reacting to a patient's stated fear is not always adequate. Some patients may not share their fears, perhaps because they are fairly certain their beliefs are accurate. Because so many myths about the pill are acccepted as facts among the general population, however, practitioners need to provide anticipatory guidance as well, identifying and addressing potential concerns, even without prompting from the patient."

References

1. The Gallup Organization. *Attitudes Toward Contraception.* A poll conducted for the American College of Obstetricians and Gynecologists. Princeton, NJ: March 1985.

2. American College of Obstetricians and Gynecologists. Poll shows women still skeptical of contraceptive safety (press release). ACOG; Washington, DC: January 20, 1994.

3. Peipert JF, Gutmann J. Oral contraceptive risk assessment: a survey of 247 educated women. *Obstet Gynecol* 1993;82:112-117.

4. Herold ES, Goodwin MS. Perceived side effects of oral contraceptives among adolescent girls. *Can Med Assoc J* 1980;123:1022-1026.

5. Grubb GS. Women's perceptions of the safety of the pill: a survey in eight developing countries. *J Biosoc Sci* 1987;19:313-321.

9.2: Contraception for Women with Medical Disorders

During the 1994 annual meeting of the Association of Reproductive Health Professionals, Kirtly Parker Jones, MD, spoke about contraceptive counseling for women with medical problems. Dr. Jones, Associate Professor of Obstetrics and Gynecology and Chief of Reproductive Endocrinology at the University of Utah Department of Obstetrics and Gynecology, discussed the importance of thoroughly assessing the risks and benefits of contraceptive options. She shared with participants a risk analysis algorithm designed to help clinicians weigh the risks of pregnancy against the risks of a method of contraception. Dr. Jones also spoke about myths concerning oral contraceptive (OC) use in certain medical conditions.

Women in their reproductive years with medical disorders have special needs with regard to contraception. Many medical conditions preclude pregnancy because they can cause serious complications in pregnancy or because pregnancy can aggravate existing medical problems. Therefore, the need to plan pregnancies and prevent unwanted pregnancies is even greater for these women than for healthy women.

Health care providers are often unsure of the best approach to contraception for women with medical disorders. Dr. Jones explained, "Most studies of contraceptives are limited to healthy women. This has led to widespread concern among health care providers that contraceptive methods that normally do not affect organ systems in healthy women may have adverse effects on women with medical diseases. The lack of available literature and data regarding the effects of a chosen contraceptive method upon a particular disease make it difficult to know the risks of exacerbating illnesses.

"The concern that a contraceptive could harm a patient leads some health practitioners to refuse to offer a method," Dr. Jones continued. Clinicians may refuse to offer a contraceptive method because they lack information about the consequences of pregnancy and the effects of a method on the disease.

Dr. Jones suggested that by acting out of the fear of the *sin of commission*, health care providers may commit the *sin of omission*. The sin of commission involves prescribing a method that results in complications for the patient and the possibility of legal action. The sin of omission involves withholding an effective contraceptive method and increasing the likelihood of a high-risk pregnancy. "By refusing to prescribe an effective method, the patient may subsequently become pregnant and suffer the often more severe medical consequences of pregnancy," she said.

Health providers need to conduct a risk-benefit analysis when recommending contraception to women with health problems. Jones and Wild developed a risk benefit algorithm to assist clinicians and patients in evaluating a contraceptive method (Figure 1).[1] The algorithm depends on assessing information from four areas: the risk of exacerbation of the disease, the risk of pregnancy, patient factors and the effectiveness of the method.

Clinicians should assess patient factors that influence the decision to use a method and consider the effectiveness of the method. Patient factors include risk-taking behavior, willingness to have an abortion and plans for future pregnancy. The patient's ability and willingness to use any particular method consistently and effectively must be taken into consideration. For example, if the patient does not think she

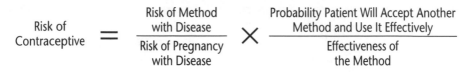

Figure 1

Risk Analysis Algorithm

$$\text{Risk of Contraceptive} = \frac{\text{Risk of Method with Disease}}{\text{Risk of Pregnancy with Disease}} \times \frac{\text{Probability Patient Will Accept Another Method and Use It Effectively}}{\text{Effectiveness of the Method}}$$

Source: Jones KP, Wild R. Contraception for patients with psychiatric or medical disorders. Am J Obstet Gynecol 1994;170:1575-1580. Reproduced with permission of Mosby-Yearbook, Inc.

will use a diaphragm consistently, then this method may not be an appropriate choice, even if it is considered safe. Effectiveness of the method also will influence contraceptive choice. The greater the risk of a pregnancy, the more desirable it is to use a highly effective method.

The algorithm developed by Jones and Wild gives practitioners a way to evaluate the appropriateness of a method. A method of contraception is deemed appropriate when the risk of pregnancy is greater than the possible risk of the contraceptive method, and the patient is unlikely to use another method effectively or refuses sterilization. Special considerations, such as the pharmacologic interactions of medications prescribed for medical conditions and contraceptive agents, must also be taken into account.

Dr. Jones presented clinical cases to illustrate how the algorithm works.

Pulmonary Hypertension

A young woman who has primary pulmonary hypertension and her husband consult with a physician to discuss contraception. Pregnancy carries a 25% to 50% risk of mortality with her condition. The woman has heavy and painful periods. Concern exists about prescribing OCs because of insufficient data on their use with this disease. Since estrogens increase total body water, there is concern that OCs might increase cardiac output and possibly compromise her already marginal right ventricle. Although the couple is aware of the risks associated with having a child, they refuse to consider sterilization. They are also ambivalent about their ability to use foam and condoms consistently, and they would not consider an abortion if the woman became pregnant.

By using the algorithm, the clinician can weigh the risks and benefits of prescribing OCs. According to the algorithm, the risk of using OCs is related to the theoretical risk of slightly increased blood volume with the method, the risk of death from pregnancy and the unlikely possibility that they would use another method more effectively. Under these conditions, OCs become a relatively good choice.

Metastatic Breast Cancer

A young woman with metastatic breast cancer is undergoing evaluation and chemotherapy in preparation for bone marrow transplantation. She is sexually active and does not want to become pregnant, as the therapy may damage a fetus or delay her bone marrow transplant. The probability exists that she will become profoundly thrombocytopenic during this therapy, and may likely develop either temporary or permanent ovarian failure secondary to chemotherapy. Uterine bleeding during her transplant therapy may be profuse. She is offered depot medroxyprogesterone acetate (DMPA), which is the hospital's standard preparation for endometrial suppression and contraception suggested by the current bone marrow transplant team. She refuses DMPA because she had used this method in the past and feels that she developed a depression.

The risk of OCs must be weighed against the significant risk of pregnancy causing a delay in her treatment. The possible risk posed by the use of OCs in breast cancer has never been documented. In fact, there is no evidence that pregnancy, with its high levels of estrogen and progesterone, hastens the course of the disease. There may be an advantage in using OCs for bleeding control during her chemotherapy. She is not likely to use another method. Because the goal of bone marrow transplant is complete cure and eradication of all cancer cells, if OCs stimulated residual cells, it would be unlikely to make a large difference in the eventual outcome. In this case, the very controversial use of OCs may be the best method. This is particularly true in light of the absence of data regarding whether OC use will exacerbate metastatic breast cancer.

Summary

In conducting a risk analysis of a contraceptive method, a thorough history of and knowledge about the patient is critical. "If a woman is not going to use condoms or a method that you have decided is 'safest' for her, then that method isn't safe. If you give her a method and she doesn't use it, then she's probably going to get pregnant. In that case, you haven't given her a safe method. Each woman and her disease make up a unique situation, and each case must be considered individually. The patient is an important partner in assessing the risks and benefits of any method," said Dr. Jones.

Many clinicians fear using hormonal methods for women with medical problems. With regard to this concern, Dr. Jones responded, "There's a dangerous myth that hormones are a risk for women with medical problems. The truth is if there's something about hormones that can make a woman's disease worse, then pregnancy is going to make it a whole lot worse. Furthermore, there are some instances in which the pill may improve disease states. For example, estrogens can sometimes help symptomatic rheumatoid arthritis.

"The pill can be taken by nearly all women," Dr. Jones continued. "That may not be a popular idea, but I'd like to point out that not so many years ago, women were not ovulating as much as they are now. It's only been in the last 100 years that we ovulated very much as a species because before that, we were usually pregnant or nursing. Women who are not on birth control pills are actually engaging in a biological experiment of their own—ovulating most of the time. In my private practice, I see many women who are suffering from the consequences of lots of ovulation. So, I'm going to suggest that maybe all women should take the pill. Women should not automatically be excluded because they have medical problems. With a proper evaluation of the risks and benefits and informed decision-making," she concluded, "the pill can be an appropriate option for many women with medical disorders."

Reference

1. Jones KP, Wild RA. Contraception for patients with psychiatric or medical disorders. *Am J Obstet Gynecol* 1994;170:1575-1580.

9.3: Contraception during Breastfeeding

The benefits of breastfeeding include transmitting important immunoglobulins from mother to infant and strengthening mother and child bonding. Although breastfeeding can provide contraceptive protection, the degree of protective effect depends on many variables. The following article describes the Lactational Amenorrhea Method, a method of birth control that capitalizes on the natural contraceptive effect of breastfeeding, as well as the advantages and disadvantages of other birth control methods for the breastfeeding woman.

Breastfeeding is the best source of infant nutrition. Breastfeeding transmits needed antibodies to the newborn, which provide protection against many infectious agents and can help prevent allergies.[1,2] Particularly in developing countries, it also helps to protect against health hazards created from misuse of infant formulas, such as incorrect dilution or dilution with contaminated water. Breastfeeding can also provide the added benefit of contraception in the early postpartum months, although the extent of protection varies according to a variety of factors.

Mechanism of Action

How does breastfeeding act to decrease fertility? After delivery, levels of progesterone and estrogen decrease, allowing the gradual return of secretion of luteinizing hormone (LH) and follicle-stimulating hormone (FSH). Ovulation and a return to fertility typically occur within 4 to 6 weeks in the nonlactating woman. However, breastfeeding extends the normal 70- to 100-day period of anovulation seen after birth. In the lactating woman, FSH levels return to normal within 30 days; however, LH levels remain suppressed.

Nipple stimulation, achieved by breastfeeding, plays an important role in suppressing ovulation. The sucking action delivers nerve impulses to the hypothalamus. These afferent neural inputs cause a local release of beta-endorphin, which depresses gonadotropin-releasing hormone (GnRH) secretion, thereby inhibiting pituitary gonadotropin secretion.[3] Since gonadotropins are critical for normal follicular development, ovulation is suppressed.[4]

The hypothalamic beta-endorphin release resulting from suckling stimuli also inhibits dopamine production. This causes an increased pituitary prolactin secretion, so both milk production and fertility suppression are mediated by the same input. Basal levels of prolactin approach 40 to 50 ng/mL with a 10- to 20-fold increase after each nursing episode in the early months of breastfeeding.[5] The high levels of prolactin produced during breastfeeding may contribute to lactational amenorrhea in one or more of the following ways: making the ovaries unresponsive to LH; suppressing the positive feedback effects of estrogen on the midcycle rise of GnRH; or directly interfering with ovarian steroid production, although there is no proof of this in the human.

Lactational Amenorrhea Method

The Lactational Amenorrhea Method of family planning, often referred to as LAM, takes advantage of the natural decline in fertility provided by breastfeeding. However, practicing this method is different than general breastfeeding. Specific guidelines are required to achieve the 98% or higher effectiveness rate that is possible with this method.[6-8]

The principle of the Lactational Amenorrhea Method is that "a woman who continues to fully or nearly fully breastfeed her infant and who remains amenorrheic during the first 6 months postpartum is protected from pregnancy during that time."[6] Nipple stimulation is crucial for effectiveness, which means the mother must be feeding frequently (including nighttime) for the method to work. Regular feeding supplementation, either formula or solids, should be avoided.

Development of the Lactational Amenorrhea Method

A consensus statement on the use of breastfeeding as a family planning method was developed during a conference of scientists held in Bellagio, Italy, in August of 1988.[7] The conference was sponsored by the Rockefeller Foundation, Family Health International (FHI) and the World Health Organization (WHO) Special Programme in Human Reproduction.

"The consensus of the group was that the maximum birth spacing effect of breastfeeding is achieved when a mother fully or nearly fully breastfeeds and remains amenorrheic. When these two conditions are fulfilled, breastfeeding provides more than 98% protection from pregnancy in the first 6 months."[7]

A second conference was held at the Georgetown University Institute for Reproductive Health in 1989 and attended by leaders in family planning programs, including representatives of International Planned Parenthood® Federation (IPPF), FHI, the Agency for International Development (AID), the Program for International Training in Health (INTRAH) and many others.

This second conference was designed to consider the Bellagio criteria and other published data and methods, in order to develop a useful, programmatic method based on science and the realities of service delivery.[8-11] The result of this second meeting was the development and naming of the Lactational Amenorrhea Method. The Lactational Amenorrhea Method adds structure and program detail to the scientific conclusions, and adds strong emphasis to the timely introduction of a complementary family planning method. The *Guidelines for Breastfeeding in Family Planning and Child Survival Programs* were the result of this meeting.

Defining Full or Nearly Full Breastfeeding

Because women and health care providers may have differing ideas as to what constitutes "full" or "nearly full" breastfeeding, the Interagency Group for Action on Breastfeeding met in 1988 in order to gain consensus on a standard nomenclature to describe patterns of breastfeeding. The researchers agreed that the term "breastfeeding" alone is inadequate to describe various patterns of breastfeeding behavior. According to Labbok and Krasovec, "exclusive" (full) breastfeeding is defined as no other liquid or solid given to the infant.[11] "Almost exclusive" breastfeeding is defined as vitamins, minerals, water, juice or feeds given infrequently in addition to breastfeeds.

Although there is a consensus that breastfeeding provides the best source of infant nutrition and should be encouraged, many clinicians do not believe that breastfeeding patterns of most U.S. women are sufficient for the practice of the Lactational Amenorrhea Method. Given the fact that many American mothers return to work approximately 6 weeks postpartum, it may be impossible for many women to adhere to the necessary guidelines.

Use of the Lactational Amenorrhea Method after 6 Months Postpartum

For breastfeeding to be effective after 6 months postpartum or after regular supplementation begins, breastfeeding demands are substantial. A study by Short et al of a group of well-nourished Australian women, members of the Nursing Mothers' Asssociation of Australia, found that contraceptive protection of lactational amenorrhea alone lasted as long as a year or more in some instances.[12] However, Gray et al, in a study of American and Filippino women, estimated that for lactational amenorrhea to be effective after the first 6 months postpartum, on average, 15 or more feedings lasting 10 minutes or more per day are required to render some degree of contraceptive protection. In addition, supplements must be limited to 10% of total intake.[13,14]

Family Planning Complementary to Breastfeeding

While the Lactational Amenorrhea Method can be an effective and reliable early contraceptive method, it is not usually the method of choice for breastfeeding women. The Lactational Amenorrhea Method is dependent upon the intensity of breastfeeding. Women in the Western world do not, as yet, practice patterns of full, on-demand breastfeeding necessary for effectiveness of the Lactational Amenorrhea Method. Therefore, complementary contraceptive options should be addressed at the time of delivery and again at follow-up.

Return of ovulation—Use of a contraceptive method is particularly important because ovulation may occur before the onset of menses in women who are less than fully breastfeeding.[13,15] A U.S. study, which assayed urine samples to determine ovulation and luteal phase adequacy, showed that two-thirds of women ovulated before signs of vaginal bleeding, although 47% of these ovulations were not accompanied by an adequate luteal phase.[15] The chance of ovulating prior to menses increases the longer a woman breastfeeds. The return of menstruation is not predictable and may occur while the woman continues to breastfeed; however, even a menstruating, nursing mother is 30% less likely to conceive as a nonnursing mother. This is probably

Use of the Lactational Amenorrhea Method for the First 6 Months Postpartum

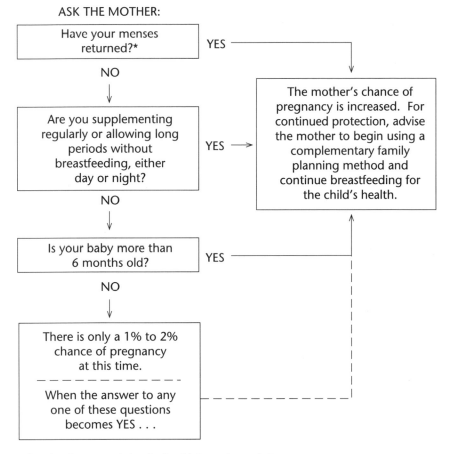

ASK THE MOTHER:

Have your menses returned?*
— YES →

NO ↓

Are you supplementing regularly or allowing long periods without breastfeeding, either day or night?
— YES →

NO ↓

Is your baby more than 6 months old?
— YES →

NO ↓

There is only a 1% to 2% chance of pregnancy at this time.

When the answer to any one of these questions becomes YES . . .

The mother's chance of pregnancy is increased. For continued protection, advise the mother to begin using a complementary family planning method and continue breastfeeding for the child's health.

*Spotting that occurs during the first 56 days not regarded as menses.

Practitioners are encouraged to adapt the language of these guidelines, as appropriate.

Source: Labbok M, et al, 1994 (see reference 8). Reproduced courtesy of the Institute of Reproductive Health, Georgetown University, Washington, DC.

due to anovulatory menses or an absent or deficient luteal phase caused by the continuing suckling stimulus.

Complementary Methods

All patients who plan to breastfeed need to be counseled regarding choice of contraceptive method, preferably before giving birth or at least by 6 weeks postpartum. Another appropriate time for additional contraceptive counseling is just prior to hospital discharge. Both hormonal and nonhormonal methods can be appropriate choices, depending on the individual woman. Nonhormonal methods include barrier

247

methods (male and female condoms, cervical cap and diaphragm), spermicides, the IUD, periodic abstinence methods and tubal sterilization. The advantages and disadvantages of each method must be considered in the context of each individual's circumstances.

Nonhormonal Methods

Condoms can be effective in preventing pregnancy if used correctly and consistently. In addition, condoms provide some protection against sexually transmitted diseases (STDs). The vagina of the nursing mother may be dryer than normal, which can make condoms irritating. Additional lubrication may be required for maximal comfort.

The cervical cap and diaphragm are barrier methods that have no effect on breast-feeding. They may be used after 6 weeks if postpartum bleeding has stopped. Refitting of caps and diaphragms may be required. Parous women may have greater failure rates with the cervical cap than nulliparous women.[16]

Spermicides may be used in the immediate postpartum period. Spermicides can alleviate the vaginal dryness and dyspareunia breastfeeding causes, although conversely, they can be an irritant for some women and men.

Intrauterine devices are very effective. There are two types of IUDs available in the U.S.—a copper-containing device and a progesterone-containing device. The copper on the copper IUD does not affect the quality or quantity of breastmilk. The progesterone-releasing IUD contains a very small amount of progesterone that is released slowly over 1 year into the uterine cavity, where it works locally rather than systemically. Although IUDs can be inserted after delivery, in the U.S. IUDs are FDA-approved for insertion only after uterine involution is complete. Interestingly, breastfeeding women who use the IUD report fewer insertion-related complaints and lower removal rates for bleeding and pain than their nonbreastfeeding counterparts.[17,18]

Periodic abstinence methods may be used during breastfeeding. The Ovulation Method and the Sympto-Thermal Method require special training and rules for the postpartum period, as well as substantial periods of abstinence; however, for certain couples, these would be the methods of choice.[8]

Tubal sterilization affects breastfeeding only by way of general anesthesia. Anesthetic agents pass into the breastmilk and can sedate the infant. Regional or local anesthetics are preferred; however, even these can diminish a sucking response in the infant. It is important that milk production be maintained by expression during any separation of the mother and child so that breastfeeding may continue.

Hormonal Methods

Progestin-only oral contraceptives ("mini-pills") are very effective contraceptives when used in combination with breastfeeding. The slightly higher failure rate associated with the mini-pill is offset by decreased fertility during lactation. A small amount of hormone passes into the breastmilk, but has no known adverse effects on the infant. In addition, certain progestins provide a modest boost to milk production; at least one study has shown that women using progestin-only OCs breastfed longer and added supplementary feeding at a later date.[19]

Combination pills containing both estrogen and a progestin are another option. In 1981, the American Academy of Pediatrics approved the use of combination oral contraceptives in women electing to breastfeed once lactation is well established. Establishing lactation is important, especially for first-time breastfeeding mothers, because estrogen may reduce the milk supply. Estrogen may pass from the mother to the infant through breastmilk; however, no detrimental effects to infants have been observed from the small amounts of transferred hormones.

In general, studies have shown that the milk supply is decreased in women who use combination OCs. However, although milk output and composition have been affected, these effects do not seem to harm infants.[20,21] The WHO Task Force on Oral Contraceptives found that although milk volume was decreased, infant growth was not adversely affected. The authors speculated that supplementary feeding or more prolonged and intense suckling episodes compensated for decreased milk volume.[20] Despite these results, WHO researchers suggested that combination OCs should not be the first-choice method for lactating women.

In addition, several Chilean studies found slower infant weight gain when mothers used combination OCs, but no adverse effects on infant health.[22-24] The longest follow-up study has been of Swedish children whose mothers used combination OCs while nursing. No adverse effects have been found on the physical, intellectual or psychological development of these children.[25]

Although many clinicians feel that combination OCs are appropriate for women once lactation has been established, others prefer the use of a nonhormonal method or the mini-pill for women who are breastfeeding. If OCs are chosen, they can be started 6 weeks postpartum. Controversy exists over whether there is an increased risk for thromboembolic events when using combination OCs immediately after childbirth.[26] Low-dose pills may have less of an effect on the risk for thromboembolism than higher-dose formulations.

DMPA does not suppress milk production. Ronald Gray, MB, BS, of The Johns Hopkins School of Hygiene and Public Health, addressed this issue at the Food and Drug Administration's (FDA) advisory meeting on June 19, 1992, which evaluated DMPA's use as a contraceptive. According to Dr. Gray, "...a whole variety of studies, including large WHO studies that I was involved in, have shown that DMPA does not suppress milk production. A number of studies in Chile found that DMPA use during breastfeeding had no particular effect. DMPA users had a somewhat longer duration of lactation than women who were not using contraception. At 4.5 years, they could find no effects on the growth and development of the children."[27-31] In fact, one study suggests that DMPA may have a beneficial effect on the quality of breast milk, as measured by fat concentration, calories, minerals, protein, lactose and immunoglobulin.[32]

Subdermal implants, which contain the progestin levonorgestrel, do not affect the growth or health of breastfed infants. In many countries, capsules are inserted immediately postpartum. In the U.S., FDA labeling suggests inserting at 6 weeks postpartum, after lactation is established.

Breastfeeding and HIV

Human immunodeficiency virus (HIV) transmission is a concern for HIV-positive women and women in high-risk categories. The virus can be transmitted *in utero*, during delivery or, less often, through breastmilk. It is thought to be more difficult to transmit the virus via breastmilk than blood, but the risk of transmission via breastmilk is still unknown.[33,34]

A 1992 review of published studies suggests infants are at risk of HIV transmission during breastfeeding.[35] Based on data from four studies in which mothers acquired HIV postnatally, researchers estimated the risk of HIV transmission was 29% (95% CI [confidence interval], 16%-42%). Based on data from five studies in which mothers were infected prenatally, "the additional risk of transmission through breastfeeding, over and above transmission *in utero* or during delivery, is 14% (95% CI, 7%-22%)."[35]

How the use of zidovudine (AZT) impacts transmission during breastfeeding is not yet known. A National Institutes of Health-sponsored study (AIDS Clinical Trials Group—Protocol 076) found AZT significantly reduces the risk of HIV transmission from mother to infant during gestation, labor and delivery, but did not assess the risk during breastfeeding (for further discussion of this study, see the section in Chapter 8 on preventing vertical HIV transmission).[36,37]

In the U.S., HIV-infected women are advised to use formula rather than breastfeed. On the other hand, breastfeeding is still recommended for women in developing countries who may have inadequate supplies of formula and/or unsanitary water conditions.

References

1. Gibson R, Makrides M, Neumann M, et al. Fatty acid status and visual function in term infants. IV International Congress of Nutrition, Adelaide, Sept. 26-Oct. 1, 1993 (abstract).

2. Laurence R. *Breastfeeding: A Guide for the Medical Professional.* St. Louis, Mo.:Mosby; 1989: 112-113.

3. Short RV. Lactational infertility in family planning. *Ann Med* 1993;25:175-80.

4. McNeilly AS. Lactational amenorrhea. *Endocrinol Metab Clin North Am* 1993;22:59-73.

5. Battin DA, Marrs RP, Fleiss PM, et al. Effect of suckling on serum prolactin, luteinizing hormone, follicle stimulating hormone, and estradiol during prolonged lactation. *Obstet Gynecol* 1985;65:785.

6. Perez A, Labbok M, Keenan JT. Clinical studies of the lactational amenorrhea method for family planning. *Lancet* 1992;339:968-970.

7. Kennedy KI, Rivera R, McNeilly AS. Consensus statement on the use of breastfeeding as a family planning method. *Contraception* 1989;39(5):477-496.

8. Labbok M, Cooney K, Coly S. *Guidelines. Breastfeeding, family planning, and the Lactational Amenorrhea Method - LAM.* Institute for Reproductive Health, Georgetown University, Washington, DC, 1994.

9. Labbok MH. Breast-feeding and contraception. *N Engl J Med* 1983;308(1):51. Letter.

10. Labbok MH, Chassell RJ. The development and use of graphically presented algorithms in community-based family planning services. *Int'l Quarterly of Community Health Education* 1987-1988;8:223-247.

11. Labbok M, Krasovec K. Toward consistency in breastfeeding definitions. *Stud Fam Plann* 1990;21(4):226-230.

12. Short RV, Lewis PR, Renfree MB, et al. Contraceptive effects of extended lactational amenorrhea: beyond the Bellagio Consensus. *Lancet* 1991;337:715-17.

13. Gray RH, Campbell OM, Apelo R, et al. Risk of ovulation during lactation. *Lancet* 1990;335:25-29.

14. Gray R. Lactational amenorrhoea. *Lancet* 1991;337:1232. Letter.

15. Campbell OM, Gray RH. Characteristics and determinants of postpartum ovarian function in women in the United States. *Am J Obstet Gynecol* 1993;169:55-60.

16. Trussell J, Strickler J, Vaughan B. Contraceptive efficacy of the diaphragm, the sponge and the cervical cap. *Fam Plann Perspect* 1993;25:100-105,135.

17. Chi IC, Wilkens LR, Champion CB, et al. Insertional pain and other IUD insertion-related rare events for breastfeeding and non-breastfeeding women—a decade's experience in developing countries. *Adv Contracept* 1989;5:101-119.

18. Farr G, Rivera R. Interactions between intrauterine contraceptive device use and breast-feeding status at time of intrauterine contraceptive device insertion: analysis of TCu-380A acceptors in developing countries. *Am J Obstet* 1992;167:144-151.

19. McCann MF, Moggia AV, Hibbins JE, et al. The effects of a progestin-only oral contraceptive (levonorgestrel 0.03 mg) on breast-feeding. *Contraception* 1989;40:635.

20. WHO Special Programme of Research, Development, and Research Training in Human Reproduction, Task Force on Oral Contraceptives. Effects of hormonal contraceptives on milk volume and infant growth. *Contraception* 1984;30(6):505-522.

21. WHO Special Programme of Research, Development, and Research Training in Human Reproduction, Task Force on Oral Contraceptives. Effects of hormonal contraceptives on breast milk composition and infant growth. *Stud Fam Plann* 1988;19(6):361-369.

22. Diaz S, Peralta O, Juez G, et al. Fertility regulation in nursing women: III. Short-term influence of a low-dose combined oral contraceptive upon lactation and infant growth. *Contraception* 1983;27(1):1-11.

23. Croxatto HB, Diaz S, Peralta O, et al. Fertility regulation in nursing women: IV. Long-term influence of a low-dose combined oral contraceptive initiated at day 30 postpartum upon lactation and infant growth. *Contraception* 1983;27(1):13-25.

24. Peralta O, Diaz S, Juez G, et al. Fertility regulation in nursing women: V. Long-term influence of a low-dose combined oral contraceptive initiated at day 90 postpartum upon lactation and infant growth. *Contraception* 1983;27(1):27-38.

25. Nilsson S, Mellbin T, Hofvander Y, et al. Long-term follow-up of children breast-fed by mothers using oral contraceptives. *Contraception* 1986;34(5):443-457.

26. WHO Task Force on Oral Contraceptives. Contraceptives during the postpartum period and during lactation: the effects on women's health. *Int J Gynecol Obstet* 1987;25S:13-27.

27. Jimenez J, Ochoa M, Soler MP, et al. Long-term follow-up of children breastfed by mothers receiving depo-medroxyprogesterone acetate. *Contraception* 1984;30:523-533.

28. Pardthaisong T, Yenchit C, Gray R. The long-term growth and development of children exposed to Depo-Provera during pregnancy or lactation. *Contraception* 1992;45:313-324.

29. World Health Organization. Effects of hormonal contraceptives on breast milk composition and infant growth. *Stud Fam Plann* 1988;19:361-369.

30. World Health Organization Task Force for Epidemiological Research on Reproductive Health. Progestogen-only contraceptives during lactation: 1. Infant growth. *Contraception* 1994;50:35-53.

31. World Health Organization Task Force for Epidemiological Research on Reproductive Health. Progestogen-only contraceptives during lactation: 1. Infant development. *Contraception* 1994;50:55-68.

32. Costa TH, Dorea JG. Concentration of fat, protein, lactose and energy in milk of mothers using hormonal contraceptives. *Ann Trop Paediatr* 1992;12:203-209.

33. WHO, Consensus Statement from the WHO/UNICEF Consultation on HIV Transmission and Breastfeeding, Geneva, 30 April-1 May 1992.

34. Oxtoby MJ. Human immunodeficiency virus and other viruses in human milk: placing the issue in broader perspective. *Pediatr Infect Dis J* 1988;7(12):825-835.

35. Dunn DT, Newell ML, Ades AE, et al. Risk of human immunodeficiency virus type 1 transmission through breastfeeding. *Lancet* 1992;340:585-588.

36. Centers for Disease Control and Prevention. Zidovudine for the prevention of HIV transmission from mother to infant. *MMWR* 1994;43:285-287.

37. Sperling RS, Shapiro DE, Coombs RW, et al. Maternal viral load, zidovudine treatment, and the risk of transmission of human immunodeficiency virus type 1 from mother to infant. *N Engl J Med* 1996;335:1621-1629.

9.4: Helping Patients to Stop Smoking

The following are excerpts from an article by Ernie J. Chaney, MD, and Joan Fox, RN.

There seems to be little debate about the desirability of quitting smoking, but a great deal of frustration as to how to help patients quit successfully. The American Academy of Family Physicians has an excellent Stop Smoking Kit for clinicians. The kit includes everything from an instruction manual and promotional materials for the hospital or office waiting area to a stop smoking manual for the patient.

The American Academy of Family Physicians stresses the importance of addressing the addiction problem at the initial visit and at each visit thereafter. Smokers are informed that stopping smoking is the single most important change they can make for their health. Patients are told they will receive a brief, gentle reminder at each visit to encourage them to quit and stay stopped. Persuasive points to make with female smokers include premature aging of the skin, the aesthetics of the habit and exposure of family members to secondhand smoke, in addition to the obvious personal health risks.

A system for marking charts of smokers is encouraged (the kit includes stickers for this purpose). This system serves as a cue to the clinician to follow-up at future visits. Smokers are encouraged to set a quit day and plan for changes in daily routines that may serve as signals to light up.

The Patient Education Coordinator sees patients who want help to stop smoking. There are usually three visits:

1. *"Getting Started"* includes the presentation of a stop smoking packet. The patient educator develops a personal plan for changes in daily routines and for handling urges to smoke during the withdrawal phase. Suggestions for coping with urges to smoke may include simple physical activities, such as a brisk walk, drinking a glass of water or brushing the teeth.

2. *"Stopping"* is a brief visit to review the plan. The patient educator also reviews instructions for nicotine gum or patches, if recommended by the physician.

3. *"Staying Stopped"* is also brief. Progress is discussed and arrangements are made for follow-up by telephone at 1, 3, 6 and 12 months.

Audiotapes and a flipchart contained in the kit are also useful. Patients who are not interested in the counseling part of the program are provided with the stop smoking packet and offered encouragement and specific tips. Those interested in a more structured approach are referred to a recognized plan, such as that of the American Cancer Society.

Additional Suggestions from the National Cancer Institute[1]:

The Four "A's" for Clinicians

1. *Ask* every patient if they smoke.

2. *Advise* all smokers in strong and personal terms about the necessity of quitting.

3. *Assist* smokers in quitting successfully—set a quit date, provide self-help materials and evaluate for nicotine replacement therapy.

4. *Arrange* for follow-up.

Five Steps to Implement in Health Care Settings

1. Appoint a clinic smoking cessation coordinator.

2. Create a smoke-free office environment.

3. Identify all patients who smoke.

4. Systematize the distribution and review of self-help materials.

5. Automatically schedule follow-up visits (especially during first 2 weeks after the quit date).

Reference

1. Glynn TJ, Manley MW. *How to Help Your Patients Stop Smoking: A National Cancer Institute Manual for Physicians.* Bethesda, Maryland: National Institutes of Health; 1990. DHHS publication NIH 90-3064.

How to Order the AAFP Stop Smoking Kit

Cost is $50 to AAFP members and $80 to nonmembers, plus $5 shipping and handling. The materials are excellent and refills are available. One special supplement addresses nicotine replacement therapy. To order toll-free, call (800) 944-0000, or fax (816) 822-0580. Or write to:

AAFP Order Dept., 8880 Ward Parkway, Kansas City, MO 64114-2797

Places You Can Call or Write for Free Information

Office of Cancer Communications National Cancer Institute
Bldg. 31, Rm. 10A24, Bethesda, MD 20892
Telephone: (800) 4-CANCER

National Heart, Lung, and Blood Institute Smoking Education Program
PO Box 30105, Bethesda, MD 20824-0105
Telephone: (301) 251-1222

American Cancer Society
1559 Clifton Rd. NE, Atlanta, GA 30329-4251
Telephone: (800) ACS-2345

Index